THE KEIL CENTRE

DEPRESSION
An integrative approach

THE MENTAL HEALTH FOUNDATION

The *Mental Health Foundation* (MHF) is Britain's leading grant making charity concerned with promoting and encouraging pioneering research and community care projects in the field of mental illness and mental handicap.

The Foundation aims to prevent mental disorders by funding and encouraging research into the causes of mental illness and mental handicap, and to improve the quality of life for mentally disordered people by funding and supporting pioneering and innovative community care schemes.

The Mental Health Foundation has several professional committees which meet at regular intervals to decide upon the allocation of funds to priority areas.

Apart from its interest in offering financial support, the MHF also runs regular seminars and conferences. These provide an arena for the exchange of information for a wide range of professionals working in the field who might otherwise find it difficult to meet.

In 1988, the MHF held a conference jointly with the Royal College of Physicians in order to assess recent advances in the prevention, treatment and care of depression. This book is loosely based upon those proceedings. Extra chapters have been commissioned in order to encompass a wider sphere of interest than would be possible during a single day's conference programme.

Eugene Paykel, Professor of Psychiatry at the University of Cambridge, is a Trustee of the MHF and also a member of the Research Committee. Dr Katia Herbst, who managed the affairs of the General Projects Committee for five years, is now Policy Development Officer for the Foundation and responsible for two of the new specialist grant giving committees.

DEPRESSION
An Integrative Approach

Edited by

KATIA R. HERBST
MA, PhD
The Mental Health Foundation, London

and

EUGENE S. PAYKEL
MA, MD, FRCP, FRCPEd, FRCPsych
Professor of Psychiatry, University of Cambridge

Heinemann Medical Books
in association with

The
Mental Health
Foundation

Heinemann Medical Books
An imprint of Heinemann Professional Publishing Ltd
Halley Court, Jordan Hill, Oxford OX2 8EJ

OXFORD LONDON SINGAPORE NAIROBI IBADAN KINGSTON

First published 1989

British Library Cataloguing in Publication Data
Depression
  1. Man. Depression. Therapy
  I. Herbst, K.   II. Paykel, E. S.
  III. Mental Health Foundation
  616.85'2706

ISBN 0 433 00090 2

Typeset by Latimer Trend & Company Ltd, Plymouth and
printed in Great Britain by Butler & Tanner Ltd, Frome.

Contents

List of contributors   vii

Preface   ix

Section 1   Introduction

1   The background: extent and nature of the disorder   3
    Eugene S. Paykel

Section 2   Causes of depression

2   Depression: a radical social perspective   21
    George W. Brown
3   Evolutionary and molecular genetic approaches to manic   45
    depression
    Hugh M.D. Gurling
4   Neuroendocrine studies of the aetiology of depression   53
    Stuart Checkley
5   Interactive models of depression: the evidence   65
    Paul E. Bebbington and Peter McGuffin
6   Drug-related depression; clinical and epidemiological aspects   81
    J. Guy Edwards

Section 3   The life cycle and depression

7   Depression in adolescence   111
    William Ll. Parry-Jones
8   Depression in the puerperium: a conceptual controversy   124
    John L. Cox
9   Depression in the elderly   140
    Elaine Murphy

Section 4   The management of depression

10 Cognitive treatment for depression   163
    J. Mark G. Williams
11 Developments in antidepressants   179
    Stuart A. Montgomery
12 Suicide and the management of suicide attempts   197
    Keith Hawton
13 The recognition, diagnosis and acknowledgement of   216
    depressive disorder by general practitioners
    André Tylee and Paul Freeling
14 The role of self–help groups in the management of   232
    depression
    Judy Wilson

Index   250

Contributors

Paul E. Bebbington
Honorary Senior Lecturer, Medical Research Council Social Psychiatry Unit, Institute of Psychiatry, London
George W. Brown
Professor of Sociology and External Scientific Staff of Medical Research Council, Royal Holloway and Bedford New College, University of London
Stuart Checkley
Consultant Psychiatrist, Maudsley Hospital, London
John L. Cox
Professor of Psychiatry, School of Postgraduate Medicine, University of Keele, Staffordshire
J. Guy Edwards
Consultant Psychiatrist, Department of Psychiatry, Royal South Hants Hospital, Southampton
Paul Freeling
Professor of General Practice and Primary Care, Department of General Practice and Primary Care, St George's Hospital Medical School, London
Hugh M. D. Gurling
Wellcome Senior Fellow in Clinical Science, Senior Lecturer and Honorary Consultant Psychiatrist, University College and Middlesex Hospital School of Medicine, London
Keith Hawton
Consultant Psychiatrist and Clinical Lecturer, University Department of Psychiatry and Warneford Hospital, Oxford
Peter McGuffin
Professor and Head of Department of Psychological Medicine, University of Wales College of Medicine, Heath Park, Cardiff
Stuart A. Montgomery
Reader in Psychiatry and Honorary Consultant, St Mary's Hospital Medical School, London
Elaine Murphy
Professor of Psychogeriatrics, United Medical and Dental Schools of Guy's and St Thomas's Hospital, Guy's Hospital, London

William Ll. Parry-Jones
Professor of Child and Adolescent Psychiatry, Department of Child and
Adolescent Psychiatry, Royal Hospital for Sick Children, Glasgow
Eugene S. Paykel
Professor of Psychiatry, Department of Psychiatry, University of Cam-
bridge, Addenbrooke's Hospital, Cambridge
André Tylee
GP principal in Sutton, Surrey. Mental Health Foundation Research
Fellow and lecturer in general practice and primary care, St Georges
Hospital Medical School.
J. Mark G. Williams
Research Clinical Psychologist, Medical Research Council Applied
Psychology Unit, Cambridge
Judy Wilson
Is leader of the Nottingham Self-Help Team, a voluntary agency funded
by Nottingham Health Authority

Preface

The Mental Health Foundation is Britain's largest fund-giving charity which concentrates solely on the promotion and support of academic research and community projects concerned with mental disorder. It does have other functions, however. One of these is to provide regular arenas for the exchange of information concerning developments in psychiatry and community services.

In 1988, The Mental Health Foundation and the Royal College of Physicians jointly sponsored a conference on depression, in London. One of the aims from the outset was to produce the focus for a book on the topic. Good conferences do not necessarily make good books as there is a limit to what can be accommodated in a single programme. Thus we commissioned extra chapters in order to encompass a wider sphere of interest.

Depression is the most common psychiatric disorder of adulthood. It effects all ages and all walks of life. It presents as much to the general practitioner, to the non-medical mental health professional and to the voluntary helper as to the specialist psychiatrist. Its effects are wide ranging and afflict not only the sufferers themselves but also their families.

We have sought in this volume to adopt a balanced and integrated approach, spanning the psychosocial and the biological antecedents to and treatments for the disorder. Several of the contributors attempt to integrate these various aspects and all the proponents of one view acknowledge the importance of the others.

The book is divided into four sections. The first section is a brief introduction to depression aimed to set the background. The second section follows with a detailed look at recent studies of causation, including social causes, molecular genetics, neuroendocrine studies, the possible iatrogenic role of drug treatments, and the interrelationship of social and familial factors. The third section focuses on three transitional points in the life cycle—adolescence, childbirth and old age—where depression may be of particular importance. The last section examines some recent developments in treatment, including cognitive therapy, antidepressant drugs, the management of suicidal behaviour, and the role of the general practitioner and self-help groups.

We hope that this book will be helpful to a variety of readers, including psychiatrists and psychiatrists in training, physicians, general practitioners, social workers, psychologists, members of helping organizations and the informed general public.

Professor Eugene Paykel
Dr Katia Herbst

SECTION 1

Introduction

1 The background: extent and nature of the disorder

EUGENE S. PAYKEL

INTRODUCTION

This chapter will discuss the epidemiology and classification of depression. It is intended as a brief introduction to set the scene for what will follow. As a review it does not aim to be comprehensive but to lay out sufficient material to set the remaining chapters into context.

EPIDEMIOLOGY

Treated disorder

The basic facts regarding rates of depression are easily summarized. About 1 per 1000 of the general population are admitted to hospital annually with depression; about 3 per 1000 are referred to psychiatrists, of whom two are treated as out-patients. However, around 3 percent of the general population are treated in this country by general practitioners and an equal number probably consult and are not recognized. The prevalance rate in the general population is about 5 percent although estimates vary considerably. Depression is therefore a kind of iceberg of which only the tip sticks up to reach the psychiatrists. The frequencies of the disorder will depend very much on how one defines it and where one studies it.

The earliest studies were based on hospital admission statistics. Although rates vary, modern figures suggest, as outlined above, that 1 per 1000 of the general population in this and similar countries are admitted to hospital annually with depression (Bebbington, 1978).

Obviously only the most severe depressives are admitted to hospital. Better figures for psychiatric care are obained by combining all kinds of treatment facilities, in-patient and out-patient, preferably using cumulative cases registers which avoid the same patient being counted twice. A number of case register studies have been reported although they tend to use different kinds of rates. Pedersen et al. (1972) in Rochester obtained a one-year prevalence of 70 per 100 000 for psychotic depressions and a first referral annual incidence rate of 33 per 1000. Juel-Nielsen *et al.* (1961) in Aarhus obtained an annual incidence rate for first and subsequent referral of all depression of 358 per 100 000. Other Scandinavian studies have produced similar figures (Boyd and Weissman, 1982). Grad de Alarcon *et al.* (1975) obtained referral rates for psychotic depression of 265 per 100 000 in Chichester and 150 per 100 000 in Salisbury, and rates for neurotic depression of 85 and 96 per 100 000 respectively. Wing and Fryers (1976) obtained figures of 295 and 240 per 100 000 for all depression in Camberwell and Salford. These studies consistently suggest psychiatric referral rates for all depression of around 3 per 1000. They are somewhat out of date, however, and may not adequately reflect increased out-patient services and more receptive attitudes to psychiatric care in recent years.

In the UK only a relatively small proportion of psychiatric problems in general practice are referred to psychiatrists. Early general practice studies suggested relatively low rates of depression (Watts *et al.*, 1964; Shepherd *et al.*, 1966), but more recent studies indicate high rates. The national morbidity survey of 1971–72 obtained an annual rate for neurotic depression of 31 per 1000, representing a 20-fold increase over a similar study 15 years earlier (Crombie, 1974), possibly reflecting both better recognition and also changed labelling habits. The most recent national morbidity survey of 1981–82 (HMSO, 1986) found rates of 26 and 2 per 1000 for neurotic and psychotic depression respectively.

The rates depend in part on the proportion of depressives who are recognized. Goldberg and Huxley (1980), based on review of a number of studies, estimated that only about half the cases of psychiatric disorder presenting to the general practitioner are recognized as such. The factors which affect the general practitioner's capacity to recognize depression are complex. Patients entering the surgery may have no disorder, a serious physical illness such as carcinoma, a minor physical illness, a psychiatric disorder presenting overtly, or one presenting in a masked way by physical symptoms. The general practitioner has a skilled and difficult task to sort this out rapidly. Freeling *et al.* (1985) compared missed and recognized depressions in general practice in London. Missed depressions were characterized by less overt and less typical symptoms, which were more closely related to physical illness. These issues are discussed further by Freeling and Tylee in Chapter 13.

General population surveys

In the long run, enumeration of all cases in the general population ought to provide the most reliable figures. However, psychiatric community surveys have faced very considerable problems and it is only in the last ten years that these have been overcome. The problems centre around the definition of what is a psychiatric case.

Early general population studies found that minor psychiatric symptoms were very common. The Midtown Manhattan Study even went so far as to suggest that a majority of New Yorkers had some psychiatric symptoms, and 23 percent were considered to show depressive symptoms (Srole *et al.*, 1962). Comstock and Helsing (1976) used the total score on a question-naire, the Center For Epidemiologic Studies Depression Scale (CES–D). An arbitrary cut-off point of 16 on this scale gave an overall prevalence of between 17 percent and 26 percent for blacks and whites in two different areas of the USA. Reviewing studies of depressive symptoms in the community, Boyd and Weissman (1982) found point prevalences of between 13 percent and 20 percent depending on the study.

The problem here is that the word 'depression' covers a variety of phenomena. It describes a normal mood which everyone will have experienced at some time, perhaps quite frequently, without it being in any way pathological. It also covers a symptom which is more severe but also common and nonspecific, recurring in a variety of psychiatric disorders.

Beyond this is a third and more specific meaning, that of disorder or illness. In establishing that a patient has a diagnosis of pathological depression, a psychiatrist usually carries out two processes: he assesses the amount of depression present and he rules out other diagnoses which might account for it. In assessing the amount of depression, he really looks for a group of disturbances that go far beyond the simple complaint of depressed mood to many other concomitants. Clinical depression is best regarded as a syndrome, with a variety of causes, in which a number of features, probably reflecting a common pathophysiology, cluster together. These include not only depressed mood, usually regarded as central, but disturbances of thought content, vegetative function such as sleep and appetite, psychomotor changes, impairment of capacity to function and changes in behaviour. The more severe the disorder, the more frequent and more severe are these symptoms.

For epidemiological studies what this requires is some definition of a disorder which is sufficiently clear-cut that it lies within the realm of the psychiatrist. The early studies went wrong either when the psychiatrist got outside his usual clinical framework and misinterpreted the presence of mild disturbance in people in the community, or when some kind of quantitative symptom scale was used but there was no real guide as to the amount of symptomatology which constituted disorder.

There have been two solutions to the problem. In this country, Wing *et al.* (1974) developed a standardized interview, the Present State Examina-tion (PSE), with defined thresholds for the presence of each of a large number of symptoms. They elaborated this using computerized decision-tree methods to produce a diagnostic schema, CATEGO, and later, based on amount and type of symptoms, an Index of Definition as to the extent to which symptoms approximate to the disorder found in psychiatric patients (Wing *et al.*, 1978). The levels of the Index of Definition include no psychiatric symptoms (1), nonspecific symptoms (2, 3), specific symptoms (4), borderline disorders (5) and definite disorders (6, 7, 8, in ascending severity). Level 5 is the crucial threshold level at which symptoms are regarded as reaching psychiatric disorder and a CATEGO diagnosis can be assigned.

In the USA, there has been a parallel set of developments. The new official American Psychiatric Association Diagnostic and Statistical Manual, 3rd edition, DSM III, contained operational criteria for each disorder. The definition for a major depressive episode in the revised schema DSM IIIR (American Psychiatric Association, 1987) includes presence of at least five symptoms. At least one of these must be consistent depressed mood, or marked loss of interest and pleasure, and the other possibilities are weight change, sleep disturbance, agitation or retardation, loss of energy, guilt, poor concentration, suicidal thoughts. Signs of certain other disorders act as excluding criteria. The classification also includes some other forms of affective disorder. A new interview schedule based on DSM III, the Diagnostic Interview Schedule (DIS; Robins *et al.*, 1981), was devised in a form which could be used by lay interviewers and from which computerized DSM III diagnoses could be made. DSM III was derived from an earlier classificatory schema, the Research Diagnostic Criteria (RDC) (Spitzer and Endicott, 1978), which employed similar depressive diagnoses, and this system has been used in some studies.

These methods have now been employed in a number of general population surveys. From these, reliable rates for depression in the general population can be derived. They are summarized in Table 1.1 which shows studies from London, Edinburgh, Canberra, Athens, several American

Table 1.1 Prevalence rates for depression in recent studies

	Site	Rates per 100		
		Men	Women	Total
PSE/ID/CATEGO (1 month)				
Henderson *et al.* (1979)	Canberra	2.6	6.7	4.1
Bebbington *et al.* (1981)	London	4.8	9.0	7.0
Dean *et al.* (1983)	Edinburgh		5.9	
Mavreas *et al.* (1986)	Athens	4.3	10.1	7.4
DSM III/RDC (6 months)				
Weissman and Myers (1978)*	New Haven	3.2	5.2	4.3
Dean *et al.* (1983)	Edinburgh		7.0	
Myers *et al.* (1984)†	Various USA	1.7	4.0	3.0
Canino *et al.* (1987)	Puerto Rico	2.4	3.3	3.0

* Point prevalence.
† Pooled data from 3 centres.
PSE rates are for CATEGO Classes D, R, N. DSM III/RDC rates are for major depression; rates for all depressive diagnoses are higher.

cities and Puerto Rico. There is some reasonable consistency from these studies as to rates, which average to approximately 4.8 percent overall: 6.4 percent in women and 3.2 percent in men.

The above studies all reported prevalences, rather than the annual episode rates which would have been comparable with the annual consultation and treatment rates presented earlier. Few studies have yet attempted to estimate episode rates in the community, because of the difficulty in timing onsets and remissions. This exercise really requires an epidemiological prevalence study followed by a second wave of interviewing after a period, to enable detection of new cases. Surtees *et al.* (1986), using such a design found an annual inception rate in women, for all disorder of 12.6 percent: about half the cases were of major depression. This may be compared with a figure of 8 percent for depression by Brown and Harris (1978), also in women, but based on retrospective reconstruction rather than repeated interviewing, and using a different case definition.

The variation in frequency across settings clearly corresponds to a range of severity. Severe depressions of the kind which are hospitalized are infrequent; mild depressions, which predominate in the community, are common. At the mild extreme, the particular criteria used may have large effects on the rates, for they probably represent arbitrary cuts on a continuum. These issues must be kept in mind in interpreting any data on frequency of depression, such as studies in the puerperium, in specific age groups or in patients in medical wards.

Associations

The aims of epidemiological studies include not just the enumeration of rates, but the search for associations which might hint at causes. For depression, the demographic associations are now fairly clear, although the aetiological inferences may be less so.

Regarding age, depression has in the past been regarded as an illness of middle and later life. However, recent samples of treated patients often show younger ages with means between 30 and 40 years. Community studies suggest similar findings. A possible reason lies in the younger age of neurotic compared with psychotic depressives found in studies of depressive classification. In the case register study of Grad de Alarcon *et al.* (1975) the peak age for psychotic depression was in the 50s and that for neurotic depression in the 30s. Over the years, as attitudes to psychiatric care have changed, out-patient services have expanded, and general practitioner recognition has improved, there has been a gradual change in the picture of treated depression towards the milder and more neurotic.

The differential sex incidence is one of the most constant findings in depression, with female predominance ranging from 2:1 to 3:1. The difference does not simply reflect help-seeking factors, as it also appears in community studies. The explanation is probably complex (Weissman and

Klerman, 1977). There is some evidence of X-linked genetic transmission in bipolar manic depressive illness, but in this disorder the sex incidence is more equal (Weissman *et al.*, 1984). Hormonal effects might be important, as reflected in such phenomena as premenstrual tension and raised incidence of post partum disorder (Pugh *et al.*, 1963; Paffenberger and McCabe, 1966; Kendell *et al.*, 1976). However, the female predominance is not limited to the post partum period and the excess in that period is far too small to explain it. The menopause does not seem to be a major cause of depression (Winokur, 1973).

Alternative explanations are psychosocial. Women do not appear to experience higher rates of life events than do men (Paykel and Rowan, 1979). Other aspects of social disadvantage might be important. High rates of affective disorder have been found among women with young children (Richman, 1977; Brown and Harris, 1978) and Brown and his colleagues, in particular, have explored the implications of social vulnerability for women. Gove (1972), reviewing studies of mental disorder in general, concluded that amongst those who were married, rates were clearly higher for women than men. However, amongst those who were single, divorced or widowed, findings were equivocal, with a tendency for higher rates in men. He suggested that being married had a detrimental effect for women, and a protective effect for men. The disadvantages for married women may include, in addition to problems with children, restriction to a single low-status role as housewife rather than an additional role in work, and dependence for finance and emotional support on the marital partner. This last may be a particular problem if the marital relationship is poor or breaks down. Grad de Alarcon *et al.* (1975) found a peak for psychotic depression in single women aged 55–64 but an additional peak for neurotic depression in married women between 25 and 34. Bebbington *et al.* (1981) found two peaks for minor psychiatric disorder in women, aged 25–34 and 45–54, and high rates in married women but unmarried men.

This is probably not the whole story. A further possibility is that it may be harder for men to acknowledge or recognize depression. Weeping and helplessness are often regarded as feminine, at least in our culture, and are more permissible in women. Some other forms of deviance, most notably alcoholism, delinquency, and adult crime, are more common in males. Winokur's studies (Winokur, 1974) indicate families with depression in the females but alcoholism and sociopathy in males, although other factors, such as hormonal differences, might also modify expression of a genotype. Suicide rates, by contrast to depression, show a male predominance, although attempted suicide occurs predominantly in young women. It is possible that in males some depression is suppressed until it reveals itself in suicide, or that distress expresses itself in different ways in the two sexes.

Regarding social class, findings are mixed. Affective disorders, in contrast to schizophrenia, were at one time regarded as more common in higher social classes. However, many studies of admission rates do not show much departure from the distribution of the general population, although there is certainly not the pronounced working-class skew which is found for schizophrenia. There is some evidence to suggest that bipolar disorder may be more common in higher social classes (Bagley, 1973). This could reflect a mixture of factors including diagnostic bias, and a possible selective advantage for some energetic personalities bordering on the hypomanic. On the other hand, community surveys tend to find higher rates in working-class subjects (Uhlenhuth *et al.*, 1974; Comstock and Helsing, 1976; Brown and Harris, 1978; Weissman and Myers, 1978; Surtees *et al.*, 1983). As community studies identify milder depression, it may be that neurotic depression and mild clinical depression show an understandable relationship to the increased social stress that might be expected in socially disadvantaged populations.

In earlier discussion of sex ratios, reference was made to suicidal behaviour. However, one must beware of basing strong inferences about depression on suicide. To some extent, depression, completed suicide and attempted suicide are three independent phenomena, although with overlap. Only about 15 percent of depressives ultimately die of suicide (Robins and Guze, 1970) and not all suicides have been depressed: the incidence of suicide, of between 10 and 20 per 100 000, is very different from that of depression. There are no definitive figures on the proportion of depressives who make suicide attempts, but available evidence suggests that up to 40 percent of those in hospital settings have made a recent or previous attempt (Paykel *et al.*, 1970; Crook *et al.*, 1975). They tend, like other suicide attempters, to be younger, female, hostile and not typical of all depressives. Likewise, about 50 percent of suicide attempters have some depressive symptoms, but these are often mild (Newson-Smith and Hirsch, 1979; Urwin and Gibbons, 1979).

CLASSIFICATION

If the last 10 years have shed great light on epidemiology, they have not done the same for classification, which has tended to become more complicated and arbitrary. Psychiatrists have always had a strong weakness for inventing classifications and arguing about them. This process reached its peak in the 19th century, and has shown signs of returning in the last 10 years. However, the wide range of severity and other features within depression, and the variation in clinical pictures, does necessitate some subgrouping. Broadly speaking, two major classifications have proved to be of lasting value in affective illness: the distinction between bipolar and unipolar disorder, and that between psychotic and neurotic (or endogenous and reactive) disorders.

Unipolar and bipolar illness
An important development in recent years has been the separation between bipolar affective disorders, with a history of mania, and unipolar disorders,

with a history of depression alone. It is assumed that any patient who has an attack of mania has bipolar disorder, irrespective of whether depression has occurred, as in follow-up studies most such patients do ultimately develop depression. Some American authors have made a distinction between Bipolar I with a history of severe mania requiring admission, and Bipolar II with a history of milder mania.

Perris (1966) and Angst (1966) showed genetic differences between the two types, with a tendency to breed true. Essentially, bipolar patients have a stronger family history, and it is virtually only bipolar patients whose relatives show bipolar disorder. Nevertheless, about half the family members of bipolar probands have unipolar disorder. There are, in addition, other differences (Andreasen, 1982; Perris, 1982). The sex incidence is more nearly equal in bipolars; age of onset tends to be earlier and course more recurrent. The possible difference in social class has already been referred to. There is also some association, far from one to one, with cyclothymic or hypomanic personality. There is clear evidence of better response to lithium, and precipitation of manic episodes by tricyclic antidepressants (Paykel, 1979). There is some rather less convincing evidence of biological abnormalities, including lower MHPG and platelet monoamine oxidase and greater augmentation of EEG-evoked responses.

Psychotic/neurotic distinction

Only a relatively small proportion of all depressions, perhaps around 10 percent, are bipolar, so that the bipolar/unipolar distinction still leaves the problem of how to divide up the remainder. Here, the well-tried psychotic/ neurotic or endogenous/reactive distinction is still of great value. Originally the bipolar/unipolar dichotomy referred only to the affective psychoses, although it is often convenient to regard unipolar depression as having psychotic and neurotic forms.

Terminology is unsatisfactory. Strictly, psychotic and neurotic depression refer to the presence or absence of a severe illness with delusions, hallucinations and lack of insight; endogenous and reactive to the absence or presence of psychological precipitants. However, the two concepts have tended to become broadened and fused with a linkage between three elements: symptom picture, precipitant stress and personality (Rosenthal and Klerman, 1966). The symptom picture of psychotic or endogenous depression is said to be one of more severe illness, without short-term mood fluctuations in response to concurrent environmental changes; with severe guilt or pessimism which may reach delusional intensity; with psychomotor retardation or agitation; more severe somatic disturbances, such as insomnia, anorexia or weight loss; with early morning wakening, and diurnal morning worsening. Neurotic depression is said to span milder illness with reactivity of mood to minor environmental changes, anxiety, self-pity, blame of others rather than self-blame, initial insomnia and evening worsening. Psychotic depressives are said to have stable personalities; neurotic depressives to show inadequacy or persisting neuroticism.

The concept has a moderately long history (Kendell, 1968) dating back to the 1920s. It received considerable empirical confirmation in a large number of multivariate statistical studies published in the 1960s and 1970s (Kendell, 1976). Factor analytic studies usually showed a factor contrasting the symptoms of endogenous and non-endogenous depression, and cluster analytic studies tended to show a group of endogenous or psychotic depressives clearly separated, but with no single group of non-endogenous depressives. The factorial dimensions were usually independent of severity although there is a partial tendency for endogenous symptoms to be associated with greater severity and to be found more commonly among in-patients (Paykel *et al.*, 1970). In the 1970s much attention was devoted to examining whether the separation was sufficiently clear-cut to produce bimodality in distribution of defining indices. Although some investigations have claimed clear separation of types the common finding is of a gradation between clear endogenous and non-endogenous depression without any sharp boundary and with mixed cases common (Paykel and Rowan, 1979).

Validation has come most convincingly from studies of physical treatment and of biological correlates. A number of studies have found the best response to electroconvulsive therapy in patients who are both severely ill and show endogenous symptoms, particularly psychomotor retardation and delusions (Paykel, 1979). The most consistent biological correlate is nonsuppression of cortisol following dexamethasone administration (Carroll *et al.*, 1981), but there appear to be associations with some other neuroendocrine markers, such as blunted growth hormone response to clonidine (Checkley *et al.*, 1984; see Chapter 4).

A number of recent studies, using careful methodology, have shown that absence of life stress and presence of the endogenous symptom pattern are at best only weakly associated (Paykel *et al.*, 1984). The depression can be endogenous in symptoms but preceded by major life stress. Presence of endogenous symptoms appears to be the more informative aspect in relation to outcome of physical treatment (Paykel, 1979) and to neuro-endocrine correlates.

There has recently been a tendency to downrate this classification, but it does have the virtue of being buttressed by a vast amount of empirical work. This includes both classificatory studies, and the studies relating it to other validating associations, including biological abnormalities, aetiology, treatment response and longer term prognosis.

DSM III and ICD 10

The two competing official diagnostic classifications at present are DSM III and the International Classification of Diseases, 10th revision (ICD 10). DSM III, the official American classification, was introduced in 1980. The classification of mood disorders in its recently revised version, DSM IIIR (American Psychiatric Association, 1987) is shown in Table 1.2. There is a separate category for bipolar disorders. A new term, major

Table 1.2 Mood disorders (DSM IIIR)

Bipolar disorders	Depressive disorders
* Bipolar disorder	* Major depression
mixed	single episode
manic	recurrent
depressive	Dysthymia
Cyclothymia	(primary, secondary)
Bipolar disorder n.o.s.	(early, late onset)
	Depressive disorder n.o.s.

* Additional specifications for severity, psychotic, in remission, melancholia, seasonal.

n.o.s.—not otherwise specified.

depression, is used for non-bipolar depressions. Neurotic depression disappeared from DSM III, but the endogenous and psychotic classifications are partly preserved because there is a subcategory of psychotic depression for depression with delusions and hallucinations, and of melancholia for depression with the endogenous pattern. The authors of DSM III abandoned the term 'endogenous' as somewhat paradoxical to describe the symptom pattern and chose instead a relatively non-loaded term, 'melancholia'. Melancholia has been slightly downgraded in DSM IIIR as not meriting separate subdigits, but it is retained. There are also other subcategories. Two other depressive disorders are included which might have been regarded as personality types: cyclothymia and dysthymia. Dysthymic disorder was a new invention in DSM III to describe a pattern of persistent fluctuating mild depression that might be virtually life-long with short intermissions. This might also have been regarded as a characterological depression or one type of chronic neurotic depression.

This classification was a very substantial innovation. It had the great advantage, for the first time in any official classification, of adopting very tightly specified definitions for the disorders, of bringing together affective disorders in one section, and of clearly separating bipolar from unipolar disorders. The category of major depression was also a considerable advance in unifying unipolar depressions, with further division kept in subcategories, of which melancholia has been used in research subsequently. Dysthymic disorder was also a valuable addition, although more novel. On the negative side, the disorders were created and defined by fiat rather than by empirical research. This problem is particularly apparent in the changes between the original DSM III and DSM IIIR, which seem more the slightly idiosyncratic views of a committee than the fruit of empirical studies.

The second official classification is the International Classification of Disease. Its 9th version was very unsatisfactory with respect to affective disorders with many alternative subcategories which were not much used and very lax definitions. A new 10th revision, ICD 10, is currently being prepared. This makes some radical changes in the direction of DSM III. The classification of affective disorders has gone through some revisions and the latest version is set out in Table 1.3. There are separate major categories for mania, bipolar affective disorder, depression, recurrent depressive disorder, persistent affective states (cyclothymia and dysthymia), and other affective episodes. Manic and depressive episodes can be subclassified.

This classification is a mixed bag. It has some of the advantages of DSM III, but lags behind in other respects. Bipolar disorders are clearly separated, but there seems little point in distinguishing single manic attacks since it is generally accepted, with good evidence, that these are part of bipolar disorder. There is not much gain in separating single and recurrent depressive disorders, since on follow-up at least 50% of the former will ultimately become the latter. The subclassification of mania

Table 1.3 ICD 10 Affective Disorders Section[1]
(Main categories and main subcategories)

Manic episode	Hypomania
	Mania without psychotic symptoms
	Mania with psychotic symptoms
	mood congruent
	mood incongruent
Bipolar affective disorder	Current episode Hypomania
	Mania (subtypes as manic episode)
	Depression (subtypes as depressive episode)
	Mixed
Depressive episode	Mild severity without somatic symptoms
	with somatic symptoms
	Moderate severity without somatic symptoms
	with somatic symptoms
	Severe without psychotic symptoms
	with psychotic symptoms
	mood congruent
	mood incongruent
Recurrent depressive disorder	Current episode as depressive disorder
Persistent affective disorder	Cyclothymia
	Dysthymia
Other mood (affective) disorders	
Affective disorder unspecified	

[1]Abridged version from ICD 10, 1989, trial Draft of Chapter V. WHO Division of Mental Health, Geneva. Copyright WHO.

appears too detailed: only the division into hypomania and mania is used in clinical practice. The subclassification of depression is also complex, in its particular way of combining severity, endogenous (somatic) and psychotic symptoms. It would have done better to ignore severity and delineate endogenous and psychotic subtypes. This classification is an advance on ICD 9: its problems appear to arise from the need to fuse too many divergent views in an international classification, and adoption of a logical symmetry, which becomes fussy when fitted to clinical reality.

CONCLUSIONS

The word depression covers a range of phenomena from a normal mood to a pathological disorder. Clinical depression is best regarded as a syndrome, with a variety of causes, in which a number of features, probably reflecting a common pathophysiology, cluster together. Modern definitions emphasize presence of mood disturbance of sufficient intensity to include many concomitant features, with an absence of primary symptoms of another disorder. Epidemiological studies show a continuum of frequency, by setting, in part reflecting severity; — with annual rates of the order of 1 per 1000 for psychiatric admission, 3 per 1000 for psychiatric referral, 3 percent for treatment in general practice and a community prevalance of around 5 percent, varying with the case definition used. Depression is associated strongly with female sex: suggested explanations include both biological and social mechanisms. Milder depression occurs across adult age groups, particularly in married females aged 20 – 40 and in working-class subjects; more severe depression tends to be found in older age groups. Although a variety of classifications has been suggested, the bipolar/unipolar and endogenous/non-endogenous classifications have been the most useful, with a significant advance in the definitions and organization of DSM III. In interpreting findings in regard of depression, the diversity in severity, type and setting, and the particular characteristics of the sample selected, should always be kept in mind.

REFERENCES

American Psychiatric Association (1987). *Diagnostic and Statistical Manual of Mental Disorders* 3rd edn, revised. Washington DC: American Psychiatric Association.

Andreasen N. C. (1982). Concepts, diagnosis and classification. In *Handbook of Affective Disorders* (Paykel E. S., ed.) Edinburgh: Churchill Livingstone, pp. 24–44.

Angst J. (1966). *The Aetiology and Nosology of Endogenous Depressive Psychoses: a Genetic, Sociological and Clinical Study*. Berlin: Springer Verlag.

Bagley C. (1973). Occupational class and symptoms of depression. *Social Science Medicine*, 7, 327–39.

Bebbington P. E. (1978). The epidemiology of depressive disorder. *Culture, Medicine and Psychiatry*, 2, 297–341.

Bebbington P. E., Hurry J., Tennant C., *et al.* (1981). Epidemiology of mental disorders in Camberwell. *Psychological Medicine*, 11, 561–79.

Boyd J. H., Weissman M. M. (1982). Epidemiology. In *Handbook of Affective Disorders* (Paykel E. S., ed.) Edinburgh: Churchill Livingstone, pp. 106–52.

Brown G. W., Harris T. O. (1978). *Social Origins of Depression*. London: Tavistock Publications.

Canino G. J., Bird H. R., Shrout P. E., *et al.* (1987). The prevalence of specific psychiatric disorders in Puerto Rico. *Archives of General Psychiatry*, 44, 727–35.

Carroll B. J., Feinberg M., Greden J. F., *et al.* (1981). A specific laboratory test for the diagnosis of melancholia: standardisation, validation and clinical utility. *Archives of General Psychiatry*, 38, 15–22.

Checkley S. A., Glass I. B., Thompson C., *et al.* (1984). The GH response to clonidine in endogenous as compared with reactive depression. *Psychological Medicine*, 14, 773–7.

Comstock G. W., Helsing K. J. (1976). Symptoms of depression in two communities. *Psychological Medicine*, 6, 551–63.

Crombie E. (1974). Changes in patterns of recorded morbidity. In *Benefits and Risks in Medical Care* (Taylor D., Ed.) London: Office of Health Economics.

Crook T., Raskin A., Davis D. (1975). Factors associated with attempted suicide among hospitalised depressed patients. *Psychological Medicine*, 5, 381.

Dean C., Surtees P. G., Sashidharan S. P. (1983). Comparison of research diagnostic systems in an Edinburgh community sample. *British Journal of Psychiatry*, 142, 247–56.

Freeling P., Rao B. M., Paykel E. S., *et al.* (1985). Unrecognised depression in general practice. *British Medical Journal*, 290, 1880–3.

Goldberg D., Huxley P. (1980). *Mental Illness in the Community: The Pathway to Psychiatric Care*. London: Tavistock Publications, pp. 57–107.

Gove W. R. (1972). The relationship between sex roles, marital status, and mental illness. *Social Forces*, 51, 34–44.

Grad de Alarcon J., Sainsbury P., Costain W. R. (1975). Incidence of referred mental illness in Chichester and Salisbury. *Psychological Medicine*, 5, 32–54.

Henderson S., Duncan-Jones P., Byrne D. G., *et al.* (1979). Psychiatric disorders in Canberra: a standardised study of prevalence. *Acta Psychiatrica Scandinavica*, 60, 355–74.

HMSO (1986). *Morbidity Statistics from General Practice: Third National Study*. London: HMSO.

Juel-Nielsen N., Bille M., Flygenring J., Helgason T. (1961). Frequency of depressive states within geographically delimited population groups. 3. Incidence. (The Aarhus County Investigation). *Acta Psychiatrica Scandinavica*, 162, 69–80.

Kendell R. E. (1968). In *The Classification of Depressive Illnesses* Maudsley Monograph No. 18. London: Oxford University Press.

Kendell R. E. (1976). The classification of depression: a review of contemporary confusion. *British Journal of Psychiatry*, 129, 15–28.

Kendell R. E., Wainwright S., Hailey A., Shannon B. (1976). The influence of childbirth on psychiatric morbidity. *Psychological Medicine*, 6, 297–302.

Mavreas V. G., Beis A., Bouyias A., *et al.* (1986). Psychiatric disorders in Athens: a community study. *Social Psychiatry*, 21, 172–81.

Myers J. K., Weissman M. M., Tischler G. L., *et al.* (1984). Six-month prevalence of psychiatric disorders in three communities: 1980–1982. *Archives of General Psychiatry*, **41**, 959–67.

Newson-Smith J. G. B., Hirsch S. R. (1979). Psychiatric symptoms in self-poisoning patients. *Psychological Medicine*, **9**, 493.

Paffenberger R. S., McCabe L. J. (1966). The effect of obstetric and perinatal events on risk of mental illness in women of childbearing age. *American Journal of Public Health*, **56**, 400–7.

Paykel E. S. (1979). Predictors of treatment response. In *Psychopharmacology of Affective Disorders* (Paykel E. S., Coppen A., eds.) Oxford: Oxford University Press, pp. 193–220.

Paykel E. S., Rowan P. R. (1979). Affective disorders. In *Recent Advances in Clinical Psychiatry* (Granville-Grossman K., ed.) Edinburgh: Churchill Livingstone, pp. 37–90.

Paykel E. S., Klerman G. L., Prusoff B. A. (1970). Treatment setting and clinical depression. *Archives of General Psychiatry*, **22**, 11–21.

Paykel E. S., Rao B. M., Taylor C. M. (1984). Life stress and symptom pattern in outpatient depression. *Psychological Medicine*, **14**, 559–68.

Pederson A. M., Barry D. J., Babigian N. M. (1972). Epidemiological considerations of psychotic depression. *Archives of General Psychiatry*, **27**, 193–7.

Perris C. (1966). A study of bipolar (manic-depressive) and unipolar recurrent affective psychoses. *Acta Psychiatrica Scandinavica*, **42**, suppl. 194.

Perris C. (1982). The distinction between bipolar and unipolar affective disorders. In *Handbook of Affective Disorders* (Paykel E. S., ed.) Edinburgh: Churchill Livingstone, pp. 45–58.

Pugh T. F., Jerath B. K., Schmidt W. M., Reed R. B. (1963). Rates of mental disease related to childbearing. *New England Journal of Medicine*, **268**, 1224–8.

Richman N. (1977). Behaviour problems in pre-school children: family and social factors. *British Journal of Psychiatry*, **131**, 523–7.

Robins E., Guze S. B. (1970). Classification of affective disorders: the primary-secondary, the endogenous-reactive, and the neurotic-psychotic concepts. In *Recent Advances in the Psychobiology of the Depressive Illnesses* (Williams T. A, Katz M. M., Shield J. A., eds.) Washington DC: US Government Printing Office.

Robins L. N., Helzer J. E., Croughan J., Ratcliff K. S. (1981). National Institute of Mental Health Diagnostic Interview Schedule: Its history, characteristics and validity. *Archives of General Psychiatry*, **38**, 381–9.

Rosenthal S. H., Klerman G. L. (1966). Content and consistency in the endogenous depressive pattern. *British Journal of Psychiatry*, **112**, 471–84.

Shepherd M., Cooper B., Brown A. C., Kalton G. W. (1966). *Psychiatric Illness in General Practice*. London: Oxford University Press.

Spitzer R. L., Endicott J. (1978). Research diagnostic criteria. Rationale and reliability. *Archives of General Psychiatry*, **35**, 773–82.

Srole L., Langner T. S., Michael S. T., *et al.* (1962). *Mental Health in the Metropolis: The Midtown Manhattan Study*. New York: McGraw-Hill.

Surtees P. G., Dean C., Ingham J. G., *et al.* (1983). Psychiatric disorder in women from an Edinburgh Community: associations with demographic factors. *British Journal of Psychiatry*, **142**, 238–46.

Surtees P. G., Sashidharan S. P., Dean C. (1986). Affective disorder amongst women in the general population: a longitudinal study. *British Journal of Psychiatry*, **148**, 176–86.

Uhlenhuth E. H., Lipman R. S., Balter M. B., Stern M. (1974). Symptom intensity and life stress in the city. *Archives of General Psychiatry*, **31**, 759–64.

Urwin P., Gibbons J.L. (1979). Psychiatric diagnosis in self-poisoning patients. *Psychological Medicine*, **9**, 501.

Watts C. A. H., Cawte E. C., Kuenssberg E. V. (1964). Survey of mental illness in general practice. *British Medical Journal*, **2**, 1351–9.

Weissman M. M., Klerman G. L. (1977). Sex differences and the epidemiology of depression. *Archives of General Psychiatry*, **34**, 98–111.

Weissman M. M., Myers J. K. (1978). Affective disorders in a United States urban community: the use of research diagnostic criteria in an epidemiological survey. *Archives of General Psychiatry*, **35**, 1204–1311.

Weissman M. M., Leaf P. J., Holzer C. E., *et al.* (1984). The epidemiology of depression: an update on sex differences in rates. *Journal of Affective Disorders*, **7**, 179–88.

Wing J. K., Fryers T. (1976). *Psychiatric services in Camberwell and Salford: statistics from the Camberwell and Salford psychiatric registers 1964–74*. London: MRC Social Psychiatry Unit.

Wing J. K., Cooper J. E., Sartorius N. (1974). *The Measurement and Classification of Psychiatric Symptoms*. Cambridge: Cambridge University Press.

Wing J. K., Mann S. A., Leff J. P., Nixon J. M. (1978). The concept of a 'case' in psychiatric population surveys. *Psychological Medicine*, **8**, 203–17.

Winokur G. (1973). Depression in the menopause. *American Journal of Psychiatry*, **130**, 92–3.

Winokur G. (1974). The division of depressive illness into depression spectrum disease and pure depressive disease. *International Pharmacopsychiatry*, **9**, 5–13.

World Health Organization (1978). *Mental Disorders: Glossary and Guide to their Classification in accordance with the ninth revision of the International Classification of Diseases*. Geneva: WHO.

World Health Organization (1987). *ICD 10 1986 Draft of Chapter V. Categories F00–F99. Mental, behavioural and developmental disorders. Clinical descriptions and diagnostic guidelines*. Geneva: WHO (Division of Mental Health).

SECTION 2

Causes of Depression

2   *Depression: a radical social perspective*

GEORGE W. BROWN

INTRODUCTION

Progress over the last 20 years in our understanding of the role of social factors in the origins of depression has been such that it is no longer a matter of whether they often play a key role. The concerns are now the degree of their importance, whether their role differs by diagnostic subgroup, and whether there are implications for prevention and treatment. Nonetheless, interest in the social origins of depression in contemporary psychiatry and psychology has been somewhat perfunctory.

There has been an immense investment in biological aspects of depression, and to a lesser extent in cognitive aspects—independently of a systematic consideration of the patient's social milieu. No one can doubt the critical importance of biological factors in bipolar conditions, nor, at times, the presence of essentially endogenous depressive conditions, nor the likely importance of neuroendocrine factors in depression once it is underway. However, almost all recent research has been carried out on patients once they are depressed and it is possible that much may prove of somewhat marginal relevance for basic aetiological processes. Except in biopolar conditions, I know of little evidence that would support the idea of some basic flaw in bodily or cognitive functions before the onset of the depressive disorder that is not a direct reflection of the social milieu—past and present. In fact, despite recent progress in biological and cognitive studies in psychology, it is possible, and perhaps useful, to take a radical sociological perspective. Leaving aside the relatively rare bipolar disorders, and considering the broad sweep of affective conditions, the most realistic conclusion, if priorities about aetiological processes were to be given at present, would be that depression is in good part a social phenomenon. There are, for example, large social class differences in rates of depression. Also low rates have been found in some populations. A recent survey in a Basque-speaking rural community found only 2 percent of women with major depression over the period of one year (Gaminde and Uria, 1987). Similarly, low rates among the elderly in Japan have been reported (Hasegawa, 1985). If these reports turn out to be correct, would we wish to put most emphasis on studies of genetic diathesis or on the exploration of differences in the quality of social support and its impact on sense of self among the elderly?

It is not a matter, here, of one perspective being right and the other being wrong. It may well be that higher rates of depression among the elderly in, say, London and New York, are, at least in part, the result of breakdowns among those predisposed to depression for genetic or constitutional reasons. It is not a matter of choosing between alternatives but of emphasis and balance. The current predeliction in psychiatry is to turn inward in its search for causes—to personality traits, long-term emotional schemata and biologically-based dispositions. But we need also to give more than lip service to an outward perspective—to the possibility that depressive conditions, in no small number, are a result of complex transactions between the individual and his or her social environment.

Recent advances in our understanding of the social influences on depression can be said to have begun with research, reported by Eugene Paykel and his colleagues in 1969, on the role of life events in the onset of the disorder among depressed *patients* (Paykel *et al.*, 1969). However, it is appropriate to give more emphasis to community-based research at this point as this avoids the problem of selective factors at work in patient samples. This, of course, requires some stand on the troublesome issue of definition of a case (Wing *et al.*, 1981). For the purpose of this chapter, the threshold for defining depression will be roughly the severity seen in everyday out-patient practice. For example, in much of the work reviewed hereafter, the Bedford College diagnostic scheme (Brown and Harris, 1978) based on the Present State Examination (PSE; Wing *et al.*, 1974) has been used. In this a person is required to have depressed mood and at least four other core symptoms of depression such as hopelessness, suicidal plans or actions, neglect due to brooding, delayed sleep and anergia (Finlay-Jones *et al.*, 1980). The threshold has been shown to be somewhat more strict than the Index of Definition Score of five (ID–5), the threshold score for the PSE-based CATEGO diagnostic system, or for major depression in the Research Diagnostic Criteria (RDC) (Spitzer *et al.*, 1977; see also Chapter 1).

The main challenge arising from recent research in the general population is that various kinds of social experience taking place at different points in time—in childhood, in early adulthood, in the months before onset and in the period immediately following any life event involved in onset—relate to an increased risk of depression. Moreover, characteristics important at one point in time tend to be fairly highly correlated with each other—for instance, low self-esteem and chronic subclinical symptomatology. Given this, it is essential to develop models and theory that take life course into account, to pay the closest attention to the temporal ordering of experience and to develop theoretical ideas to guide the task of sorting out the complex interplay of experiences, both external and internal.

The present review will concentrate on women. Women have been studied far more often than men, but studies of men do indicate that current aetiological ideas are broadly applicable to them, despite their apparent lower prevalence of depression (Bebbington *et al.*, 1981; Murphy, 1982; Eales, 1988; Bolton and Oakley, 1987). All recent aetiological enquiries have placed central emphasis on the study of life events. Most of the studies to be reviewed utilized the Bedford College Life Event and Difficulty Schedule (LEDS), based on intensive interviewing and subsequent consensus ratings designed to eliminate bias (Brown and Harris, 1988). When this instrument is used, only events with severe long-term threat have proved to be critical for depression, and these events have provided the basis for more detailed exploration of aetiological processes. To be included as a severe event, such threat (in contrast to short-term threat) had still to be present some 7 to 10 days after the occurrence of the event. Also associated with onset have been *major* difficulties (persisting stressful social situations rather than recent new events or changes) lasting at least 2 years.

The results of the original population survey in Camberwell concerning severe life events have been replicated on at least ten occasions (see Table 2.1, column 2). When such events and difficulties are taken into account, their impact is considerable. Expressed in terms of an epidemiological measure, the population attributable risk, which gives the proportion of onsets of depression related to prior event or difficulty and allowing for their juxtaposition by chance, the average percentage is 73 percent. For severe events alone the average is 54 percent.

Findings concerning the aetiological role of difficulties have been less consistent than those for events. However, in a number of studies *major* difficulties (defined as above) have made an additional contribution to risk of depression (Table 2.1, columns 2, 3 and 4). The term *provoking agent* will be used to refer to the presence of either a severe event or a major difficulty. In spite of this evidence, though, there must be some uncertainty at present about the exact role of such difficulties. This issue will be returned to again below.

The most common way of viewing life events differs a good deal from the one used in these studies. Events have usually been collected by checklists, and have been seen as discrete happenings that can be added together to arrive at an estimate of overall adversity or strain. The same 'score' is given to, say, birth of a child, whether it involved a single mother living in deprived circumstances or a married couple eager to have a child. Such an approach, which deals with events as components to be equated and added (and perhaps subtracted), ignores that events occur in settings and are therefore usually an integral part of our lives and concerns. Our sense of self largely derives from such settings, together with the roles and purposes associated with them and the history of activity that has gone before. But, as plans and fantasies about the future can also be involved, a

Table 2.1 Summary of population studies using LEDS** of women in the 18 – 65 age range giving relationship of severe events and major difficulties to onset of caseness of depression (chronic cases of depression excluded)

Studies (random sample unless stated)	Length of period studied	Onset cases			Non-cases
		Severe events %†	Major difficulty %†	Severe event or major difficulty %†	Severe event or major difficulty %†
Brown and Harris (1978): Camberwell	38 weeks	25/37 68	18/37 49	33/37 89	115/382 30
Brown and Prudo (1981): Lewis, Outer Hebrides	1 year	11/16 69	6/16 38	13/16 81	42/171 25
Costello (1982): Calgary, Alberta	1 year	18/38 47	20/38 53	—	—
Campbell et al. (1983): Oxford (working-class with child)	1 year*	6/11 55	6/11 55	10/11 91	21/60 35
		5/12 42	5/12 42	9/12 75	17/52 33
Cooper and Sylph (1973): London (general practice)	3 months	16/34 47	—	—	—

Study	Period									
Finlay-Jones and Brown (1981): London (general practice)	1 year	27/32	84	6/32	19	27/32	84	32/119	27
Martin (1982, 1988): Manchester (pregnant women)	1 year	13/14	93	4/14	29	13/14	93	25/64	39
Brown *et al.* (1986a): Islington	6 months	29/32	91	15/32	47	30/32	94	92/271	34
(working-class with child)		25/33	76	14/33	42	28/33	85	107/323	33
Parry and Shapiro (1986): Sheffield (working-class with child)	1 year	12/20	60	3/20	15	14/20	70	62/172	36
Bebbington *et al.* (1984): Camberwell	10 months	—	—	—	—	13/21	62	45/131	34
TOTAL		212/312	68	107/279	38	218/261	84‡	558/1745	32‡

* Sample seen on two occasions 12 months apart.
**Bedford College Life Events and Difficulty Schedule (Brown and Harris, 1989).
† Percent with at least one event/difficulty.
‡ Average population attributable = 73.1 percent.

sense of self can go beyond such a history. In fact the origins of depression appear to be often intimately linked to loss of hope about some plan and fantasy.

There are, of course, difficulties in translating such a perspective into effective measurement—but the LEDS has made an attempt, albeit crude, to do this. The 'threat' ratings so far utilized are *contextual* measures— ratings that attempt to take account of setting and the event's relevance for ongoing plans. However, the concept of a plan (or some similar notion such as motive, purpose, or goal) is not ideal, because it conveys striving or awareness of some desirable future state. The most neutral term *concern* is perhaps preferable, because it suggests that the motivational background can be largely silent until the event has occurred (Klinger, 1977; Frijda, 1986). It is in so far as life events generate meaning in this way that they are important for understanding depression.

The most recent study to use this approach was carried out in Islington in North London. It was longitudinal and aimed to recontact women after a follow-up period of 1 year to find out about any onset of a depressive disorder. Working-class women with a child at home and single mothers were selected as earlier research had suggested they were the women most likely to develop depression. At the first contact, measures of the quality of personal ties, support received, and measures of 'self', such as self-esteem, were collected, together with an account of psychiatric disorder both at the time of interview and in the preceding 12 months. The second-phase interview covered details of any psychiatric disorder and of life events and difficulties occurring during the follow-up year, together with actual social support received during any significant crisis as well as the women's response to it (Brown *et al.*, 1985; Brown *et al.*, 1986a). Three-hundred and three women, who had not had a depressive condition at first contact, were followed up. Among the 32 women subsequently developing depression, 29 had a severe event not long before onset, giving a population attributable risk of 81 percent.

The majority of these severe events involved a loss or failure (see Brown *et al.*, 1987; Brown, 1988), and most had occurred within a few weeks of onset. There has been a general agreement in the literature about the critical importance for depression of loss (e.g. Paykel, 1974; Finlay-Jones and Brown, 1981; Miller and Ingham, 1983; Dohrenwend *et al.*, 1987). The nature of the severe events in Islington occurring before onset of depression fall into three roughly equal categories in terms of loss and disappointment. For 12 of the 29 women, the event presented a threat to their identity as a wife or mother, and one about which they could do very little—at least in the immediate future. For most of them, it was part of a long history of difficulty or failure in one or both of these roles—children getting into some kind of serious difficulty was particularly common.

A second set of eight women had a more diverse set of experiences, but what appeared to be in common was that they felt imprisoned in a non-rewarding and deprived setting, with the event itself underlining how little they could do about extracting themselves—that any way forward appeared to be blocked. Five of the eight had experienced events concerning poor housing, or debt, or both. However, there were usually wider ramifications: for example, one woman, a single mother, lived in poor housing with an extremely hyperactive child. Of the remaining three women in this second category, two experienced events concerned with severe physical handicap—one involving a husband and one the woman herself. Some of this second group of women also had reason to feel a failure in terms of some aspect of their core identity, and doubtless some at least of the 12 in the first category saw themselves as trapped. The distinction between the two categories is therefore one of degree.

The final nine women were all involved in the loss of a core person they had known for some time—in most instances a relative. Some incidents merely involved a break in the contact but, in most, the women had reason to feel rejected. Six in fact continued the theme of failure and rejection— for example, a husband leaving home, or the death of a child in circumstances that might convey some element of failure on the woman's part. The remaining three experienced a death (a mother, husband, and friend respectively), but there was no obvious reason for the woman to feel in any way responsible or, for that matter, rejected.

FURTHER REFINEMENTS OF THE CONCEPT OF SEVERE EVENTS

Studies using the LEDS have consistently shown that only about 1 in 5 of women experiencing a severe event go on to develop a depressive disorder. The Islington research has increased the strength of this link by refining the definition of severe events in a number of ways. The first is of particular interest, given the somewhat uncertain status of the link between long-term difficulties and onset of depression. Difficulties were considered if they had lasted at least 6 months at the point of first interview. For each severe event occurring in the follow-up period a straightforward judge- ment was made about whether there was a 'link' between the event and such an ongoing marked difficulty. For example, did the threat of eviction because of rent arrears match the difficulty present at first interview concerning such payments? If there were such a link, the events were known as matching *D-events*. The majority were related to the ongoing difficulty in a straightforward sense—for example, a husband leaving home in the context of marital disputes over his heavy drinking and violence, or a difficulty with a child (such as misbehaviour at school) involving an event with the same child (say referral to a Child Guidance Clinic). There was a three-fold greater risk of depression among those with such a D-event (Table 2.2A). Eales (1988), in a study of unemployed men, has established an apparently similar effect: unemployment was far more likely to lead to depression of caseness severity among men who had had a previous history

Table 2.2 Onset among women with a 'severe event' in Islington (130) by whether it 'matched' certain first interview measures

A. Severe event matching prior difficulty of 6 months or more (D-Event)		B. Severe event matching prior commitment (C-Event)		C. Either severe event matching prior difficulty of 6 months or more, or prior commitment (D-Event or C-Event)	
	% onset		% onset		% onset
Yes	46 (16/35)	Yes	40 (16/40)	Yes	37 (24/65)
No	14 (13/95)	No	14 (13/90)	No	8 (5/65)
TOTAL	22 (29/130)	TOTAL	22 (29/130)	TOTAL	22 (29/130)
$p < 0.001$		$p < 0.01$		$p < 0.001$	

of financial or employment difficulties. There is some suggestion in the Islington data that women were more likely, following a D-event, to respond with profound feelings of hopelessness—a reaction proposed earlier as forming an integral part of the development of a depressive disorder (Brown *et al.*, 1987).

A second way of dealing with severe events concerns matching with an earlier conflict—in this case *R-event* stands for role conflict at the time of the first interview. Conflicting demands of work and domestic responsibilities were most often involved. As there is a great deal of overlap with D-events, a combined *D/R event* category will be used in the final overview of results.

A third way of refining severe events proved to be quite independent of these forms of matching. Severe events matching high commitment in areas such as marriage, children and employment, were known as *C-events* and women with one of these were three times more likely to develop depression than those with another severe event (Table 2.2B). The greater risk of depression appears to reflect the fact that marked commitment increases the saliency of a loss or disappointment.

These results are methodologically impressive because the 'soft' material used as a basis for matching was collected at first interview before the occurrence of either severe event or depression; they underline the central role of meaning of events. However, despite the welcome increase in ability to predict depression, fewer than half the women who experienced such a matching severe event went on to develop depression. In other words, there were still plenty of women with children in Islington who had an important loss or disappointment but did not develop depression. To go further, it is necessary to consider ongoing vulnerability and quality of support.

Vulnerability may be defined as any characteristic of a person, or an environment, that increases risk *only in the presence of provoking agent.*

Various factors were isolated, in the first inquiry in Camberwell to use the LEDS, and it was speculated then that low self-esteem might provide a common explanation for their link with increased risk of depression (Brown and Harris, 1978). In Islington, low self-esteem, when judged on the basis of the negative comments a woman made about herself at the time she was first interviewed, did appear to play such a role. Among women with a provoking agent, rate of onset was increased, almost threefold in the presence of such low self-esteem (see Table 2.3).

Again, the result is methodologically impressive as self-esteem was measured before the follow-up period and reporting could not have been contaminated by any depressive disorder developing after it. Furthermore, another longitudinal enquiry has recently produced consistent findings (Ingham *et al.*, 1986, 1987; Miller *et al.*, 1987). However, the exact role of self-esteem remains to be settled, and this cannot be done without taking into account its quite high correlation with the quality of social support from core ties (namely a husband, lover, or anyone described as 'very close' in response to direct questioning at the time of our first interview).

SOCIAL SUPPORT

The notion of support has been closely linked with that of vulnerability. In the Camberwell survey, lack of confiding and intimacy with a husband or lover was much the most important vulnerability factor, and this finding has now been replicated on many occasions (see Table 2.4). However, the intimacy measure contains an important ambiguity: it takes account both of the other person's behaviour during any crisis leading to depression, and of behaviour before this. Such behaviour is not necessarily of one piece and in a cross-sectional study it is difficult to separate the relative contributions of past and present. In the Camberwell survey, the two were in fact amalgamated in the overall rating of intimacy, although where there was an obvious discrepancy, most weight was given to behaviour at the time of the crisis.

Table 2.3 Low self-esteem at 1st interview (negative evaluation of self) and onset depression (303 Islington women)

Low self-esteem	Provoking agent	
	Yes—% onset	*No*—% onset
Yes	33 (18/54)	4 (1/27)
No	13 (12/96)	1 (1/126)
	$p < 0.01$	not significant

Table 2.4 Onset of 'caseness' depression, intimacy with husband and presence of a severe event or major difficulty

	Provoking agent			No provoking agent		
	No intimacy (% onset)	Intimacy (% onset)		No intimacy (% onset)	Intimacy (% onset)	
(A) Severe events or major difficulty						
Strict replication of Camberwell survey						
Brown and Harris (1978): Camberwell	32 (24/76)	10 (9/88)	p < 0.001	3 (2/62)	1 (2/193)	n.s.
Campbell *et al.* (1983): Oxford	46 (12/26)	13 (3/23)	p < 0.02	12 (2/17)	2 (1/44)	n.s.
Brown and Prudo (1981): Lewis	36 (8/22)	15 (5/33)	n.s.	5 (2/40)	1 (1/92)	n.s.
Bebbington *et al.* (1984): Camberwell	22 (8/37)	24 (5/21)	n.s.	11 (5/45)	6 (3/49)	n.s.
Parry and Shapiro (1986): Sheffield	31 (8/26)	10 (5/49)	p < 0.05	10 (2/19)	5 (5/98)	n.s.
Finlay-Jones[a]: Regents Park area, London	45 (24/53)	17 (4/23)	p < 0.05	8 (3/36)	3 (1/39)	n.s.
Brown and Andrews (1985): Islington	26 (23/90)	12 (7/60)	p < 0.05	3 (1/38)	1 (1/115)	n.s.
(B) Severe events only						
Costello (1982): Calgary	57 (8/14)	21 (5/24)	p < 0.05	7 (4/56)	5 (14/292)	n.s.
Martin *et al.* (1989)[b]: Manchester	73 (8/11)	14 (2/14)	p < 0.01	40 (2/5)	4 (2/47)	p < 0.01
TOTAL	35 (123/355)	13 (45/335)	—	7 (23/318)	3 (30/969)	—
Closely related studies						
Paykel *et al.* (1980)[c]: South London	82 (9/11)	24 (8/34)	p < 0.001	14 (1/7)	12 (6/52)	n.s.
Murphy (1982)[d]: North London	35 (6/17)	11 (10/90)	p < 0.02	0 (0/19)	3 (2/74)	n.s.
OVERALL TOTAL	36 (138/383)	14 (63/459)	—	7 (24/344)	3 (38/1095)	—

The values shown are percentages, with the numbers of subjects in parentheses.
[a] R. A. Finlay-Jones (personal communication).
[b] A study of a series of women covering a pregnancy and a birth in every instance.
[c] Study of post-partum women: one or more undesirable events and poor communication with husband.
[d] Elderly sample of both sexes: severe event or major difficulty. Low intimacy = no confiding with anyone, i.e. not only husband.
n.s. — not significant.

As the Islington survey was based on a longitudinal design, it was possible to contrast measures of support at two points in time. It turned out that if the two differed, it was support at the point of crisis that was critical. The results are complex, but Table 2.5, dealing with married women, illustrates the basic finding. It shows that women who did confide at this earlier point in time and who failed to obtain support in a subsequent crisis were particularly likely to develop depression. *Crisis support* was defined by three criteria: confiding in the other person, receiving active emotional support from the same person, and lack of a negative reaction on the person's part at some point in the crisis. Women who failed to receive support that they might reasonably have expected on the basis of the level of confiding at the time of the first interview were defined as *let down*. It is possible that their high risk was due, at least in part, to the fact that being let down may have contributed to a fall in self-esteem over and above any fall resulting from the provoking crisis itself— that is a two-step lowering of self-esteem.

Married women were particularly prone to be let down by either a husband or someone they had named as 'very close' at first interview—that is someone other than a husband or child under 16 living at home. By contrast, single mothers practically always received crisis support from those they had named as very close and with whom they had been confiding. Their high risk of depression was related much less to being let down and more to the fact of lacking support in the first place (Brown *et al.*, 1986a). When a woman was let down, support from some other core tie in the crisis did not relate to a reduced risk of depression. However, earlier research was confirmed which suggested that, even when support from a husband or lover was missing, support from others could, at times, be protective. For married women, for example, crisis support from a person living outside the household (usually a woman), who had been named as very close, was highly related to reduced risk (that is, as long as she had not been let down by her husband).

Table 2.5 Confiding in husband at first interview, crisis support during the follow-up year and onset of depression among those with a provoking agent (98 married Islington women)

Confiding in husband at first interview	Crisis support from husband during follow-up		
	Yes—% onset	*No*—% onset	*Total*—% onset
Yes	4 (1/28)	37 (7/19) 'let down'	17 (8/47)
No	25 (2/8)	24 (10/42)	24 (12/50)

Crisis support not known for three subjects.

PRIOR PSYCHIATRIC SYMPTOMATOLOGY

Critics of a psychosocial view of depression frequently cite the importance of prior depressive symptoms in determining subsequent disorder, and the role of such ongoing symptomatology needs to be considered (see Akiskal, 1985). Does such symptomatology play a role in the putative aetiological processes so far outlined, and if so, what is involved?

In Islington, chronic subclinical symptomatology was in fact an important predictor of subsequent onset (Brown *et al.*, 1986b). All conditions were present at the time of the first contact with the women and almost all involved anxiety or depression—a few non-depressive conditions at a caseness level were, however, included with them. The key question arising from this result is the likely aetiological mechanism involved, bearing in mind that chronic subclinical symptoms, as much as low self-esteem, may reflect the quality of a woman's core relationships. Indeed, it is just such a link that appears to explain their effectiveness as a predictor: such symptoms showed no association at all with subsequent depression *unless they were also accompanied at the time of the first interview by a marked social difficulty*. Furthermore, this increased risk was entirely the result of the occurrence of D-events, arising out of such difficulties. There was therefore nothing to suggest that chronic subclinical symptoms raised the risk except in the presence of ongoing difficulties, which presumably had often played a role in their perpetuation (and perhaps onset) in the first place.

These Islington results are unambiguous, but need to be replicated. Given this caveat, there is at present no reason to believe that a chronic depressive or anxiety condition before the onset of a frank depressive disorder is a threat to the validity of the psychosocial perspective so far outlined. Indeed, given the established role of ongoing difficulties in the aetiological process, it is just the kind of link that would be expected. At the same time, there are no grounds for asserting that such symptoms may not at times also be related to biological processes which are independent of psychosocial influences (see also Chapter 5).

AN OVERALL VIEW

The Islington material suggests that once a difficulty is underway it will usually require a change in the ongoing situation to bring about onset of depression—a change that provokes some kind of reassessment of the person's sense of self and future. Absence or presence of social support can be expected to interact with such experiences in quite complex ways to increase or reduct risk. Support from husband, lover or someone named as very close was highly correlated with high self-esteem at the time of the first contact. Leaving aside the kind of complicated interplay that is likely between the two, it is important to recognize that self-esteem can fall dramatically, perhaps in a matter of hours, with any failure of social support (Harris, 1987).

Social support appears to play four major roles in onset. As a first possibility, we have seen that a close tie can place a person in jeopardy— once a crisis has occurred it is possible to be *let down* and thereby experience a double loss. Second, an ongoing situation of poor support may induce feelings of low self-esteem and thereby make a person *vulnerable* to depression once a major loss has occurred. Third, irrespective of these two possibilities, another source of support from a close tie may offer *protection*. This could arise if a woman, say, in a poor marriage, received effective support from a female friend during a crisis concerning her husband. A fourth possibility has not so far been discussed. A situation of generally poor support can raise the risk of subsequent losses and disappointments. (For example, a poor marriage may lead to a legal separation, to serious violence and so on.) This is a matter of *event production* and is best considered in terms of an overall aetiological model.

Enough has been reviewed to suggest that any such model will need to take account of a person's social milieu both before and at the time of any crisis. The instrument used for this purpose in the Islington enquiry—the Self-Evaluation and Social Support Schedule (SESS)—deals not only with external manifestations of current life structure in areas such as marriage and motherhood, but with how activities are internally represented in terms of ideas and feelings about self (O'Connor and Brown, 1984). In order to obtain an index of the quality of a women's life, scales dealing with objective aspects of her life—such as the amount of tension in her marriage—were considered. The resulting *Index of Negative Elements in Core Relationships* was constructed in terms of the effectiveness of the ratings to predict low self-esteem. For married women, the main items were negative interaction with children, negative interaction with husband, lack of primary quality in her relationship with him, and the security-diminishing characteristics of her housewife role (a measure largely reflecting shortcomings in the practical and financial help provided by her husband). It should also be emphasized that the *Negative Elements in Core* Relationship Index encompassed a wide range of situations, ranging from the obviously grossly disturbing to somewhat subtle shortcomings, say, in the quality of the marital relationship. It is of interest in the light of what is to follow that it was just such more minor negative features that at times predicted major problems in the follow-up year. For example, one woman was included in the index because of a 'moderate' rating on the negativity of interaction with husband despite a 'marked' rating for positive interaction, many other favourable ratings, and no other negative ratings on the index itself. The 'moderate' rating was based on the woman's comment that there 'can be tension when we go out together and he's in one of his moods'. 'He sometimes gets on my nerves when we are home together and I want to get on with work'. (He was unemployed.) 'He's very quick-tempered.' During the follow-up year he became very disturbed as part of a paranoid disorder, and it turned out that the woman had underplayed the difficulty his selfish and unreasonable behaviour had brought to the marriage a year before our first interview with her. It needs therefore to be emphasized that the index is an atheoretical one that will eventually require explication. It almost certainly represents a range of phenomena including at times some component of dissatisfaction and irritability on the women's part, attempts to downplay a potentially difficult situation, as well as a fairly sensitive device for picking up the early signs of serious trouble in core relationships. For the most part its predictive importance in terms of subsequent onset of depression probably lies in what its title reflects, but it would be misleading to present it simply in these terms. Its present importance probably lies in the fact that it conveys that the seeds of the post-event situation were often present well before its occurrence.

Once low self-esteem and this new index were taken into account, only one other measure made at first interview predicted onset. This was the presence of chronic subclinical symptoms already discussed, and it had therefore also been taken into account. The most notable finding is that neither of the two internal measures (i.e. low self-esteem or subclinical symptoms), nor the index concerning negative elements in core relationships, were associated with onset of depression without the presence of the other—thus it is only the combination of negative elements in core relationships with one or the other of the two internal measures that predicted onset (Table 2.6). Under these circumstances once a provoking agent occurred the risk of depression was considerable—44 percent (25/57) and 5 percent (5/93) respectively for those with and without such an agent.

As this set of results will now be used to discuss an aetiological model of depression, a less cumbersome way of referring to the factors is desirable. The presence of either low self-esteem or chronic subclinical symptoms will be referred to as *discomfiture* and the presence of discomfiture *and*

Table 2.6 Basic results concerning conjoint negative index: negativity of core relationships *and* discomfiture

A. Women with negative elements in core relationships and discomfiture		B. Negative elements in core relationships and *discomfiture* at onset			C. Total onsets associated with negative elements in core relationships and *discomfiture*	
% onset		Both	One or other (% onset)	None	% onset	
26	(80/303)	33 (26/80)	4 (4/104) $p < 0.001$	2 (2/119)	81	(26/32)

negative elements in core relationships will be sufficient to rate on a negative *Conjoint Index*. Using this index as the core of the analysis, I will deal only with the 150 of the 303 women in Islington who experienced a provoking agent because, as already noted, they contained practically all the onsets of depression (30/150 vs. 2/153).

The first component of the resulting aetiological model has already been anticipated. The Conjoint Index predicted the occurrence of matching D/R-events. This association is hardly surprising given that, by definition, such severe events had to be linked with prior difficulties or sources of conflict. This means that the important process of 'event production' is restricted to such D/R-events. Here it is important to note that on its own, the fact that the Conjoint Index led to D/R-events did not in itself contribute to a raised risk of depression. The Conjoint Index *also* acted as a *vulnerability factor*, and it was by playing by this dual role that it was associated with practically all the onsets following a D/R-event (17 out of 18; Fig. 2.1).

A second model is sufficient to deal with the rest of the women, namely those experiencing a provoking agent which does not involve a D/R-event. The model is simpler as it lacks an event-production component: in this second model it is only when the Conjoint Index and severe events happen to occur together that they act synergistically to increase risk. Here again, most of the onsets are the outcome of the resulting vulnerability effect (Fig. 2.2).

The central importance of a woman's current life, as represented by the Conjoint Index, is therefore clear. However, there are still two issues that need to be incorporated in any overview—adequacy of support in a crisis, and early experience, as exemplified by lack of care.

THE ROLE OF SUPPORT IN OVERVIEW

Inadequacy of support, following the earlier discussion, will be defined in terms of lack of crisis support *or* being 'let down'. It is highly correlated with the three factors of the Negative Conjoint Index—negative elements

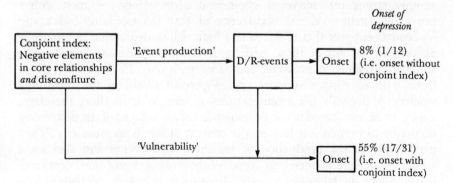

Fig. 2.1 *Vulnerability and event production—for those with D/R events*

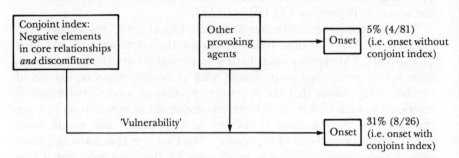

Fig. 2.2 *Vulnerability only—for those with provoking agents other than D/R events*

in core relationships, low self-esteem and chronic subclinical symptoms. In this sense, its critical role in the development of depression can be seen as underlining the tightness of the links already discussed. The degree of overlap between inadequacy of support and the Conjoint Index is to be expected, given that the common theme throughout this review has been the critical importance for depression of shortcomings in core relationships. In effect, such lack of support serves as a central mediating factor, linking the internal and external factors of the Negative Conjoint Index with onset; in practice, lack of crisis support often confirmed what was fairly obvious from the situation described by the woman at the time of first interview (Fig. 2.3).

Because the association between the negative Conjoint Index and subsequent inadequate support is high, the actual changes in numerical terms brought about by its inclusion model are relatively modest (Brown, 1989, appendix 2). Inadequate support can, without too much simplification, be seen as simply mediating the vulnerability mechanism reflected in the Conjoint Index. In terms of actual results, what in fact occurs is yet another strong interactive or synergistic effect. Among women with a provoking agent it is the occurrence of *both* the Conjoint Index and inadequate support that is linked to a high risk or depression. As many as 58 percent (23/40) of those with both Conjoint Index and inadequate support developed depression, compared with only 15 percent (4/26) of those with only poor support, and 4 percent (3/80) of the remaining women. A person's life circumstances at one point in time, therefore, appear to be implicated in the development of a good deal of the depression occurring to women—at least in the context of life in an inner city. They play a role in the production of matching D/R-events and also via a vulnerability effect once any type of provoking agent has occurred. Furthermore, in Islington at least, those most at risk of depression in a given year formed a surprisingly small proportion of the total population.

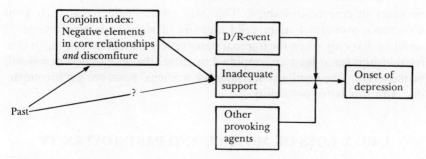

Fig. 2.3 *Intervening role of support*

Three-quarters of onsets (25/32) occurred among just over a quarter of the women (26 percent—80/303) who at the time of first interview were positive on this Index and who had not already depression at a caseness level.

With this degree of overlap between the factors in the model, the role of low self-esteem requires some comment. It still plays a central role, but only in conjunction with negative elements in of core relationships, and its exact effect is difficult to unravel because of its correlation with chronic subclinical symptoms. These results are compatible with it playing no direct role in key causal processes. For example, it seems probable that an ongoing difficulty in some way leads to a subsequent D-event, quite irrespective of the presence of low self-esteem, with which such difficulties are correlated. In a similar manner, low self-esteem may be the result of difficulties in a core relationship, and it is this difficult relationship that results in inadequate support in a crisis. But these possibilities do not rule out that low self-esteem may at the same time play a role—for example, in the sense that a woman's low self-esteem in response to a difficult relationship my serve to make that tie even more difficult. It may also make a quite independent contribution. It may, for example, influence the degree of hopelessness felt in response to events—and thus contribute to the critical final pathway in our model.

Several other possibilities could be given and it is therefore possible that low self-esteem plays a critical role in explaining the impact of the factors in the model. However, given their correlation with self-esteem, this cannot at present be unequivocally demonstrated. Therefore, in spite of obtaining exactly the result that had been predicted and despite the use of a longitudinal enquiry, arguments for the inclusion of low self-esteem as an important part of the aetiological process must at the moment depend on what is theoretically plausible. The possibility that it does play a key role is, in fact, reasonably compelling, and it would be shortsighted to rule out a central role for it.

It will be recalled, however, that neither low self-esteem nor chronic subclinical symptoms related to risk of depression without negative elements in core relationships. This may merely reflect that their joint occurrence provides a more valid measure of relevant internal states. It could be that only when the internal states reflect some shortcoming in core relationships (or at least are amplified by them) that risk of depression will be increased. The results concerning the womens' pasts are not incompatible with this latter possibility.

EARLY LOSS OF MOTHER AND PAST ADVERSITY

The aetiological model isolated in the original Camberwell enquiry included loss of mother before the age of 11, due to either death or a separation of at least one year. Such loss was associated with a raised risk of depression once a provoking agent had occurred. Along with this increase in incidence went a greater prevalence of depression at a caseness level (Brown *et al.*, 1977). There has been a good deal of controversy about the findings (Crooke and Eliot, 1980; Tennant *et al.*, 1980; Brown and Harris, 1986; Harris *et al.*, 1986). Nonetheless, two further population studies have produced equally clear evidence. An enquiry in Walthamstow screened a large number of women to provide instances of such loss; those with early loss of mother, by death or separation, had a much higher rate of current depression, and this also held for losses between the ages of 11 and 17 (Brown *et al.*, 1986c; Harris *et al.*, 1986, 1987). In the Islington survey, a high rate of depression again occurred among those losing a mother between age 11 and 17, suggesting that the original cut-off at age 11 may have been rather too hastily adopted (Bifulco *et al.*, 1987).

The mode of the impact of early loss of mother for women is undoubtedly complex, and on the basis of the recent research the role of untoward experiences *after* the loss has been emphasized, rather than the loss itself (Brown *et al.*, 1986c; Harris *et al.*, 1986, 1987; Bifulco *et al.*, 1987). In order to throw light on this link, it is necessary to trace the history of the person from the early loss itself to later depression, through a series of experiences from which it is possible to gain some sense of a person's life trajectory. But such an exercise should not be approached in any spirit of determinism: it is quite clear that intervening experiences can serve to reduce as well as increase risk in adult life. Attempting to chart this chain of circumstances, we became aware that certain early life events were particularly associated with a raised risk of provoking agents and vulnerability factors in the current environment (Harris *et al.*, 1986, 1987). More important than early loss of the mother itself in setting a person on such a life-course trajectory of depression was the quality of replacement parental care after the loss. If this was judged inadequate (in terms of an index of parental indifference and lax control, termed *lack of care*), the risk of current depression was doubled.

Another factor which turned out to play a critical mediating role was the experience of a premarital pregnancy, and, like lack of care itself, this was found to be associated with experience of a provoking agent in the year of the survey (Brown, 1988). A pregnancy of this kind involved any conception before legal marriage, irrespective of whether marriage or a live birth followed. What seemed to be crucial about these premarital pregnancies was that they often trapped women in relationships which they might well not otherwise have chosen and which had become a source of provoking agents—for example, housing and financial problems consequent upon a couple starting a family too young to have built up adequate savings, or marital difficulties with undependable partners. These women also emerged as less upwardly mobile, in terms of social class, than their peers without such premarital pregnancies. In interpreting this complex of experiences leading to depression, a conveyor belt of adversities was outlined, on which some women were moved inexorably from one crisis to another, starting with lack of care in childhood and passing via premarital pregnancy to current working-class status, lack of social support, and high rates of provoking agents. We were, however, fully aware that to attribute this chain of circumstances solely to environmental factors might prove short-sighted. Although it was often hard to see from the women's accounts of their lives how they could have left this conveyor belt, once their childhood had located them on it, a more personal element could almost have played a role.

This kind of early experience finally needs to be incorporated into the overall picture. An *Index of Early Inadequate Parenting* based largely on the experience of 'lack of care' from a key carer is quite highly related to the Negative Conjoint Index (namely negative elements in core relationships and discomfiture). However, in terms of the link between past environment and present provoking agents, the current situation appeared to be critical. The past was entirely unassociated, for example, with the occurrence of a D/R-event (so heavily implicated in onset), unless there was also the relevant event-producing life structure represented by the Conjoint Index.

However, in terms of the second key aetiological factor, *inadequate support*, there was a modest but statistically significant link with early inadequate parenting adversity that was independent of the Conjoint Index, and there is a possibility that a personality factor linked to early experience may play a direct part in a woman's ability to develop effective social ties (Andrews and Brown, 1988). This does not, however, imply that personality plays a role outside the confines of the model that has been outlined. It seems most likely that its main impact on risk of depression is via lack of support, and that such a factor is important in so far as it contributes to this. (For further discussion on the possible roles of personality in predisposition to depression see Chapter 5).

RECOVERY FROM DEPRESSION

So far, I have dealt with the issue of onset, but one of the most significant public health problems presented by depression is that half of those suffering from it at any one time, at a caseness level, are *chronic* sufferers. In other words, the episode has lasted for at least one year and usually a good deal longer. The role of psychosocial factors both in perpetuating depression and in recovery has therefore also to be considered.

Material collected over a 2-year period in Islington has confirmed a finding from the earlier Camberwell research that ongoing difficulties play a significant role in perpetuating depression. However, the most interesting finding is that recovery (including any major improvement) in women with chronic depression at a caseness level was related either to significant reduction in the overall experience of ongoing difficulties or to a *fresh start event*—a new concept. Such events involve the idea of starting again, and while this often goes with a reduction in a difficulty, this is by no means always so. Fresh start events appear to make a contribution to recovery over and above that made by any reduction in difficulties. Moreover, they quite often involve a significant degree of threat (a quarter were rated severe events). The important thing about them is that they convey some hope that things will be better (Brown *et al.*, 1988). The majority recovering from chronic depression had either experienced difficulty-reduction or a fresh start event, and in this sense, the general importance of a cognitive-affective approach to depression is again underlined. The study can only be seen as exploratory, but there have been other suggestive studies (Surtees and Ingham, 1980; Tennant *et al.*, 1981; Parker *et al.*, 1985; Miller *et al.*, 1987), and the recent data are enough to make a preliminary case that the process of recovery in general is often the mirror-image of the psychosocial processes leading to onset—at least for those with depression that had been in existence for some time.

A QUESTION OF DISTRESS VERSUS DISEASE

Unfortunately, it is only possible to sketch a reply to a common response, on the part of psychiatrists at least, to the findings that have been outlined—that those concerned are, on the whole, not depressed in a true clinical sense. This may well be so if one has in mind patients suffering from manic-depression or severe melancholic forms with psychotic features (although it is now well established that the latter frequently have provoking agents before onset—see Katschnig *et al.*, 1986). However, such severely disturbed, depressed patients are not typical of the general run of patients seen by psychiatrists—especially in an out-patient clinic. Certainly research so far indicates that the kind of model of depression outlined in this chapter is probably relevant for the majority of depressed patients seen by psychiatrists—although for a somewhat smaller proportion than those selected at random in the general population.

There is still, however, a great deal to be done. Published research has been unsatisfactory in its specification of just which psychiatric patients have been studied—for example, what about the large number seen by psychiatrists only once? It has also, by and large, failed to consider the role and effect of powerful selective factors which channel only some people but not others into psychiatric services (Goldberg and Huxley, 1980). In Islington only 13 percent of women suffering from depression at a caseness level saw a psychiatrist; and, although those that were seen apparently did not differ in severity of depression, they did more often try to harm themselves or were also heavy drinkers or drug users. In other words, psychiatrists often appeared to be seeing women who were both depressed and showing behaviour likely to be worrying for a general practitioner. It is of interest that two studies have now shown that such attempts at self-harm are closely linked to early separation from mothers but *not* to loss by death (Brown *et al.*, 1985). In short, we need to explain the role of social factors in *symptom-formation* as well as aetiology and course, and also to bear in mind the way such selective factors may influence thinking among psychiatrists about the nature of depression itself. It is possible, for instance, that thinking about 'neurotic' forms of depression has been highly influenced by such selective factors.

Such issues would require another review. Much has still to be established and there is an urgent need to carry out psychosocial and biological measures on the same population of depressed individuals. Perhaps here the area of sleep architecture is the most promising (Kupfer, 1986). However, sufficient is already known for there to be some confidence in the notion that differences in the role of the social environment in the onset and course of depressive disorder in the patient and in the general population will be of degree rather than of kind.

REFERENCES

Akiskal H. S. (1985). Interaction of biologic and psychologic factors in the origin of depressive disorders. *Acta Scandinavica Supplement*, **319**, (71) 131–9.

Andrews B., Brown, G. W. (1987). Social support, onset of depression and personality: an exploratory analysis. *Social Psychiatry*, **23**, 99–108.

Bebbington P., Hurry, J., Tennant, C., *et al.* (1981). Epidemiology of mental disorders in Camberwell. *Psychological Medicine*, **11**, 561–79.

Bebbington P., Sturt E., Tennant C., Hurry J. (1984). Misfortune and resilience: a replication of the work of Brown and Harris. *Psychological Medicine*, **14**, 347–63.

Bifulco A., Brown G. W., Harris T. O. (1987). Childhood loss of parent and adult psychiatric disorder: the Islington study. *Journal of Affective Disorders*, **12**, 115–28.

Bolton W., Oatley, K. (1987). A longitudinal study of social support and depression in unemployed men. *Psychological Medicine*, 17, 453–60.

Brown G. W., Harris T.O., Copeland J.R. (1977). Depression and loss. *British Journal of Psychiatry*, 130, 1–18.

Brown G. W. (1989). Aetiology and course of depression—a social perspective. In *Community Psychiatry* (Bennett D. H., Freeman H., eds.).

Brown, G. W., Andrews B. (1985). *Comparison of Camberwell and Islington intimacy ratings* (unpublished).

Brown G. W. (1989). Stressor, vulnerability and depression: a question of replication. *Psychological Medicine*, 16, 739–44.

Brown G. W., Harris T. O. (1978). *Social Origins of Depression: A Study of Psychiatric Disorder in Women*. London: Tavistock Publications; New York: Free Press.

Brown G. W., Harris T. O. (1988). Life Events and Measurement. In *Life Events and Illness* (Brown G. W., Harris T. O., eds.) New York: Guildford Press.

Brown G. W., Prudo R. (1981). Psychiatric disorder and physical illness. *Journal of Psychosomatic Research*, 25, 461–73.

Brown G. W., Craig T. K. J., Harris T. O. (1985). Depression: disease or distress? Some epidemiological considerations. *British Journal of Psychiatry*, 147, 612–22.

Brown G. W., Andrews, B., Harris, T. O., *et al.* (1986a), Social support, self-esteem and depression. *Psychological Medicine*, 16, 813–31.

Brown G. W., Bifulco A., Harris T. O., Bridge L. (1986b) Life stress, chronic psychiatric symptoms and vulnerability to clinical depression. *Journal of Affective Disorders*, 11, 1–19.

Brown G. W., Harris T. O., Bifulco A. (1986c). Long-term effect of early loss of parent. In *Depression in Childhood: Developmental Perspectives* (Rutter M., Izard C., Read P., eds.) New York: Guildford Press.

Brown G. W., Bifulco A., Harris T. O. (1987). Life events, vulnerability and onset of depression: some refinements. *British Journal of Psychiatry*, 150, 30–42.

Campbell E. (1982). *Vulnerability to depression and cognitive predisposition: psychosocial correlates of Brown and Harris vulnerability factors*. Paper presented to the British Psychological Society Annual Conference.

Campbell E., Cope S., Teasdale, J. (1983). Social factors and affective disorder: an investigation of Brown and Harris' model. *British Journal of Psychiatry*, 143, 548–53.

Cooper B., Sylph J. (1973). Life events and the onset of neurotic illness: an investigation in general practice. *Psychological Medicine*, 3, 421–35.

Costello C. G. (1982). Social factors associated with depression: a retrospective community study. *Psychological Medicine*, 12, 329–39.

Crooke T., Eliot J. (1980). Parental death during childhood and adult depression: a critical review of the literature. *Psychological Bulletin*, 87, 252–9.

Dohrenwend B., Shrout P., Link B., *et al.* (1987). Overview and initial results from a risk-factor study of depression and schizophrenia. Reprinted from *Mental Disorders in the Community* (Barrett J. E., Rose R. M., eds.) New York: Guildford Press.

Eales M. J. (1988). Affective disorders in unemployed men. *Psychological Medicine*, 18, 935–46.

Finlay-Jones R., Brown, G. W. (1981). Types of stressful life event and the onset of anxiety and depressive disorders. *Psychological Medicine*, 11, 803–15.

Finlay-Jones R., Brown, G. W., Duncan-Jones, R., *et al.* (1980). Depression and anxiety in the community. *Psychological Medicine*, 10, 445–54.

Frijda N. H. (1986). *The Emotions*. New York: Cambridge University Press.

Gaminde I., Uria, M. (1987). *Desorderes affectivos y factores sociales en la comunidad autonoma Vasca—3 Comarco de Tolosa*. Bilbao: Report to the Basque Government.

Goldberg D., Huxley P. (1980). *Mental Illness in the Community: the Pathway to Psychiatric Care*. London: Tavistock Publications.

Harris T. O. (1987). Recent developments in the measurement of life events. In *Psychiatric Epidemiology: Progress and Prospects* (Cooper B., ed.) London: Croom Helm.

Harris T. O., Brown G. W., Bifulco A. (1986). Loss of parent in childhood and adult psychiatric disorder: The Walthamstow study 1. The role of lack of adequate parental care. *Psychological Medicine*, 16, 641–59.

Harris T. O., Brown G. W., Bifulco A. (1987). Loss of parent in childhood and adult psychiatric disorder: the role of social class position and premarital pregnancy. *Psychological Medicine* 17, 163–83.

Hasegawa K. (1985). The epidemiology of depression in late life. *Journal of Affective Disorders*, Suppl. 1, 53–6.

Ingham J. G., Kreitman N. B., Miller P. McC. *et al.* (1986). Self-esteem, vulnerability and psychiatric disorder in the community. *British Journal of Psychiatry*, 148, 375–85.

Ingham J. G., Kreitman N. B., Miller P., *et al.* (1987). Self-appraisal, anxiety and depression in women—a prospective enquiry. *British Journal of Psychiatry*, 151, 643–51.

Katschnig H., Pakesch G., Egger-Zeidner E. (1986). Life stress and depressive subtypes: a review of present diagnostic criteria and recent research results. In *Life Events and Psychiatric Disorders: Controversial Issues* (Katschnig H., ed.) Cambridge: Cambridge University Press.

Klinger E. (1977). *Meaning and Void: Inner Experience and the Incentives in People's Lives*. Minneapolis: University of Minnesota Press.

Kupfer, D. J. (1986). The sleep EEG in diagnosis and treatment of depression. In *Depression: Basic Mechanisms, Diagnosis and Treatment* (Rush, A. J. Altshuler, KZ. eds.). New York: Guildford Press.

Martin C. J., Brown G. W., Brockington I. F., Goldberg, D. (1989). Psychosocial stress and puerperal depression. *Journal of Affective Disorders*, 16, 283–93.

Miller P. McC., Ingham J. G. (1983). Dimensions of experience. *Psychological Medicine*, 13, 417–29.

Miller P. McC., Ingham J. G., Kreitman N. B., *et al.* (1987). Life events and other factors implicated in onset and in remission of psychiatric illness in women. *Journal of Affective Disorders*, 12, 73–8.

Murphy E. (1982). Social origins of depression in old age. *British Journal of Psychiatry*, 141, 135–42.

O'Connor P., Brown G. W. (1984). Supportive relationships: fact or fancy? *Journal of Social and Personal Relationships*, 1: 159–75.

Parker G., Tennant C., Blignault I. (1985). Predicting improvement in patients with non-endogenous depression. *British Journal of Psychiatry*, 146: 132–9.

Parry G., Shapiro D. A. (1986). Life events and social support in working-class mothers: stress-buffering or independent effects. *Archives of General Psychiatry*, 43, 315–23.

Paykel E. S. (1973). Life events and acute depression. In *Separation and Depression*, Publication 94, (Scott J. P., Senay E. C., eds.) Washington DC: American Association for the Advancement of Science.

Paykel E. S. (1974). Recent life events and clinical depression. In *Life Stress and Illness* (Gunderson I. K. E., Rahe R. D., eds.) Illinois: Charles C. Thomas.

Paykel E. S., Myers J. K., Dienelt M. N., *et al.* (1969). Life events and depression: a controlled study. *Archives of General Psychiatry*, 21, 753–60.

Paykel E. S., Emms E. M., Fletcher J., Rassaby E. S. (1980). Life events and social support in puerperal depression. *British Journal of Psychiatry*, 136, 339–46.

Spitzer R. L., Endicott J., Robins E. (1977). *Research Diagnostic Criteria for a Selected Group of Functional Disorders*, edn 3. New York: Biometrics Research Division, New York State Psychiatric Institute.

Surtees P. G., Ingham J. G. (1980). Life stress and depressive outcome: application of a dissipation model to life events. *Social Psychiatry*, 15, 21–31.

Tennant C., Bebbington P., Hurry J. (1980). Parental death in childhood and risk of adult depressive disorders: a review. *Psychological Medicine*, 10, 289–99.

Tennant C., Bebbington P., Hurry J. (1981). The short-term outcome of neurotic disorders in the community: the relation of remission to clinical factors and to 'neutralizing' life events. *British Journal of Psychiatry*, 139, 213–20.

Wing J. K., Bebbington P., Robins L.N. (1981). *What is a Case?* London: Grant McIntyre.

Wing J. K., Cooper J. E., Sartorius N. (1974). *The Measurement and Classification of Psychiatric Symptoms*. Cambridge: Cambridge University Press.

3 Evolutionary and molecular genetic approaches to manic depression

HUGH M. D. GURLING

GENETIC RESEARCH INTO MANIC DEPRESSION

Segregation analyses of manic depressive kindreds using modern methods (O'Rourke et al., 1983; Pauls, 1985; Rice et al., 1987) have consistently shown that the observed familial patterns of recurrence of both unipolar and bipolar disorders are compatible with a single major genetic locus causing the disorder within families. However it has only recently become possible to systematically develop this area of research in psychiatry using methods to map genes by linkage (Gurling, 1985, 1986). Such methods have been very informative because they have been able to detect underlying heterogeneity caused by mutations being localized to different chromosomes which the previous segregation analyses were not able to detect. (Further genetic inputs of depression not involving linkage are discussed in Chapter 5.)

Research published in 1969 (Winokur et al., 1969) was suggestive of an X-linked type of manic depression. However, only in 1987 have molecular genetic and other types of linkage markers successfully confirmed this finding. The most convincing proof of X-linked dominant gene transmission in manic depression has come from the study of large Israeli families and from Belgium (Baron et al., 1987; Mendlewicz et al., 1987). Such confirmation depends on a statistical probability called the lod score. Simply stated this is the $\log_{10}$ of the odds for linkage between marker and disease loci against non-linkage. When this is above 3.00 in two separate studies then the linkage result is accepted.

The lod scores for X-linked manic depression computed by Baron and co-workers in Israel, using the colour blindness and glucose-6-phosphate dehydrogenase loci as linkage markers, and also by Mendlewicz and his colleagues in Belgium, using the taq I DNA polymorphism at the factor IX locus, combine to give a lod score of over 12.00. A chromosome 11 linkage for manic depression has also been reported by Egeland et al. (1987) but with a lod score that has not reached the status of a confirmed result. In contrast, work in London (Hodgkinson et al., 1987a, 1987b) and in the

USA (Detera Wadleigh *et al.*, 1987), also using the same diagnostic instruments, has failed to confirm chromosome 11 linkage and has rejected this locus as being responsible in six extended kindreds. Work on an Irish family in Dublin (Gill, 1988) has produced another negative chromosome 11 result. So far, therefore, there are seven families without chromosome 11 linkage and one with. Probably about 1 in 3 to 1 in 20 families are X-linked (Baron *et al.*, 1987).

CLINICAL HETEROGENEITY AND GENOTYPIC FORMS OF MANIC DEPRESSION

The finding of linkage heterogeneity for manic depression has complicated the outlook for future linkage studies. It will now be necessary to apply statistical tests for heterogeneity when conducting studies on relatively small family units where no single family provides enough statistical power. Diagnosis in the recent genetic linkage studies was uniformly made using the Research Diagnostic Criteria (RDC) of Spitzer and Endicott (1978). In order to determine whether certain clinical features of manic depression are specific to the recently determined genetic subtypes, I and my colleagues (see Acknowledgements) carried out a comparison across the published linkage studies.

For purposes of comparison, schizo-affective cases together with bipolar I and bipolar II cases were counted. Only those individuals over the age of 18 were counted as being at risk. The largest sample was that of the Israeli study. The proportion of those at risk who received affective disorder diagnoses is highest in Iceland and lowest in the Amish ($\chi^2 = 6.71$, d.f. $= 1$, $p < 0.01$). This could be due to differences in age distribution within the families or due to environmental and polygenic background effects. The proportion of cases of depression who are schizo-affective or bipolar (as opposed to unipolar) was highest in the Amish (74 percent) and lowest amongst the Icelandic (46 percent), but the differences did not reach statistical significance ($\chi^2 = 3.24$, d.f. $= 1$, $p < 0.1$) even when cases of unipolar depression complicated by alcoholism were excluded. It is of note that alcoholism combined with unipolar depression was confined to the Icelandic kindreds. When the rates of unipolar depression, uncomplicated by alcoholism, were compared between the Icelandic kindreds and the non-alcohol drinking Sephardic Jewish families, similar incidences were found. Schizo-affective mania was found rarely in both the X-linked as well as the non-11/non-X forms.

It is interesting that the pedigrees published by Hodgkinson *et al.* (1987b) and by Baron *et al.* (1987) show specific families both in Iceland and in Israel in which the bipolar rather than the unipolar type of expression is predominant (Gurling *et al.*, 1988). It is possible, therefore, that there may be genetic or environmental familial factors influencing penetrance which are more important than the role of a specific mutation.

The analysis is preliminary, and statistical work to examine differences in age-related penetrance for the genotypically defined forms of manic depression is being carried out. Even though genetic linkage has not yet brought about a subclassification of manic depression on clinical grounds, considerable benefit could be obtained from precisely defining all the mutations causing the illness. Below are described some of the evolutionary theories concerning manic depression in an attempt to understand the clinical phenomena of the disease and how they relate to the presence of single gene mutations.

EVOLUTIONARY THEORIES OF MANIC DEPRESSION

The mutant alleles causing manic depression have persisted throughout evolution even though the illness would appear to decrease fitness. Therefore, a number of authors have hypothesized that the tendency to develop manic depression must have originally conferred some selective advantage when the trait was only partially expressed. John Price (1967, 1972; Price and Sloman, 1987), who drew heavily on the observations of ethologists, has proposed the concept of a social dominance hierarchy. This schema proposes that dominant individuals would feel elated from their high social position but show irritability and aggression to their inferiors and that inferiors would, in turn, show anxiety to superiors. Excesses of these two tendencies in either direction might lead to mental illness.

From clinical observation it is clear that mobility in the depressed patient may vary from a frozen state or stupor to incessant restless activity. Price (1972) also postulated that such extremes may serve different functions with regard to the geographical dispersion of the population and he calls these 'stay put' and 'move on' depressions. Depressions of the 'move on' type, expressed as restless overactivity, may have been an advantage to nomadic peoples. Another possible adaptive function could have been in the formation of the pair bond, particularly husband–wife bonding, where elation with its associated sociability, self-confidence and raised libido increased the chances of finding a mate. During separations, 'stay put' depressions functioned to reduce libidinal attachments thus maintaining the pair bond until the physical separation ended.

Other concepts of the possible adaptive functions of mental illness have been suggested: these include the conservation of energy (Frank, 1954); and the hypothesis that it might prevent incapable and rejected members from rejoining the herd or group, so that depression was adaptive for the group as a whole rather than for the individual (Rodger, 1961). Farley (1976) has developed a somewhat different hypothesis suggesting that psychosis is a 'release' phenomenon. He proposes that the genetically determined component in the clinical presentation derives from phylo-genetic adaptations released from their normal learnt constraints and displayed in inappropriate, incomplete forms. Farley describes innate behaviour as having a massive survival value, facilitating adaptation to the environment, but at the same time maintaining a genetically determined diversity of behaviour which may help populations survive environmental and cultural change. In this scenario, deviant personalities thrown up by the random segregation of genes may be the agents of social change and creativity. Personality disorder and psychosis, therefore, represent the price that man pays for change.

Most of the theories outlined above share common themes and, by the same token, similar criticisms may be made of them. Clearly none of them may be tested very easily or directly. In addition, the role of evolutionary adaptive mechanisms in modern society in terms of advantage to the individual is unclear. It is possible that modern cultural and social factors may have an influence on the expression of the manic-depressive genotype that has made it more or less penetrant than before. Some evidence that penetrance for manic depression has increased since 1940 has recently emerged (Gershon *et al.*, 1987). A simpler and preferable explanation for the survival of the manic-depressive phenotype could be that it arises as a number of random, mutational events at various loci, with relatively late expression in the life cycle, which have not affected fertility and fitness very much. The phenotype as a whole could be the result of such a mutation interfering with the brain systems controlling mood and activity, but in itself the mutation has not played a role in the evolutionary development of these behavioural systems as a whole. A proportion of cases may of course be new mutations, and chromosomal 'hot spots' for such mutations may exist at specific loci.

The effect of a specific mutation will be modified by other genes, an effect known as epistasis. Such epistasis may involve many genes or single genes. Recent work in drosophila genetics has found the unexpected effect that the variance of a trait may increase rather than decrease after there has been an experimentally induced restriction of the number of alleles (genetic bottleneck) in a breeding population (Bryant, 1986). Using the definition of epistasis current in population and quantitative genetics, where it refers to all non-allelic gene interactions, it seems possible, therefore, that relatively isolated populations such as the Amish may demonstrate epistatic effects not seen in more heterogeneous populations.

FROM LINKAGE TO LOCUS: RECOMBINANT DNA APPROACHES TO DEFINE THE MUTATIONS CAUSING MANIC DEPRESSIVE PSYCHOSIS

The mutations responsible for manic depression may be deletions, base-pair mutations or some type of genetic rearrangement such as gene conversion. Techniques to define deletions have successfully been used in the study of Duchenne muscular dystrophy (DMD) and chronic granulo-tomatous disease (CGD). Kunkel *et al.* (1985) made use of an unusual

DMD patient who had an interstitial deletion on the short arm of the X chromosome at Xp 21.1. As a result of using the phenol-enhanced reassociation technique (PERT), one clone detected genomic DNA deletions in some DMD patients and was closely linked to the disorder. Chromosome 'walking' identified further DNA in this region. Non-repetitive DNA segments which were highly conserved in many species were identified using 'zoo' blots by Monaco *et al.* (1985) and these were used to find candidate mRNA transcripts for the DMD gene. Such an approach could work for manic depression if such a deletion was identified. Our own survey of the cytogenetic studies of manic depression has not revealed a single reported instance of a case associated with a chromosomal abnormality.

Chronic granulotomatous disease is another disorder with a chromosomal deletion mapping to the X chromosome. The deletion was identified cytogenetically in a combined CGD/DMD patient by Francke *et al.* (1985). Genomic clones generated by Monaco *et al.* (1985) that mapped to the DMD deletions also mapped to the deletion found in CGD. B-cell lymphoblastoid lines created from a patient with CGD and a cytogenetic deletion were used to prepare mRNA. After subtractive screening with complementary DNA (cDNA) prepared from mRNA from normal phagocytic cells, the resultant cDNA clones were hybridized with the deletion clones. One clone identified a phagocyte-specific mRNA that was absent from some patients and which exhibited a deletion in others (Royer-Pokora *et al.*, 1986). Such an approach could not easily be accomplished in manic depression because of the complexity of brain mRNA and also because mRNA is not readily available except at post-mortem examination where it may have become degraded.

An example of a molecular approach where there was no apparent cytogenetic deletion, but where the disease locus was shown to be on chromosome 7 by the DNA linkage markers MET and J3.11, is that which has been applied to cystic fibrosis (CF). In this instance, the critical finding that enabled successful fine mapping was the observed linkage disequilibrium between one of the linkage markers and the disease mutation. Normally linkage marker polymorphisms are randomly associated with mutations even when they are close enough to show linkage in genetic studies. However, if they are sufficiently close to each other so that very little recombination between the two has taken place during evolution, then both mutation and polymorphism will remain linked together and show up as a population association between marker and disease amongst unrelated affected individuals. This is known as linkage disequilibrium or allelic association.

Estivill *et al.* (1987) used physical mapping procedures to show that MET and J3.11 were very close to the disease locus and created cell lines that contained transgenomes including them. From these lines, a non-methylated CpG rare cutter cosmid library was created. This enabled the isolation of Hpa II tiny fragments (HTF) islands which identified coding sequences. Clones were then selected on the basis of showing strong linkage disequilibrium with CF. 'Zoo' blots were used to select clones that were highly conserved across species and these in turn were used to screen lung cDNA libraries for candidate genes.

Such an approach will of course only be feasible in manic-depressive disorder when the localization of the disease locus is known and when markers sufficiently close to be in linkage disequilibrium with the disorder are identified. The problems of genetic heterogeneity must be considered carefully when attempting to establish such disequilibrium. One approach is the prior establishment of a manic-depressive individual's genetic subtype by linkage analysis of the patient's family followed by association analysis across unrelated cases who share a common subtype. Another approach is to obtain a sufficiently large sample of affected cases from many different families and then to hope that linkage disequilibrium for a particular subtype will show through the 'noise'. The success of the latter approach depends on just how heterogeneous manic depression turns out to be.

Despite the problems of heterogeneity, molecular biology seems poised to increase our understanding of manic depression both at the level of mutations in the human genome and also in terms of the expression of specific genes.

ACKNOWLEDGEMENTS

The author is a Wellcome Senior Fellow in clinical science. The research was funded by the Wellcome Trust and the Rothschild Schizophrenia Research Fund. I gratefully acknowledge the kind assistance of Icelandair and the NATO science committee for support enabling international collaboration, and also the contribution to this research and writing made by my colleagues R. P. Sherrington, J. Brynjolfsson, M. Potter, M. McInnis, S. Hodgkinson and H. Petursson.

REFERENCES

Baron M., Risch N., Hamburger R., *et al.* (1987). X chromosome markers and bipolar affective illness. *Nature*, **326**, 289–92.

Bryant E. H. (1986). The effect of an experimental bottleneck upon quantitative genetic variation in the housefly. *Genetics*, **114**, 1191–7.

Detera Wadleigh S. D., Berretini W. H., Goldin R. R., *et al.* (1987). Close linkage of C Harvey-ras 1 and the insulin gene to affective disorder is ruled out in three North American pedigrees, *Nature*, **325**, 783–7.

Egeland J., Gerhard D. S., Pauls D. L., *et al.* (1987). Bipolar affective disorders linked to DNA markers on chromosome 11. *Nature*, **325**, 783–7.

Estivill X., Farrall M., Scambler P. J., *et al.* (1987). A candidate for the cystic fibrosis locus isolated by selection for methylation-free islands. *Nature*, **326**, 840–5.

Farley J. P. (1976). Phylogenetic adaptations and the genetics of psychosis. *Acta Psychiatrica Scandinavica*, **53**, 173–92.

Francke U., Ochs H. D., De Martinville B., *et al.* (1985). Minor Xp21 chromosome deletion in a male associated with expression of Duchenne muscular dystrophy, chronic granulomatous disease, retinitis pigmentosa and McLeod Syndrome. *American Journal of Human Genetics*, **37**, 250–67.

Frank R. L. (1954). The organized aspects of the Depression-Elation Response. In *Depression* (Hock P. H., Zubin J., eds.) New York: Brunne and Stratton, pp. 51–65.

Gershon E. S., Hamovit J. H., Guroff J. J., Nurnberger J. I. (1987). Birth-cohort changes in manic and depressive disorders in relatives of bipolar and schizo-affective patients. *Archives of General Psychiatry*, **44**, 314–9.

Gill M., McKeown P., Humphries P. (1988). Linkage analysis of manic depression in an Irish family using H-Ras 1 and INS DNA markers. *Journal of Medical Genetics*, **25**, 634–5.

Gurling H. M. D. (1985). Application of molecular biology to mental illness. Analysis of genomic DNA and mRNA. *Psychiatric Developments*, **3**, 257–73.

Gurling H. M. D. (1986). Candidate genes and favoured loci: strategies for molecular genetic research into schizophrenia, manic depression, autism, alcoholism and Alzheimer's disease. *Psychiatric Developments*, **4**, 289–309.

Gurling H. M. D. Sherrington R. P., Potter M., *et al.* (1988). Molecular genetics, heterogeneity and the evolution of manic depression. *Molecular Neurobiology*, **2**, 1–7.

Hodgkinson S., Gurling H. M. D., Marchbanks R. M., *et al.* (1987a). Minisatellite mapping in manic depression, *Journal of Psychiatric Research*, **21**, 589–96.

Hodgkinson S., Sherrington R., Gurling H. M. D., *et al.* (1987b). Molecular genetic evidence for heterogeneity in manic depression. *Nature*, **325**, 805–6.

Kunkel K. M., Monaco A. P., Middlesworth W., *et al.* (1985). Specific cloning of DNA fragments absent from the DNA of a male patient with an X chromosome deletion. *Proceedings of the National Academy of Sciences USA*, **82**, 4778–82.

Mendlewicz J., Simon P., Sevy S., *et al.* (1987). Polymorphic marker on X chromosome and manic depression. *Lancet*, **8544**, 1230–1.

Monaco A. P., Bertelson W., Middlesworth W., *et al.* (1985). Detection of deletions spanning Duchenne muscular dystrophy locus using a tightly linked DNA segment. *Nature*, **316**, 842–5.

O'Rourke D. H., McGuffin P., Reich T. (1983). Genetic analysis of manic depressive illness. *American Journal of Physical Anthropology*, **62**, 51–9.

Pauls D. (1985). *Segregation analysis of bipolar and unipolar disorders in the US Amish*. 4th. World Congress in Biological Psychiatry, Philadelphia, USA.

Price J. (1967). The dominance hierarchy and the evolution of mental illness. *Lancet*, **2**, 243–6.

Price J. (1972). Genetic and phylogenetic aspects of mood variation. *International Journal of Mental Health*, **1**, 124–44.

Price J., Sloman L., (1987). Depression versus yielding behaviour: an animal model based on Schjelderup-Ebbe's pecking order. *Ethology and Sociobiology* (Suppl.) **7**, 53–66.

Rice J., Reich, T., Andreasen N. C., Endicott J., *et al.* (1987). *Archives of General Psychiatry*, **44**, 441–7.

Rodger T. F. (1961). The Anglo–Saxon approach to depression. *Acta Psychiatrica Scandinavica*, **162** (Suppl.) 201–9.

Royer-Pokora B., Kunkel L. M., Monaco A. P., *et al.* (1986). Cloning the gene for an inherited human disorder-chronic granulomatous disease, on the basis of its chromosomal location. *Nature*, **322**, 32–8.

Spitzer R. L., Endicott J. (1978). *Critical Issues in Psychiatric Diagnosis.* New York: Raven Press.

Winokur G., Clayton P. J., Reich T. (1969). *Manic Depressive Illness.* St. Louis: C. V. Mosby.

4 *Neuroendocrine studies of the aetiology of depression*

STUART CHECKLEY

HYPOTHALAMIC PITUITARY ADRENAL FUNCTION IN DEPRESSION

The longest established neuroendocrine change in depression is over activity of the hypothalamic pituitary adrenal (HPA) axis (Gibbons, 1964). The normal circadian rhythm of plasma cortisol is preserved in endo genous depression and, at all times of the day and night, plasma cortisol concentrations are elevated (Halbreich *et al.*, 1985; Linkowski *et al.*, 1985; Pfohl *et al.*, 1985; Rubin *et al.*, 1987). Depressed patients with hypercorti-solaemia are the ones who resist cortisol suppression with dexamethasone (Rubin *et al.*, 1987), which activates the negative feedback mechanism through which cortisol normally controls the secretion of adrenocortico-trophic hormone (ACTH).

Recent studies have done much to explain the neuroendocrine mechan-isms underlying overactivity of the HPA axis in endogenous depression. The following observations indicate a central activation of the HPA axis with an increased secretion of the hypothalamic hormone, corticotrophin-releasing factor (CRF). An apparently paradoxical finding is that plasma ACTH concentrations may not be raised in patients with elevated cerebrospinal fluid (CSF) CRF and plasma cortisol concentrations. It is thought that the paradox is explained by a negative feedback restraint by high cortisol levels on ACTH secretion. The argument that CRF is overproduced but that its effects on ACTH secretion are restrained by hypercortisolaemia is based on the following observations:

1. CSF concentrations of CRF are elevated in patients with endogenous depression (Nemeroff *et al.*, 1984).
2. The pattern of hypercortisolaemia with preservation of circadian rhythm that is seen in endogenous depression may be due to increased CRF secretion as this pattern can be reproduced in normal volunteers treated with prolonged infusions of ovine CRF (Schulte *et al.*, 1985).
3. In endogenous depression the ACTH response to CRF is reduced (Gold *et al.*, 1984; Holsboer *et al.*, 1984). The fact that the size of this

response is inversely proportional to the baseline plasma cortisol concentration (Gold *et al.*, 1984) suggests that cortisol may be restraining ACTH secretion under these conditions.

4. In endogenous depression the cortisol response to ACTH is increased (Amsterdam *et al.*, 1983). This finding indicates a hyper-responsive adrenal cortex in patients with endogenous depression.

While presenting some of these findings, Gold *et al.*, (1984) also reviewed the results from animal studies. These showed that some of the behavioural features of depression can be reproduced in animals by treatment with CRF. However, the suggestion that an overproduction of CRF causes depression is questioned by the observation that CRF overproduction is also found in patients with anorexia nervosa (Gold *et al.*, 1987) and possibly in patients with anxiety disorder (Roy-Byrne *et al.*, 1988). Rather than being the cause of depression, CRF overproduction is more likely to be one of several disturbances of hypothalamic function. The neuroceptor control of CRF secretion requires further study and may involve an α_1-adrenergic mechanism.

NEUROENDOCRINE TESTS OF α_1-ADRENOCEPTOR FUNCTION IN PATIENTS WITH ENDOGENOUS DEPRESSION

The first evidence that α_1-adrenoceptors might regulate HPA function was the demonstration that the cortisol response to methylamphetamines could be reduced by the selective α_1-antagonist thymoxamine (Rees *et al.*, 1970). Subsequently it was shown that this response is reduced in depressed as compared to recovered depressives (Checkley and Crammer, 1978). It is also reduced in endogenous as compared to non-endogenous depressives (Checkley, 1979). These results, together with the subsequent finding of abnormal cortisol responses to *d*-amphetamine (Sachar *et al.*, 1981), have been interpreted as evidence of altered responsiveness of α_1-adrenoceptors in neuroendocrine systems in patients with endogenous depression.

However, amphetamines release dopamine as well as noradrenaline and even though dopamine may not influence the HPA axis in man (Checkley, 1979) a more selective probe of the α_1-adrenoceptor is required. The ACTH and cortisol response to the selective α_1-agonist methoxamine is a better measure of α_1-adrenoceptor function, particularly as this response is blocked by the selective α_1-antagonist, thymoxamine (Al-Damluji *et al.*, 1987 a,b). Studies are now underway to measure this response in patients with endogenous depression.

NEUROENDOCRINE MEASURES OF α_2-ADRENOCEPTOR FUNCTION IN PATIENTS WITH ENDOGENOUS DEPRESSION

Considerable evidence supports the view that the growth hormone (GH) response to clonidine depends upon the stimulation by α_2-adrenoceptors in the hypothalmus:

1. The response is inhibited by a variety of selective and non-selective α_2-antagonists (Eriksson *et al.*, 1982; Kruhlich *et al.*, 1982; Cella *et al.*, 1983, 1984; McWilliam and Meldrum, 1983).
2. The receptors mediating this response are within territory of the carotid rather than the vertebral arteries (Rudolph *et al.*, 1980) and they are closer to the third than to the fourth cerebral ventricle (Lovinger *et al.*, 1976).
3. At least some of the receptors must be in the arcuate nucleus of the hypothalamus as the GH response to clonidine is abolished by lesions of the arcuate nucleus (Katakami *et al.*, 1984). Furthermore, the arcuate nucleus is the main site of growth hormone releasing factor (GRF) in the human brain (Bloch *et al.*, 1983) and the GH response to clonidine involves GRF because it is abolished by GRF antisera (Miki *et al.*, 1984).

Four groups have independently reported that the GH response to clonidine is reduced in patients with endogenous depression (Matussek *et al.*, 1980; Checkley *et al.*, 1981; Charney *et al.*, 1982; Siever *et al.*, 1982). A fifth group did not find reduced responses in patients with endogenous depression but they did find reduced responses in depressed patients with dexamethatone resistance (Horton *et al.*, 1986): dexamethatone resistance is itself particularly common in endogenous depression. In the largest series reported to date, significant correlations were found between the size of the GH response to clonidine and several measures of endogenous depression (Checkley *et al.*, 1984).

A reduced GH response to clonidine could be due to a defect at α_2-adrenoceptors, a defect in GRF secretion, or a defect in the pituitary response to GRF. However, GH responses to apomorphine are normal in depression (Casper *et al.*, 1977; Garver *et al.*, 1977; Maany *et al.*, 1979; Jimerson *et al.*, 1984) even in the same depressed patients who have impaired GH responses to clonidine (Corn *et al.*, 1984a). Not only do these findings of normal GH responses to apomorphine suggest a lesion at the α_2-adrenoceptor, they also make it unlikely that nonspecific dietary or metabolic factors have caused the reduced response to clonidine.

Although the reduced GH response to clonidine may indicate a defect at α_2-adrenoceptors in endogenous depression, depression cannot be caused by a generalized defect at all central α_2-adrenoceptors because other effects of clonidine (on sedation and blood pressure), which are known to depend on the stimulation of central α_2-adrenoceptors, are normal in depression

(Checkley *et al.*, 1981); reduced GH responses to clonidine have been reported in psychiatric conditions which overlap with depression, such as obsessional neurosis (Siever *et al.*, 1983) and agoraphobia (Uhde *et al.*, 1986); and desipramine, which is known to down-regulate α_2-adrenoceptors in animals, reduces the GH response to clonidine both in depressed patients (as they recover) and in normal volunteers (whose mood does not change as they receive desipramine; Corn *et al.*, 1984b). For these reasons a reduced responsiveness at α_2-adrenoceptors cannot be the primary biochemical cause of depression. Rather, it may represent one of several neuroreceptor changes within the hypothalamus of patients with endogenous depression and in patients with some other conditons.

NEUROENDOCRINE TESTS OF 5-HT RECEPTOR FUNCTION IN PATIENTS WITH ENDOGENOUS DEPRESSION

There are not yet well-developed neuroendocrine tests for investigating the functional status of the subtypes of the 5-hydroxytryptamine (5-HT) receptor in man. However, there are several indirect measures of the excitatory 5-HT control of prolactin (PRL) secretion. The prolactin response to tryptophan involves 5-HT mechanisms as it is increased by the 5-HT uptake inhibitor, chlomipramine (Anderson and Cowen, 1986) and it is reduced by the non-selective 5-HT antagonist, methergoline (McCance *et al.*, 1987). The prolactin response to tryptophan infusion is reduced in depressed patients (Heninger *et al.*, 1984), at least in those without conspicuous weight loss (Cowen and Charing, 1987). With the development of more selective agonists, such as gepirone for the $5HT_{1A}$ receptor and *m*-chlorophenylpiperazine for the $5HT_{1B}$ receptor, it may be possible to develop neuroendocrine tests of the functional status of some of these receptors.

NEUROENDOCRINE STUDIES OF THE EFFECTS OF TRICYCLIC ANTIDEPRESSANTS UPON MONOAMINERGIC NEUROTRANSMISSION IN DEPRESSED PATIENTS

Tricyclic antidepressants, which are the drugs of first choice in the physical treatment of depression, have multiple effects both upon monoamine uptake and upon monoaminergic receptors (Charney *et al.*, 1981). These effects have been described in experimental animals and so the first task for clinical research is to determine whether or not similar changes occur in man. Neuroendocrine challenge tests provide one of the very few ways in which central monoaminergic receptor function can be studied in man.

The second task for clinical research is to determine the net effect of tricyclic antidepressants upon monoaminergic neurotransmission. Again neuroendocrine models are the most appropriate for answering this question.

The third task is to test whether or not there is a causal relationship between antidepressant response and change in monoaminergic neuro-transmission.

Clinical studies of inhibition of noradrenaline uptake

In animal, tricyclic antidepressants inhibit the re-uptake of noradrenaline into noradrenergic terminals (Iversen, 1965). In man, noradrenergic neurotransmission can be monitored by measuring changes in melatonin secretion. The secretion of melatonin from the pineal depends upon its noradrenergic innervation because the loss of these fibres as a result of illness or an experimental lesion results in the abolition of melatonin secretion (Checkley and Park, 1988). The tricyclic antidepressant, desipra-mine, which is a relatively selective inhibitor of noradrenaline uptake, increases the secretion of melatonin in man (Checkley *et al.*, 1985) as does the highly selective inhibitor of noradrenaline uptake, oxaprotiline. Oxa-protiline exists as two enantiomers, (+)- and (−)-oxaprotiline, and of these only (+)-oxaprotiline inhibits noradrenaline uptake (Mishra *et al.*, 1982). The fact that only (+)-oxaprotiline increases melatonin secretion, while (−)-oxaprotiline does not (Checkley *et al.*, 1985), is therefore strong evidence that the effect of oxaprotiline on melatonin secretion is due to the inhibition of noradrenaline uptake.

Blockade of a_1-adrenoceptors

In experimental animals, single doses of tricyclic antidepressants, such as desipramine, block α_1-adrenoceptors (U'Pritchard *et al.*, 1978). Similar effects have been demonstrated in the human pupil in which the ability of the α_1-agonist to dilate the pupil was blocked by treatment with desipra-mine (Shur and Checkley, 1982). The fact that the resting pupil diameter was still increased, however, showed that the functional significance of noradrenaline uptake inhibition was greater than that of α_1-adrenoceptor blockage.

A similar conclusion can be drawn from the fact that desipramine increases melatonin secretion in man. For whereas the effect of noradrena-line uptake blockade is to increase melatonin secretion (Checkley *et al.*, 1985) the effect of α_1-adrenoceptor blockage with prazosin is to reduce melatonin secretion (Palazidou *et al.*, 1989).

Clinical studies of chronic effect of antidepressant drugs upon noradrenergic receptors

In experimental animals, chronic treatment with tricyclic antidepressants results in adaptive changes at α_1-, α_2- and β_1-adrenoceptors (Charney *et al.*, 1987). The responsiveness of α_1-adrenoceptors is increased while that of α_2- and β_2-adrenoceptors is decreased. Clinical studies are needed to determine whether or not similar changes occur in man.

As has already been discussed, the GH response to clonidine is a measure of the responsiveness of α_2-adrenoceptors. If tricyclic antidepressants cause adaptive changes at α_2-adrenoceptors, then they should cause corresponding changes in the GH response to clonidine. Consistent with this prediction, we have reported changes in the GH response to clonidine in depressed patients treated with desipramine (Glass *et al.*, 1982). After one week of treatment, the response was increased, but over the second and third weeks of treatment the response became significantly reduced. Similar changes were subsequently reported in normal volunteers (Corn *et al.*, 1984b). Furthermore, the GH responses to clonidine remained attenuated for at least three weeks after discontinuation of desipramine treatment (Corn *et al.*, 1984b). Further evidence that changes in the GH response to clonidine during desipramine treatment are due to changes at α_2-adrenoceptors comes from the finding that in rats similar changes are produced by prolonged treatment with clonidine and with desipramine, whereas chronic treatment with the α_2-antagonist, yohimbine, increases the GH response to clonidine (Eriksson *et al.*, 1982). Taken together the above findings provide the strongest evidence so far that tricyclic antidepressants modify central monoamine receptors in man.

FUNCTIONAL SIGNIFICANCE OF ANTIDEPRESSANT-INDUCED RECEPTOR CHANGES

The question now arises as to the functional significance of such changes at monoaminergic receptors. An increase in noradrenergic neurotransmission is to be expected from inhibition of noradrenaline uptake, from any reduced responsiveness of presynaptic α_2-adrenoceptors and from any enhanced responsiveness of α_1-adrenoceptors. However, down-regulation of postsynaptic β-adrenoceptors will reduce noradrenergic neurotransmission, as will the down-regulation of postsynaptic α_2-adrenoceptors.

Sulser has proposed that down-regulation at β-adrenoceptors is the dominant action of antidepressant treatments as a result of which they reduce noradrenergic neurotransmission. He has reported a reduced number or function of central β-adrenoceptors following three weeks of treatment with ECT, tricyclic antidepressants, monoamine oxidase inhibitors and some of the newer antidepressants (Sulser, 1984). Although down-regulation of β-adrenoceptors is a common effect of an impressively wide range of antidepressant treatments, it remains to be shown whether or not noradrenergic neurotransmission is reduced as a result.

The noradrenergic control of melatonin secretion in the pineal is a convenient neuroendocrine model with which to answer this question—both in experimental animals and in man. The noradrenergic supply of the pineal has a noradrenaline uptake mechanism (Klein, 1985) and prejunctional α_2-adrenoceptors (Pelayo *et al.*, 1977). The melatonin-secreting pinealocytes are endowed with β_1- and α_1-adrenoceptors, both of which influence the secretion of melatonin (Klein, 1985). There is clinical evidence that α_1-, α_2- and β_1-adrenoceptors have a similar influence on melatonin secretion in man (Checkley and Park, 1988). Consequently, the secretion of melatonin can be considered as the physiological output from a typical noradrenergic system both in experimental animals and man. If antidepressants reduce noradrenergic neurotransmission, then they will reduce melatonin secretion; and if they increase noradrenergic neurotransmission, melatonin secretion will be correspondingly increased.

In experimental animals, chronic imipramine treatment results in down-regulation of pineal β-adrenoceptors and in a corresponding decrease in the synthesis of melatonin (Friedman *et al.*, 1984). In man, however, melatonin secretion is not reduced by chronic treatment with tricyclic antidepressants. In most studies, melatonin secretion has been increased by desipramine (Thompson *et al.*, 1985; Sack and Lewy, 1986). In no human study has melatonin secretion yet been reduced by antidepressant treatment. Even though down-regulation at β-adrenoceptors may occur in the human pineal, noradrenergic neurotransmission is not reduced.

Whether there is a causal relationship between the antidepressant effect of desipramine and its effect upon noradrenaline is not known, but the studies which have been described provide a basis for testing this possibility. If desipramine acts by increasing noradrenergic neurotransmission then its antidepressant action should be enhanced by its combined administration with drugs which enhance its action upon noradrenaline and melatonin. We have shown that melatonin secretion is increased by a phosphodiesterase inhibitor (Checkley *et al.*, 1984) and by an α_2-antagonist (Palazidou *et al.*, 1989). Phosphodiesterase inhibitors enhance noradrenergic neurotransmission by increasing the availability of the second messenger, cyclic AMP. Alpha$_2$-antagonists increase noradrenergic neurotransmission by blocking an autoreceptor-mediated, negative feedback control of noradrenaline release. Each type of drug should therefore augment the effect of desipramine and noradrenaline and melatonin, and each type of drug should therefore enhance the antidepressant action of desipramine. These predictions are being tested at present.

CONCLUSIONS

The present review leads to the following conclusions:

1. Antidepressant drugs increase noradrenergic and serotonergic neuro-transmission in man. It follows that the functional disorder in depression could either be within monoaminergic systems or could be distal to the monoaminergic projections.
2. The following suggest that the disorder is more likely to be distal to the monoaminergic projections:
   (a) despite intensive study no consistent monoaminergic defects have been found in post-mortem studies of the brains of depressed patients;
   (b) selective inhibitors of noradrenaline and 5HT uptake have identical antidepressant effects, a fact most readily explained by assuming that the primary disturbance is at a site distal to both noradrenaline and 5HT projections;
   (c) if antidepressant drugs act by increasing monoaminergic neuro-transmission then the delay in onset of antidepressant action cannot be due to changes at receptors which will reduce neurotransmission. The delay in onset remains unexplained but would be due to events distal to the monoamine projections.
3. If the lesion in depression is distal to the monoamine projections then might it be within the hypothalamus? Relevant to this:
   (a) the range of the neuroendocrine changes in depression as reviewed in this chapter is greater than that reported for any functional psychiatric disorder;
   (b) none of these neuroendocrine changes could, of themselves, be the cause of depression, because they can be found in non-depressed patients or volunteers;
   (c) it is therefore more likely that the site of the primary disturbance in depression lies at some point distal to the monoamine projections but proximal to the hypothalamic nuclei, such as in the arcuate and the paraventricular whose function is clearly altered in depression.

REFERENCES

Al-Damluji S., Cunnah D., Perry L., *et al.* (1987a). The effect of alpha adrenergic manipulation on the 24 hour pattern of cortisol secretion in man. *Clinical Endocrinology*, **26**, 61–6.

Al-Damluji S., Perry L., Tomlin S., *et al.* (1987b). Alpha adrenergic stimulation of corticotrophin secretion by a specific central mechanism. *Neuroendocrinology*, **45**, 68–6.

Amsterdam J. D., Winokur A., Abelman E., *et al.* (1983). Cosyntropin (ACTH 1-24) test in depressed patients and healthy subjects. *American Journal of Psychiatry*, **140**, 907–9.

Anderson I. M., Cowen P. J. (1986). Chlomipramine enhances prolactin and growth hormone responses to L-tryptophan. *Psychopharmacology*, **89**, 131–3.

Bloch B., Brazeau P., Ling N., *et al.* (1983). Immunohistochemical detection of growth hormone releasing factor in brain. *Nature*, **301**, 607–8.

Casper R. C., Davis J. M., Pandey G. N., *et al.* (1977). Neuroendocrine and amine studies in affective illness. *Psychoneuroendocrinology*, **2**, 105–8.

Cella S. G., Picotti C. B., Muller E. E. (1983). Adrenergic stimulation enhances growth hormone secretion in the dog. *Life Sciences*, **32**, 2785–92.

Cella S. C., Picotti G. B., Morgese M., *et al.* (1984). Presynaptic α_2 adrenergic stimulation leads to growth hormone release in the dog. *Life Sciences*, **34**, 447–54.

Charney D. S., Menkes D. B., Heninger G. R. (1981). Receptor sensitivity and the mechanism of action of antidepressant treatment. *Archives of General Psychiatry*, **38**, 1160–80.

Charney D. S., Heninger G. R., Sternberg D. E., *et al.* (1982). Adrenergic receptor sensitivity in depression. Effects of clonidine in depressed patients and healthy subjects. *Archives of General Psychiatry*, **39**, 290–4.

Checkley S. A. (1979). Corticosteroid and growth hormone responses to methylamphetamine in depressive illness. *Psychological Medicine*, **9**, 107–15.

Checkley S. A., Crammer J. L. (1978). Hormonal responses to methylamphetamine in depression: a new approach to the noradrenaline deficiency hypothesis. *British Journal of Psychiatry*, **131**, 582–6.

Checkley S. A., Park S. B. G. (1988). The psychopharmacology of the human pineal. *Journal of Psychopharmacology*, **1**, 109–25.

Checkley S. A., Slade A. P., Shur E. (1981). Growth hormone and other responses to clonidine in patients with endogenous depression. *British Journal of Psychiatry*, **138**, 51–5.

Checkley S. A., Glass I. B., Thompson C., *et al.* (1984). The growth hormone response to clonidine in endogenous as compared to reactive depression. *Psychological Medicine*, **14**, 773–7.

Checkley S. A., Thompson C., Burton S., *et al.* (1985). Clinical studies of the effect of ($+$) and ($-$) oxaprotiline upon noradrenaline uptake. *Psychopharmacology*, **87**, 116–8.

Corn T., Hale A. S., Thompson C., *et al.* (1984a). A comparison of the growth hormone responses to clonidine and apomorphine in the same patients with endogenous depression. *British Journal of Psychiatry*, **144**, 636–9.

Corn T., Thompson C., Checkley S. A. (1984b). Effects of desipramine treatment upon central adrenoceptor function in normal subjects. *British Journal of Psychiatry*, **145**, 139–45.

Cowen P. J., Charing E. M. (1987). Neuroendocrine responses to intravenous tryptophan in major depression. *Archives of General Psychiatry*, **44**, 958–66.

Eriksson E., Eden S., Modigh K. (1982). Up- and down-regulation of central post synaptic $alpha_2$ receptors reflected in the growth hormone response to clonidine in reserpine pretreated rats. *Psychopharmacology*, **77**, 327–31.

Friedman E., Yocca F. D., Cooper T. B. (1984). Antidepressant drugs with various pharmacological profiles alter pineal beta adrenergic mediated function. *Journal of Pharmacology and Experimental Therapeutics*, **228**, 545–9.

Garver D. L., Pandey G. N., Hengeveld C., Davis J. M. (1977). Growth hormone response and central aminergic systems in affective diseases. *Psychopharmacology Bulletin*, **13**, 61–3.

Gibbons J. L. (1964). Cortisol secretion rate in depressive illness. *Archives of General Psychiatry*, 10, 572–5.

Glass I. B., Checkley S. A., Shur E., Dawling S. (1982). The effect of desipramine upon central adrenergic functions in depressed patients. *British Journal of Psychiatry*, 141, 372–6.

Gold P. W., Chrousos G. P., Kellner C. H., *et al.* (1984). Psychiatric implications of basic and clinical studies with corticotrophin-releasing factor. *American Journal of Psychiatry*, 141, 619–27.

Gold P. W., Kling M. A., Calabrese J. R. *et al.* (1987). Physiological diagnostic and pathophysiological implications of corticotrophin releasing hormone. In *Handbook of Clinical Endocrinology* (Nemeroff C. B., Loosen P. T., eds.). Chichester: John Wiley and Sons, pp. 85–108.

Halbreich U., Asnis G. M., Shindledecker R., *et al.* (1985). Cortisol secretion in endogenous depression. II Time related functions. *Archives of General Psychiatry*, 42, 909–14.

Heninger G. R., Charney D. S., Sternberg D. E. (1984). Serotonin function in depression. Prolactive response to intravenous tryptophan in depressed patients and healthy subjects. *Archives of General Psychiatry*, 44, 398–402.

Holsboer F., Genken H., Stalla G. K., Muller G. H. (1984). Blunted ACTH responses to human CRH in depression (letter). *New England Journal of Medicine*, 311, 1127.

Horton R. W., Katona C. L. E., Theodorou A. E., *et al.* (1986). Platelet radioligand binding and neuroendocrine challenge tests in depression. In *Antidepressants and Receptor Function* (Murphy D. L., ed.). Chichester: John Wiley and Sons.

Iversen L. L. (1965). *The Uptake and Storage of Noradrenaline in Sympathetic Nerves.* Cambridge: Cambridge University Press.

Jimerson D. C., Cutler N. R., Post R. M., *et al.* (1984). Neuroendocrine responses to apomorphine in depressed patients and healthy control subjects. *Psychiatry Research*, 13, 1–12.

Katakami H., Kato Y., Matsushita N., Imura H. (1984). Effects of neonatal treatment with monosodium glutamate on growth hormone release induced by clonidine and prostaglandin E, in conscious male rats. *Neuroendocrinology*, 38, 1–5.

Klein D. C. (1985). Photoneural regulation of the human pineal gland. In *Photoperiodism, Melatonin and the Pineal Gland*, CIBA Foundation Symposium, 117. (R.V. Short, ed.) London: Pitman, pp. 38–51.

Kruhlich L., Mayfield M. A., Steele M. K., *et al.* (1982). Differential effects of pharmacological manipulations of central alpha₁ and alpha₂ adrenergic receptors on the secretion of thyrotrophin and growth hormone in male rats. *Endocrinology*, 110, 796–804.

Linkowski P., Mendlewicz J., Leclercq R., *et al.* (1985). The 24-hour profile of adrenocorticotrophin and cortisol in major depressive illness. *Journal of Clinical Endocrinology and Metabolism*, 61, 429–37.

Lovinger R., Holland J., Kaplan S., *et al.* (1976). Pharmacological evidence for stimulation of growth hormone secretion by a central noradrenergic system in dogs. *Neuroscience*, 1, 443–50.

Maany I., Mendels J., Frazer A., Brunswick D. (1979). A study of hormone release in depression. *Neuropsychobiology*, 5, 282–5.

Matussek N., Achenheil M., Hippius H., *et al.* (1980). Effect of clonidine on growth hormone release in psychiatric patients and controls. *Psychiatry Research*, **2**, 25–36.

McCance S. L., Cowen P. J., Grahame-Smith D. G. (1987). Methergoline attenuates the prolactin response to 1-tryptophan. *British Journal of Clinical Pharmacology*, **23**, 607–8.

McWilliam J. R., Meldrum B. S. (1983). Noradrenergic regulation of growth hormone secretion in the baboon. *Endocrinology*, **112**, 254–9.

Miki N., Ono M., Shizume K. (1984). Evidence that opiatergic and alpha-adrenergic mechanisms stimulate rat growth hormone release via growth hormone releasing factor. *Endocrinology*, **114**, 1950–2.

Mishra R., Gillespie D. D., Lovell R. A., et al. (1982). Oxaprotiline: induction of central noradrenergic subsensitivity by its (+)-enantiomer. *Life Sciences*, **30**, 1747–55.

Nemeroff C. B., Widerlou E., Bissette G., et al. (1984). Elevated immunoreactive corticotrophin-releasing hormone in depressed patients. *Science*, **244**, 1342–4.

Palazidou E., Stahl S., Franey C., et al. (1989). Evidence for an alpha$_1$ adrenoceptor control of melatonin in man. *Psychoneuroendocrinology* (in press).

Pelayo F., Dubocovich M. L., Langer S. Z. (1977). Regulation of noradrenaline release in the rat pineal through a negative feedback mechanism mediated by presynaptic alpha adrenoceptors. *European Journal of Pharmacology*, **45**, 317–8.

Pfohl B., Sherman B., Schlechte J., Stone R. (1985). Pituitary–adrenal axis rhythm disturbances in psychiatric depression. *Archives of General Psychiatry*, **42**, 897–903.

Rees L., Butler P. W. P., Gosling C., Besser G. M. (1970). Adrenergic blockade and the corticosteroid and growth hormone response to methylamphetamine. *Nature*, **228**, 565–6.

Roy-Byrne P. P., Uhde T., Post R. M., et al. (1989). Blunted ACTH response to ovine CRH in panic–anxiety disorder. *American Journal of Psychiatry* (in press).

Rubin R. T., Poland R. E., Lesser I. M., et al. (1987). Neuroendocrine aspects of primary endogenous depression. I. Cortisol secretory dynamics in patients and matched controls. *Archives of General Psychiatry*, **44**, 328–36.

Rudolph C. D., Kaplan S. L., Ganong W. F. (1980). Sites at which clonidine acts to affect blood pressure and the secretion of renin, growth hormone and ACTH. *Neuroendocrinology*, **31**, 121–8.

Sachar E. J., Halbreich U., Asnis G. M., et al. (1981). Paradoxical cortisol responses to dextroamphetamine in endogenous depression. *Archives of General Psychiatry*, **38**, 1113–7.

Sack R. L., Lewy A. J. (1986). Desmethylimipramine treatment increases melatonin production in humans. *Biological Psychiatry*, **21**, 406–16.

Schulte H. M., Chrousos G., Gold P. W., et al. (1985). Continuous infusion of CRF in normal volunteers. Physiological and pathophysiological implications. *Journal of Clinical Investigation*, **75**, 1781–5.

Shur E., Checkley S. A. (1982). Pupil studies in depressed patients: an investigation of the mechanism of action of desipramine. *British Journal of Psychiatry*, **140**, 181–4.

Siever L. J., Uhde T. W., Silberman E. V., et al. (1982). Growth hormone response to clonidine as a probe of noradrenergic receptor responsiveness in affective disorder patients and controls. *Psychiatry Research*, **6**, 171–83.

Siever L. J., Thomas R. I., Himeson D. C., et al. (1983). Growth hormone response to clonidine in obsessive-compulsive patients. *British Journal of Psychiatry*, **142**, 184–7.

Sulser F. (1984). Regulation and function of noradrenaline receptor systems in brain. Psychopharmacological aspects. *Neuropharmacology*, **23**, 255–61.

Thompson C., Mezey G., Corn T. H., *et al*. (1985). The effect of desipramine upon melatonin and cortisol in depressed and normal subjects. *British Journal of Psychiatry*, **147**, 389–93.

Uhde T. W., Vittone B. J., Siever L. J., *et al*. (1986). Blunted growth hormone response to clonidine in panic disorder patients. *Biological Psychiatry*, **21**, 1077–81.

U'Pritchard D. C., Greenberg D. A., Sheehan P. P., Snyder P. H. (1978). Tricyclic antidepressants: therapeutic properties and affinity for alpha noradrenergic binding sites in the brain. *Science*, **199**, 197–8.

5 *Interactive models of depression: the evidence*

PAUL E. BEBBINGTON AND PETER McGUFFIN

CALAMITY, CONSTITUTION AND THE ORIGINS OF DEPRESSION

The study of social causation in affective disorder has now reached the stage where both its methods and its findings are widely accepted, as demonstrated by Brown in Chapter 2. It seems clear that the psychosocial environment has a major influence on the manifestation of these disorders. On the other hand, the idea that certain categories of mood disturbances can be usefully regarded as illnesses carries with it the implication that there are contributions from factors other than the purely social (Bebbington, 1987). Biological and genetic research into affective disorders also show increasing sophistication (see Chapters 3, 4 and 6); indeed the evidence for a genetic contribution to severe depression is compelling.

It is clear that unpleasant events, even of calamitous proportions, do not inevitably result in a depressive reaction and it therefore seems likely that constitutional or 'endogenous' factors need to be incorporated along with psychosocial factors in any complete account of the origins of depression. Biopsychosocial models of affective disorder have certainly plumped for interactive (see definition below) effects of social and biological influences (Akiskal and McKinney, 1975; Akiskal, 1979; Depue *et al.*, 1979). However, such models are largely conjectural and drawn from separate biological and social studies. There have been, in fact, very few studies that have attempted to examine both types of influences directly and it is our purpose in this chapter to review them.

Statistical and genetic models usually distinguish between additive and non-additive combinations of factors. Strictly speaking, only non-additive combinations are called interactions. Here the terms 'interaction' and 'interactive' will be used in a more general, less technical sense to cover both the additive co-action of two or more factors and non-additive interactions.

The issue of interaction between variables at the psychosocial and biological levels is closely tied to ideas about the pattern of depressive symptoms. It is a common and time-honoured notion that only the more severe, 'endogenous' cases of depressive disorder are likely to connote important biological changes. Where biological changes are of importance, it might be argued that psychosocial influences would be less so. Two consequences should follow: psychosocial variables will be of less account in the explanation of the more severe depressive disorders; and conditions appearing to arise from social circumstances will be less associated with potential biological causes and correlates.

In this chaper, we will concentrate on life events and social difficulties and on the two types of 'constitutional' variables that have been used in interactive studies. These are neuroendocrine status, particularly as measured by the dexamethasone suppression test (DST), and a familial loading for depression.

Each of these variables is a somewhat crude marker of what it purports to represent. Life events and social difficulties comprise only part of the realm of psychosocial stress, and in order for analysis to be possible at all, each must be dragooned into rigid categories or omitted because their inclusion would carry too great a risk of spuriousness. The DST is likewise a crude and partial measure of the neuroendocrine dysfunction in depressive illness, and some of this dysfunction may in any case be secondary rather than an intrinsic part of the depressive process. Finally, a family history of depression may arise by chance or through shared culture, rather than from a genetic heritage. Nonetheless, these variables share the distinct virtue that we actually have some data on which to base our inferences.

The first topic to be discussed therefore is the relationship between these variables and the form of the symptoms of depressive disorder. We might expect from what had been said so far that there would be associations between both familiality and neuroendocrine disturbance and a severe or endogenous pattern of depression and this is largely borne out by the literature (McGuffin and Katz, 1986; see also Chapter 4). But what of neurotic or milder forms of depression, do they show a particular association with adversity?

ADVERSITY AND THE FORM OF DEPRESSION

Reports of the relationship between the depressive symptom pattern and the experience of psychosocial adversity show a curious schism. On one hand, multivariate studies almost invariably find that the absence of adversity discriminates endogenous from neurotic symptom pictures as powerfully as any of the so-called 'endogenous' symptoms (Hamilton and White, 1959; Kiloh and Garside, 1963; Carney *et al.*, 1965; Rosenthal and Klerman, 1966; Rosenthal and Gudeman, 1967; Mendels and Cochrane, 1968; Garside *et al.*, 1971; Feinberg and Carroll, 1982). Paykel (1971) reported findings similar to those quoted above, but suggested that effects of age might account for the results of this and other studies. Depression in older people is more likely to be of endogenous type, and life events are rarer in older subjects.

The results of multivariate studies stand in contrast to those specifically designed to test the association of adversity with different symptom patterns in depression. Even without controlling for age, the experience of preceding adversity in endogenous and reactive groups is usually similar (see, for example Hudgens *et al.*, 1967; Leff *et al.*, 1970; Thompson and Hendrie, 1972; Brown and Harris, 1978; Benjaminsen, 1981; Katschnig *et al.*, 1981, 1986; Katschnig, 1984; Paykel *et al.*, 1984; Brugha and Conroy, 1985; Dolan *et al.*, 1985; Roy *et al.*, 1986), although some more recent studies do provide support for an association between adversity and a neurotic symptom picture (Roy *et al.*, 1985; Zimmerman *et al.*, 1986). Approaching the problem in a slightly different way, Nelson and Charney (1980) showed that depressive states reactive to social stresses were much less likely to fulfil the criteria for primary affective disorder.

The contrasting results described above could arise from various differences of method (Katschnig *et al.*, 1986). More importantly, the findings of the multivariate studies may be an artefact. Clinical psychiatrists make the distinction between endogenous and reactive depression on grounds both of characteristic symptoms and of the relationship with potential psychosocial stressors (Katschnig *et al.*, 1981). As clinicians' judgements are used as the basis for validating the multivariate functions, or in the claim that the psychosocial history is relevant to onset, it is not surprising that the relationship with preceding adversity appears highly significant. In some studies, the discriminant function actually included the clinician's judgement of whether there had been significant social precipitants.

On the other hand, many of the direct comparison studies have used periods of analysis for preceding life events which may have been too long. It has been suggested that the period which seems to be important if events are to lead to 'normal' affective responses is limited to two to three months before onset (Brown and Harris, 1978; Bebbington *et al.*, 1981). Comparison on the basis of longer preceding periods may obscure differences between groups. However, Katschnig (1984) analysed his data in a manner identical to that of the community study of Bebbington and his colleagues (1981) but failed to find differences in the history of adversity between symptomatic groups. At most, the literature therefore provides only slender and inconsistent evidence for 'pure' endogeneity in endogenous depression.

THE GENETIC CONTRIBUTION

Perhaps the most consistent clue to the puzzling aetiology of depressive illness is its tendency to run in families. Kraepelin (1922) was among the first to emphasize the importance of hereditary factors in manic depressive insanity. There is good agreement that no matter how probands are selected, their relatives tend to be more often affected than do members of the general population. Modern studies show a consistent pattern with an average lifetime risk of affective illness of just under 10 percent in the first degree relatives of unipolar probands and about 19 percent in the first degree relatives of bipolar probands (reviewed by McGuffin and Katz, 1986).

Familiality does not necessarily imply that a disorder is genetic. However, twin and adoption studies of affective disorder do suggest that genetic factors play a large part (Reich *et al.*, 1982), and the analysis of twin data assuming a multifactorial threshold model suggests that genes, rather than family environment, are responsible for most of the variation in liability (McGuffin and Katz, 1986). Adoption studies confirm the importance of genes in bipolar disorder (Mendlewicz and Rainer, 1977). In unipolar disorder, however, the genetic component is more modest (Wender *et al.*, 1986; Von Knorring *et al.*, 1983).

Among the unipolar conditions, the genetic evidence is most clear-cut for typical Kraepelinian or 'endogenous' patterns of illness, and where only neurotic or non-endogenous cases are considered, twin studies suggest that genetic influences are small and indirect. Only two published studies of neurotic depression provide family data in adequate detail, and both suggest that depression is somewhat more common in the first degree relatives of neurotically depressed probands that in the general population. Stenstedt (1966) found a morbid risk of depression of 5.4 percent in the relatives of neurotic depressives, while the estimated population morbid risk was around 3 percent. The data here were based almost entirely on family history, and so may have provided an underestimate. Indeed, the more recent study of Perris *et al.* (1982), using case records of relatives, found a morbid risk of depression of 9 percent in the first degree relatives of neurotic depressives. Thus neurotic depression would appear to be somewhat less familial than the more severe forms.

Furthermore, twin studies suggest that the major source of familial aggregation in neurotic depression is not genetic. Slater and Shields (1969) found zero concordance for narrowly defined depression in the co-twins of neurotically depressed probands and, like the latter study of Torgersen (1985), were able to find little difference between monozygotic (MZ) and dizygotic (DZ) concordance even after taking a much broader diagnostic perspective. On the other hand, Shapiro (1970) did find higher concordances in MZ than in DZ twins, but his series of so-called 'non-endogenous' depressives was ascertained through probands who had all been treated as in-patients, and certainly an admixture of probands suffering from what in Denmark is called reactive depressive psychosis.

NEUROENDOCRINE CHANGES

The hypothalamic–pituitary–adrenal axis has an endogenous circadian rhythm: secretion begins at midnight and wanes through the day from a maximum at the end of the night. A normal subject given 1 mg of dexamethasone at 23.00 h will secrete virtually no cortisol the next day. In at least some depressed patients this negative feedback is suppressed, almost certainly as a result of changes directly consequent on the development of depression (Checkley, 1984).

It seems likely that the changes flagged by the DST are strongly associated with the endogenous type of depression. Certainly, delusional depression is said to be almost always associated with an abnormal DST, and Carroll and his colleagues have consistently claimed that abnormal DST results are almost exclusively seen in those with clinical diagnoses of endogenous depression (Carroll *et al.*, 1981). The use of standardized criteria attenuates this finding somewhat (Checkley, 1984), but the conclusion must be that the more severe forms of depression, distinguished by endogenous symptoms, are indeed less likely to show suppression.

However well they distinguish endogenous and non-endogenous symptom patterns, the abnormal findings with the DST appear to be state dependent—with recovery they become less common (Checkley, 1984).

INTERACTIONAL STUDIES

The earliest hints about interactions between social and biological influences emerge from genetic studies. Stenstedt (1952) suggested that those patients whose illnesses seemed related to obvious environmental factors had fewer family members affected than did those where there was no clear precipitant. An attempt to follow up this suggestion has been reported by Pollitt (1972), who considered the roles of both familial diathesis and potential stresses together. Pollitt found that the morbid risk of depression among relatives of the depressed proband whose illness arose 'out of the blue' was higher, at about 21 percent, than when the proband's illness was 'justifiable', where the morbid risk in relatives was between 6 and 12 percent. 'Justifiable' illnesses comprised those following either a severe physical stress or some psychological trauma. It is only much more recently that there have been attempts to study social and neuroendocrine factors in combination.

SOCIAL FACTORS AND ENDOCRINE CHANGES

Calloway, Dolan and their colleagues (Calloway *et al.*, 1984a, 1984b; Dolan *et al.*, 1985; Calloway, 1988) have conducted a neuroendocrine and psychosocial study of 72 depressed patients. All subjects fulfilled Research

Diagnostic Criteria (Spitzer *et al.*, 1978) for primary major depression. Two-fifths were in-patients, and two-fifths were male. A third were in their first episode and only two patients failed to reach Index of Definition level 5, suggesting they were reasonably severe. Assessment of mental state was based on the Present State Examination (PSE; Wing *et al.*, 1974) the Hamilton Depression Scale (Hamilton, 1960) and the Newcastle criteria for distinguishing categories of neurotic and endogenous depression (Carney *et al.*, 1965). Patients could also be allocated to categories of neurotic and endogenous depression using the CATEGO, a computer-program which provides a classification based on PSE data (Wing and Sturt, 1978; also see below), permitting an alternative way of dividing them into endogenous and neurotic types, identical to that used in our own studies. There was a roughly even spread between the endogenous and neurotic categories. All in all, this sample of patients sounds very similar in severity and category to that of the index cases in our own social and familial study described below.

The neuroendocrine status of the patients was assessed in a variety of ways. Assessments included a 1 mg DST, 24 h urinary cortisols, the thyrotrophin-releasing hormone (TRH) test and the Free Thyroxine Index (FTI). Life events and chronic difficulties were elicited by the semi-structured life events and difficulties schedule (LEDS) of Brown and Harris (1978; discussed in Chapter 2) and were rated on severity of threat, focus and independence, although it is not clear whether the ratings were made by a panel 'blind' to mental state findings, as Brown and Harris recommend, or by the interviewer. Life events were restricted in the usual manner for the purpose of analysis to those rated 'independent' and 'possibly independent' (Calloway, 1988). The date of onset of the depression was established, and life events were included if they had occurred within the six months before onset. For some analyses of the neuroendocrine assays, life events in the six months before the test were also evaluated. Only *severe* events (Brown and Harris, 1978) were included. *Marked* difficulties, that is, those enduring for a year before onset, were also analysed. In addition, any family history of depression was established from interviews with the patient and an informant, and from case records.

Two-fifths of the sample were non-suppressors, and a similar proportion had experienced severe life events; a quarter suffered marked difficulties, and over half had a history either of a life event or of a difficulty. There were no differences between the patients with or without a family history of depression in their experience of life events or of difficulties. Nor were there differences between suppressors and non-suppressors on the DST. However, the 24 h urinary cortisol before the DST was *raised* in those with life events and difficulties. It is possible, therefore, that this measure reflects a reactive neuroendocrine change, whereas the resetting of the system, as indicated by the DST, is not a stress-related phenomenon. This makes a nice tale: clearly the only way of substantiating it is through further social-biological studies of this type. Unfortunately, so far, there is no confirmatory evidence and the study of Roy *et al.* (1988) failed to show an association between urinary cortisol and life events.

The results concerning hypothalamic–pituitary–thyroid axis functioning (Calloway *et al.*, 1984b) are confusing. It appears that blunted responses to the TRH test were more likely in those who were experiencing social difficulties (but were not, apparently, related to life events). Moreover, those with blunted responses and marked difficulties had higher FTI than those who only had blunted responses. It is possible that prolonged stress induces a subclinical hypothyroidism, but that the mechanism of blunting in those without stress is different, perhaps operating at the pituitary level. However, this really does seem far-fetched. While separate neuroendocrine systems might display different responses to stress and to the development of depressive illness, it is significant that five of the six patients with delusional depression showed abnormalities of DST, urinary free cortisol (UFC), TRH response and FTI.

The results for family history were also strange. Those with a family history of depression (presumably a marker for a depressive diathesis) were *more* likely to have normal TRH response, but *less* likely, albeit nonsignificantly so, to show suppression following dexamethasone.

Roy *et al.* (1986) have also examined the relationship between certain biological markers of depression and exposure to antecedent life events. All the patients met the DSM-III criteria (American Psychiatric Association, 1980) for Major Depressive Episode, and two-thirds also met the criteria for melancholia. Onset was dated and the experience of life events in the preceding six months was established, using Paykel's interview (Paykel *et al.*, 1969) which is based on a checklist of events rather than a semi-structured interview. There was no difference in Hamilton score or in the proportion with melancholia between those with and without antecedent life events. However, those without life events had significantly lower levels of cerebrospinal-fluid homovanillic acid and 5-hydroxyindole acetic acid (5-HIAA), and were more likely to be non-suppressors on the dexamethasone suppression test. Roy *et al.* (1986) believe that the presence of life events serves to distinguish separate biological types. However, their findings are based on only 20 cases.

SOCIAL AND FAMILIAL FACTORS

Our own study, the Camberwell Collaborative Depression Study, was an investigation of 76 female and 54 male cases of recent onset depression, and of their first degree relatives. The design and methods of the study are described in detail elsewhere (Bebbington *et al.*, 1988; McGuffin *et al.*, 1988a, 1988b). The probands were sampled on the basis of an initial or renewed out-patient contact, although a substantial proportion had previous or subsequent in-patient treatment. Clinical status was established through the PSE, and the LEDS of Brown and Harris (1978) was used by a separate interviewer to establish a history of life events and difficulties in the 6-month period before onset. Events and onset were carefully dated. Events were rated for threat, independence and focus, using the panel method of Brown and Harris (1978).

Attempts were made to contact the first degree relatives of the probands. In 83 families at least one first degree relative was interviewed, yielding 244 such interviews in total. Good information from two or more informants, and case notes where applicable, were acquired on a further 71 relatives. The current mental state was again established through the PSE, and past episodes were identified using the Past History Schedule as decribed by McGuffin and Katz (1986). The LEDS was again used to derive a 6-month history of life events, before onset in current cases, before interview for current non-cases, and before datable past episodes.

The CATEGO program was used to provide a classification for each subject. CATEGO uses three categories for depressive disorders: D (delusional depression), R (retarded depression) and N (neurotic depression). Psychiatrists tend to allocate the R class evenly between ICD-296.2 and ICD-300.4 (World Health Organization, 1978). In addition, some of our cases of depression were allocated to the A (anxiety) class, although all had the symptom of depression. For our purposes, we divided the cases into a combination of classes D and R and a combination of classes N and A, to give an approximate 'endogenous'/'neurotic' split.

A variety of analyses were carried out to test the proposition that the experience of life events and difficulties would successfully discriminate between those endogenous and neurotic categories. In fact there was no difference. This is best illustrated in Figs. 5.1 and 5.2, which show that an excess of both mild and more serious events is seen equally in neurotic and in endogenous sub-types. This excess is highly significant in comparison with the rate of events experienced in the general population (Bebbington

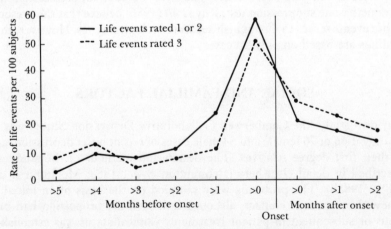

Fig. 5.1 *Life events and the onset of neurotic depression*

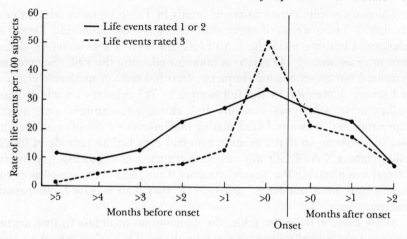

Fig. 5.2 *Life events and the onset of 'endogenous depression'*

et al., 1981). It is possible that the pre-onset rise occurs earlier and reaches a lower level in the endogenous depressives, but it is not clear that much can be made of this.

We have not, therefore, shown any association between a neurotic pattern of symptoms and reactivity to adversity. This contrasts with the findings of the earlier Camberwell Community Survey (Bebbington *et al.*, 1981) but, as we have seen, is in keeping with the predominantly negative results of studies elsewhere. What then of the relationship between pattern of illness, adversity and familiality of depression? Based on received wisdom, we could put forward two hypotheses. First, familial aggregation of depression will be much more pronounced where the probands (index cases) have an endogenous pattern of symptoms than when the illness is of the neurotic type. Second, familial aggregation will be most marked where the proband's illness has arisen without any obvious precipitants than where the proband has become ill in the face of threatening life events or chronic difficulties. Let us first examine our results of the relationship between familiality and pattern of symptoms.

As described above, we divided the probands into neurotic and endogenous categories on the basis of PSE/CATEGO classes. However, from the point of view of a family–genetic study, a 'lifetime ever' classification is of greater interest than purely a classification based upon the index episode of illness. Thus where probands have had multiple episodes of illness, a hierarchical approach was adopted to combine CATEGO classes, the simple rule being that endogenous illness takes priority over neurotic disorder. Hence, some probands whose current CATEGO class was in the neurotic category, but who had had previous episodes of an endogenous type, were reclassified as endogenous.

The main results are summarized briefly in Table 5.1 (after McGuffin *et al.*, 1987). Here we used three different ways of classifying illness in relatives. First, we used the CATEGO ID level 5 and above to define current cases among 244 relatives interviewed using the PSE. Second, we examined the age-corrected frequency (morbid risk) of moderately severe and severe depression in the full sample of 315 relatives on whom good quality information was available and, third, we examined only severe depression in this group. In calculating morbid risk we considered 'lifetime ever' depression, so that a relative who had ever had an episode of illness falling into a CATEGO depression category and requiring psychiatric referral was placed in the 'severe' category if they had been treated as an in-patient and in a 'moderate' category if they had received out-patient treatment only.

As we can see from the table, the distribution of illness in first degree relatives only partially fits with our hypothesis. Thus when we take a very broad definition of current 'cases' there is actually much more illness among the first degree relatives of probands with neurotic depression. This is the reverse of the predicted direction and, indeed, current cases among the relatives of endogenous probands are only slightly more common than the previously reported rate of 11 percent in the general population (Bebbington *et al.*, 1981). Lifetime expectancy, or morbid risk, has greater interest from the point of view of the geneticist but even here there is little difference between the relatives of neurotic and endogenously depressed probands when we consider fairly broadly defined depression. Both groups of relatives show a high morbid risk to age 65 of moderate depression compared with the general population. However, it is only when we consider severe depression in relatives that we obtain a result in a predicted direction—with illness of sufficient severity to warrant in-patient treatment being nearly twice as common among the relatives of endogenous probands as among those of neurotic probands.

The implications of these findings from the point of view of genetic

Table 5.1 Frequency (%) of depression in the first degree relatives of probands with neurotic or endogenous depression (from McGuffin *et al.*, 1987)

	Proband type		General population
	Neurotic	*Endogenous*	
Prevalence of current 'cases'	23.5	12.7	11.1**
Morbid risk* of moderate plus severe depression	23.7	25.7	8.9***
Morbid risk* of severe depression	7.9	14.7	2.6***

* to age 65; ** from Bebbington *et al.* (1981); *** from Sturt *et al.* (1984).

studies are important. They demonstrate that not only is depressive illness an irregular and clumsy phenotype but it is also one which is highly elastic. It becomes difficult to make any firm pronouncements about the transmission of 'depression' unless we are prepared to give a full and explicit answer to the question 'Which depression?' The problem is of course widespread in psychiatric research. For example, it might be argued that schizophrenia is a more readily defined condition but a recent study showed that heritability estimates based on twin concordance varied from 0 to over 80 percent depending on which definition of the disorder was used (McGuffin *et al.*, 1984).

In considering depression and adversity in the relatives of depressed probands, our findings were also contrary to expectation. We were unable to show an inverse relationship between antecedent stress in the proband and familial diathesis in terms of frequency of depression in first degree relatives. Indeed, the morbid risk in relatives for moderate plus severe depression was slightly higher where the proband had experienced life events or chronic difficulties in the 3-month period prior to the onset of depression. The highest life-time prevalence of depression was found in the relatives of probands who had experienced both life events and chronic difficulties preceding the onset of their disorder, but neither difference between the groups of relatives classified according to these proband characteristics proved to be significant (McGuffin *et al.*, 1988b). These findings cannot be regarded as completely contradictory to those of Pollitt (1972) because the majority of precipitants of disorder in Pollitt's justifiable group of depressed probands consisted of infections or other physical stressors. In our series, none of the 83 probands appear to have important physical factors contributing to the onset of the depression. Nevertheless, our results do present a serious challenge to dividing depression into familial/non-reactive and non-familial/reactive categories. This corresponds to our failure, discussed above, to demonstrate a difference in the association of life events with onsets of 'endogenous' or 'neurotic' patterns of depression (Bebbington *et al.*, 1988).

To examine the relationship between familiality of depression and life events in greater detail, we compared the personally interviewed, first degree relatives with a representative sample from the community from whom data had been collected using virtually identical methods of assessment (Bebbington *et al.*, 1981). These findings are briefly summarized in Table 5.2. There are three main points to note. First, as we have already observed, current cases were significantly more frequent among first degree relatives than in the community. Second, the association between recent life events and current disorder in the community sample is marked and striking, whereas in first degree relatives the association is weak. Third, we have found that not only does current illness appear to aggregate in families, but so also do recent life events. The increased rate of life events among first degree relatives compared with the community sample is highly significant and remains so even when all potentially

Table 5.2 Current depression and recent life events in first degree relatives of depressed probands compared with a community sample (data from McGuffin *et al.*, 1988b)

	Subjects with recent life events %	Cases among subjects with recent life events %	Cases among subjects with no recent life events %	Total cases %
Community sample (*n* = 289)	7.3	57.1	7.5	11.1
First degree relatives (*n* = 244)	28.7	21.4	15.5	17.2

confounding proband–related events are removed. Furthermore, when we plotted life events over time in the relative sample (McGuffin *et al.*, 1988b), we did not find a peak of life events in close proximity to the proband's onset of illness. It therefore seems unlikely that the high rate of events (all of which were judged to be 'independent' or 'possibly independent' by our panel of raters) was associated either with the turmoil created by the onset of the proband's disorder or by certain life events which impinged both upon the proband and other family members. A logistic regression analysis, taking current disorder as the response variable, showed that both the experience of life events and being a first degree relative had significant effects, but there was also a highly significant relative × life event interaction. This was because, as we have already pointed out, the effect of recent life events on current illness is large in the general population but small for those who are a first degree relative of a depressed proband.

These findings are extremely complex and require careful interpretation. Our simple starting hypothesis was that both family loading and threatening life events have a causal relationship with depression and that there would be an inverse relationship between the two. However, our findings oblige us to reject this. We might, therefore, consider alternative and more radical hypotheses—for example, that a common familial factor predisposes both to depression and to a propensity to experience (or report) life events. It would then be tempting to speculate that the association between life events and depression, which has been repeatedly observed in community studies, is a spurious one induced by the fact that both affective illness and tendency to experience life events are caused by the same familial factor. However, this does not fit well with our findings based on the proband sample alone, where there is a clear temporal relationship between life events and subsequent onsets of depression.

We are left with the conclusion that the tendency to experience (or to report) life events and the tendency to experience depressive symptoms are both familial. These tendencies appear to be inextricably bound up with each other so that given our present data, no simple model readily explains the relationship. One obvious familial explanatory variable might be social class. However, not only is there a lack of relationship between depression and social class in our data but there is a lack of relationship between frequency of adversity and social class. We are currently exploring the relationship between life events, depression and personality (including cognitive factors and attributional style). However, preliminary results (Katz and McGuffin, 1987) do not suggest a relationship between propensity to experience life events and conventional dimensions such as those measured on the Eysenck Personality Questionnaire (Eysenck and Eysenck, 1975).

It is now traditional for reviewers to conclude with a plea for more research. This is also our plea, but we feel that it is here a particularly well-founded one. Much space in the literature has been devoted to the elaboration of interactive, 'biopsychosocial' theories of psychiatric conditions in general and of affective disorders in particular (Slater and Cowie, 1971; Akiskal and McKinney, 1975; Akiskal, 1979; Depue *et al.*, 1979). These models have been postulated almost entirely on the basis of research from the separate realms of genetic, biological, social and psychological study. The complexity and uncertainty of the findings from the few truly interactive studies reviewed here suggest that these models have far to travel, from a pleasing face validity and the support of circumstantial evidence to a proper corroboration.

REFERENCES

Akiskal H. S. (1979). A biobehavioural approach to depression. In *The Psychobiology of Depressive Disorders: Implications for the Effect of Stress* (Depue R. A., ed.). New York: Academic Press.

Akiskal H. S., McKinney W. T. (1975). Overview of recent research in depression: Integration of ten conceptual models into a comprehensive clinical frame. *Archives of General Psychiatry*, 32, 285–305.

American Psychiatric Association (1980). *Diagnostic and Statistical Manual*, 3rd edn. (DSM-III). Washington: American Psychiatric Association.

Bebbington P. E. (1987). Misery and beyond: the pursuit of disease theories of depression. *International Journal of Social Psychiatry*, 33, 13–20.

Bebbington P. E., Tennant C., Hurry J. (1981). Life events and the nature of psychiatric disorder in the community. *Journal of Affective Disorders*, 3, 345–66.

Bebbington P. E., Brugha T., MacCarthy B., *et al.* (1988). The Camberwell Collaborative Depression Study. I. Depressed probands: Adversity and the form of depression. *British Journal of Psychiatry*, 152, 754–65.

Benjaminsen S. (1981). Primary non-endogenous depression and features attributed to reactive depression. *Journal of Affective Disorders*, 3, 245–59.

Brown G. W., Harris T. O. (1978). *Social Origins of Depression*. London: Tavistock.

Brugha T., Conroy R. (1985). Categories of depression: Reported life events in a controlled design. *British Journal of Psychiatry*, **147**, 641–6.

Calloway S. P. (1988). Endocrine changes and clinical profiles in depression. In *Life Events and Illness* (Brown G. W., Harris T., eds.). London: Guildford Press.

Calloway S. P., Dolan R. J., Fonagy P., *et al.* (1984a). Endocrine changes and clinical profiles in depression: I. The dexamethasone suppression test. *Psychological Medicine*, **14**, 749–58.

Calloway S. P., Dolan R. J., Fonagy P., *et al.* (1984b). Endocrine changes and clinical profiles in depression: II. The thyrotropin-releasing hormone test. *Psychological Medicine*, **14**, 759–66.

Carney M. W. P., Roth M., Garside R. F. (1965). The diagnosis of depressive syndromes and the prediction of ECT response. *British Journal of Psychiatry*, **111**, 659–74.

Carroll B. J., Feinberg M., Greden J. F., *et al.* (1981). A specific laboratory test for the diagnosis of melancholia. *Archives of General Psychiatry*, **38**, 15–22.

Checkley S. (1984). Endocrine changes in mental illness. In *Scientific Principles of Psychopathology* (McGuffin P., Shanks M. F., Hodgson R., eds.). London: Academic Press, pp. 137–50.

Depue R. A., Monroe S. M., Shackman S. L. (1979). The psychobiology of human disease: Implications for conceptualising the depressive disorders. In *The Psychobiology of the Depressive Disorders: Implications for the Effects of Stress* (Depue R. A., ed.). New York: Academic Press.

Dolan R. J., Calloway S. P., Fonagy P., *et al.* (1985). Life events, depression and hypothalamic-pituitary-adrenal axis function. *British Journal of Psychiatry*, **147**, 429–33.

Eysenck H., Eysenck S. B. G. (1975). *Manual of the Eysenck Personality Questionnaire*. London: Hodder and Stoughton.

Feinberg M., Carroll B.J. (1982). Separation of subtypes of depression using discriminant analysis: I. Separation of unipolar endogenous depression from non-endogenous depression. *British Journal of Psychiatry*, **140**, 384–91.

Garside R. F., Kay D. W. K., Wilson I. C., *et al.* (1971). Depressive syndromes and the classification of patients. *Psychological Medicine*, **1**, 333–8.

Hamilton M. (1960). A rating scale for depression. *Journal of Neurology, Neurosurgery and Psychiatry*, **23**, 56–66.

Hamilton M., White J.M. (1959). Clinical syndromes in depressive states. *Journal of Mental Science*, **105**, 985–98.

Hudgens R. W., Morrison J. R., Barchka R. (1957). Life events and onset of primary affective disorders. A study of 40 hospitalised patients and 40 controls. *Archives of General Psychiatry*, **16**, 134–45.

Katschnig H. (1984). (Commentary to) Paul Bebbington, Inferring causes: some constraints in the social psychiatry of depressive disorders. *Integrative Psychiatry*, **2**, 77–9.

Katschnig H., Brandl-Nebehay A., Fuchs-Robetin G., Seelig, P., *et al.* (1981). *Lebensverändernde Ereignisse, Psychoziale Dispositionen und Depressive Verstimmungzustände*. Wien, Abteilung Für Sozialpsychiatrie und Dokumentation. Psychiatriche Universitätsklinik.

Katschnig H., Pakesh G., Egger-Zeidner E. (1986). Life stress and subtypes of depression. In *Life Events and Psychiatric Disorders: Controversial Issues* (Katschnig H., ed.). Cambridge: Cambridge University Press.

Katz R., McGuffin P. (1987). Neuroticism in familial depression. *Psychological Medicine*, 17, 155–61.

Kay D. W. K., Garside R. F., Beamish P., Roy J. R. (1969). Endogenous and neurotic syndromes of depression—a factor analytic study of 104 cases. Clinical Features. *British Journal of Psychiatry*, 115, 377–88.

Kiloh L. G., Garside R.F. (1963). The independence of neurotic depression and endogenous depression. *British Journal of Psychiatry*, 119, 415–63.

Kraepelin E. (1922). *Manic Depressive Insanity and Paranoia* (Barclay R. M., translator). Edinburgh: E. & S. Livingstone.

Leff M. H., Roach J. F., Bunney W. E. (1970). Environmental factors preceding the onsets of severe depressions. *Psychiatry*, 33, 293–311.

McGuffin P., Farmer A. E., Gottesman I. I., *et al.* (1984). Twin concordance for operationally defined schizophrenia: Confirmation of familiality and heritability. *Archives of General Psychiatry*, 41, 541–5.

McGuffin P., Katz R. (1986). Nature, nurture and affective disorders. In *The Biology of Depression* (Deakin J. F. W., ed.). Royal College of Psychiatrists Special Publication, London: Gaskell Press, pp. 26–52.

McGuffin P., Katz R., Aldrich J. (1986). Past and Present State Examination: The assessment of 'lifetime ever' psychopathology. *Psychological Medicine*, 16, 461–6.

McGuffin P., Katz R., Bebbington P. E. (1987). Hazard, heredity and depression. A family study. *Journal of Psychiatric Research*, 21 (4), 365–75.

McGuffin P., Katz R., Aldrich J., Bebbington P. E. (1988a). The Camberwell Collaborative Depression Study. II. The investigation of family members. *British Journal of Psychiatry*, 152, 766–74.

McGuffin P., Katz R., Bebbington P. E. (1988b). The Camberwell Collaborative Depression Study. III. Depression and adversity in the relatives of depressed probands. *British Journal of Psychiatry*, 152, 775–82.

Mendels J., Cochrane C. (1968). The nosology of depression—the endogenous reactive concept. *American Journal of Psychiatry*, 124 (suppl.), 1–11.

Mendlewicz J., Rainer J. D. (1977). Adoption study supporting genetic transmission in manic-depressive illness. *Nature*, 268, 326–9.

Nelson C. J., Charney D. S. (1980). Primary affective disorder criteria and the endogenous-reactive distinction. *Archives of General Psychiatry*, 37, 787–93.

Paykel E. S. (1971). Classification of depressed patients: a cluster analysis derived grouping. *British Journal of Psychiatry*, 118, 275–88.

Paykel E. S., Myers J. K., Dienelt M. N., *et al.* (1969). Life events and depression: a controlled study. *Archives of General Psychiatry*, 21, 753–60.

Paykel E. S., Rao B. M., Taylor C. N. (1984). Life stress and symptom pattern in out-patient depression. *Psychological Medicine*, 14, 559–68.

Perris C., Perris H., Ericsson U., Von Knorring L. (1982). The genetics of depression. A family study of unipolar and neurotic-reactive depressed patients. *Archiv für Psychiatrie und Nervenkrankheiten*, 232, 137–55.

Pollitt J. (1972). The relationship between genetic and precipitating factors in depressive illness. *British Journal of Psychiatry*, 121, 67–70.

Reich T., Cloninger C. R., Suarez B., Rice J. (1982). Genetics of the affective psychoses. In *Psychosis of Uncertain Aetiology Handbook of Psychiatry* vol. 3 (Wing J. K., Wing L., eds.). Cambridge: Cambridge University Press.

Rosenthal S. H., Klerman G. L. (1966). Content and consistency in the endogenous depressive pattern. *British Journal of Psychiatry*, 112, 471–84.

Rosenthal S. H., Gudeman J. E. (1967). The endogenous depressive pattern. *Archives of General Psychiatry*, **16**, 241–9.

Roy A., Breir A., Doran A. R., Pickar D. (1985). Life events and depression: Relation to subtypes. *Journal of Affective Disorders*, **9**, 143–8.

Roy A., Pickar D., Douillet P., Linnoila, M., Karoum, P. (1986). Urinary monoamines and monoamine metabolites in subtypes of unipolar depressive disorder and normal controls. *Psychological Medicine*, **16**, 541–8.

Roy A., Linnoila M., Karoum F., Pickar D. (1988). Urinary-free cortisol in depressed patients and controls: relationship to urinary indices of noradrenergic function. *Psychological Medicine*, **18**, 93–8.

Shapiro R.W. (1970). A twin study of non-endogenous depression. *Acta Jutlandica XLII* (publication of the University of Aarhus).

Slater E., Cowie V. (1971). *The Genetics of Mental Disorders*. London: Oxford University Press.

Slater E., Shields J. (1969). Genetical aspects of anxiety. In *Studies of Anxiety* (Lader, M. H., ed.). British Journal of Psychiatry, Special Publication No. 3. Ashford: Headley Brothers.

Spitzer R. L., Endicott J., Robins E. (1978). Research Diagnostic Criteria: Rationale and reliability. *Archives of General Psychiatry*, **35**, 773–82.

Stendstedt A. (1952). A study in manic depressive psychosis: clinical, social and genetic investigations. *Acta Psychiatrica* (suppl.) **79**.

Stenstedt A. (1966). Genetics of neurotic depression. *Acta Psychiatrica Scandinavica*, **42**, 392–409.

Sturt E., Kumakura N., Der G. (1984). How depressing life is. Life-long morbidity risk for depressive disorder in the general population. *Journal of Affective Disorders*, **7**, 109–22.

Thompson K. C., Hendrie H. C. (1972). Environmental stress in primary depressive illness. *Archives of General Psychiatry*, **26**, 130–2.

Torgersen S. (1985). Genetic factors in moderately severe and mild affective disorders. *Archives of General Psychiatry*, **43**, 222–6.

Von Knorring A. L., Cloninger C. R., Bohman M., Sigvardsson S. (1983). An adoption study of depressive disorders and substance abuse. *Archives of General Psychiatry*, **40**, 943–50.

Wender P. H., Kety S. S., Rosenthal D., *et al.* (1986). Psychiatric disorders in the biological and adoptive families of adopted individuals with affective disorders. *Archives of General Psychiatry*, **43**, 923–9.

Wing J. K., Cooper J., Sartorius N. (1974). *The Measurement and Classification of Psychiatric Symptoms*. Cambridge: Cambridge University Press.

Wing J. K., Sturt E. (1978). *The PSE-ID-CATEGO System Supplementary Manual* (Medical Research Council mimeo). London: Institute of Psychiatry.

World Health Organization (1978). *Mental Disorders: Glossary and Guide to their Classification in accordance with the Ninth Revision of the International Classification of Diseases*. Geneva: World Health Organization.

Zimmerman M., Coryell W., Pfohl B., Strangel D. (1986). The validity of four definitions of endogenous depression: II. Clinical, demographic, familial and psychosocial correlates. *Archives of General Psychiatry*, **43**, 234–44.

6 Drug-related depression: clinical and epidemiological aspects

J. GUY EDWARDS

Whitlock and Evans (1978) pointed out that about 200 drugs have been alleged to cause depression and many more have been considered as possibly contributing to this disorder. Even when the list is limited to those drugs reported in the literature as a cause of depression on four or more occasions, it still contains 80 single substances or compound preparations. It is essential to study the evidence for and against these many allegations in order to help understand the causes of depression in individual cases, to ensure that prescribed treatments are not adding to patients' suffering, and to avoid discontinuing suspect drugs needed for the treatment of serious medical conditions. Such an inquiry assists also in the search for a pharmacological model of depression. The discovery of such a model could advance understanding of the aetiology of depressive illness—an illness that afflicts millions of people, causes indescribable suffering and wreaks havoc with their lives. It is also important, for medicolegal reasons, to be aware of which drugs cause depression; this is especially so in the case of suicide.

If we are to believe current biological theories of the cause of depression, it seems incredible that so many different drugs, of so many different categories, should act through similar neurophysiological or neurochemical mechanisms. It is probable, therefore, that some drugs, at least, have been wrongly incriminated. In this chapter the evidence that has been put forward in support of the idea that certain categories of drugs cause depression will be reviewed. But first let us look at the clinical features of drug-related 'depression'.

PHENOMENOLOGY

It is clear that depression is a highly complex phenomenon; there are no clear-cut definitions and the word means different things to different people. There are no entirely objective tests for diagnosing depression, despite the enthusiasm of some for markers such as the dexamethasone suppression test (see Chapter 5). We therefore have to rely almost entirely on phenomenology. With a penetrating phenomenological approach, a skilled interview technique and a reliable operational definition, clinicians and researchers can achieve a high level of inter-observer agreement in the recognition of depressive illness. However, such methodology is rarely applied to depression occurring during general medical treatment because skilled phenomenologists do little liaison with psychiatry and general physicians are not usually trained to elicit the finer details of affective symptoms. These considerations must make us consider whether or not reports of 'depression' occurring during drug treatments of physical disorders really do refer to depression in the psychiatric sense of the word.

Much of the depression allegedly caused by drugs appears to be a mixture of lethargy, apathy, tiredness, drowsiness and feeling 'sluggish' or slowed down. Such symptoms may be accompanied by other features of a drug-induced toxic reaction, including confusion and psychotic phenomena. Naturally, patients having to tolerate these troublesome unwanted effects and being unable to function properly are unlikely to be in the brightest of spirits—but is this depression? Surely not, if the word is to have a specific psychiatric meaning, and certainly not in the context of the symposium upon which this book is based.

CAUSE AND EFFECT

The second problem which has to be faced is that of establishing a causal connection between drug and depression. In many reports there is the overt suggestion or tacit assumption that depression, even when convincingly present, is mediated by pharmacological mechanisms. This, however, many not necessarily be the case for the following reasons.

Firstly, the depression may be purely coincidental. Depression is one of the most common phenomena encountered in the whole of medical practice. Apart from normal depression, which is universal, depressive symptoms have been found in nine community studies carried out in England and the USA between 1957 and 1979 to have a point prevalence ranging from 13 to 20 percent (Boyd and Weissman, 1982). Using various structured screening instruments, including the Present State Examination (PSE; Wing *et al.*, 1974) and the Schedule for Affective Disorders and Schizophrenia (Spitzer and Endicott, 1978), and diagnostic criteria such as the Research Diagnostic Criteria (Spitzer *et al.*, 1978a, b), the point prevalence for non-bipolar depression in industrial countries was found to be 3.2 percent in the adult male, and 5.2–9.3 percent in the adult female, population. Being such a commonly found condition, depression must occur as a coincidental phenomenon during the course of treatment with many drugs.

Secondly, the depression may be a symptom of the illness being treated or of a concurrent, diagnosed or undiagnosed, psychiatric or non-psychiatric disorder. It can occur in most psychiatric illnesses—even in mania. A high incidence of depression has also been said to occur in a wide range of diseases: these include primary dementias (including Huntington's disease), brain tumours, multiple sclerosis, epilepsy, thyroid dysfunction, hyperparathyroidism, Cushing's disease, Addison's disease, rheumatoid arthritis, cancer, protein and vitamin B deficiency, viral disease (particularly influenza, infectious mononucleosis and human immunodeficiency virus disease) and myocardial infarction. The depression may be a reaction to the mental or physical disability caused by the disease or may result from concern and fear over its outcome.

Thirdly, the depression may be the result of a psychic reaction to the drug or other treatments that the patient is receiving. As such it may be a reaction to unwanted effects—for example, severe toxicity in the case of cytotoxic agents or over-sedation due to psychotropic drugs. The psychic response may be superimposed on the toxic reaction. Although over-sedation is not in itself as distressing as severe toxic reactions, it can have a profound effect on patients' ability to function normally and their sense of purpose in life. Depression may also result from loss of hope when the treatment does not seem to be achieving its aims. The total effect is, of course, always the sum of the drug's pharmacological actions, the nonspecific (placebo) response and such specific psychogenic reactions as those referred to.

Fourthly, the depression may be due to some other drug the patient has been prescribed, has bought over the counter or has taken illegally. Communication between doctors often leaves much to be desired and each of us may be unaware of what the other is prescribing for the patient. Depression may also be due to drug interactions or withdrawal from previous medication. Depression as a benzodiazepine-withdrawal symptom is a common example of the latter and is frequently overlooked.

Finally, the depression may be related to another non-pharmacological treatment the patient has received. It may, for instance, follow a mastectomy (McGuire *et al.*, 1978) or hysterectomy operation (Barker, 1968) or it may emerge during psychotherapy given alongside drug treatment.

Thus, the occurrence of depression during treatment with a drug does not necessarily mean that it is caused by the drug and it should not be attributed to the pharmacological properties of the drug as readily as it has been in the past. Instead, more greater should be made to learn more about patients and what their illness and its treatment means to them—their perception of the disease, their concern over its outcome and their thoughts as to what effects the drug is having on them. A careful check should also be made as to what substances the patient is, and has been, taking in addition to the suspect agent.

METHODS OF REPORTING

There are many methods of reporting adverse drug reactions. Isolated case reports in the literature are important in drawing attention to a possible unwanted effect, but cannot be accepted as proof of a causal connection between drug and reaction. The same holds true, although to a lesser extent, in the case of series of cases and reports to drug regulatory authorities such as the British Committee on the Safety of Medicines (CSM). Frequently occurring reactions can be identified during clinical drug trials, but even here the method of relating effect to drug is often inadequate.

For these reasons, more sophisticated methods have been adopted. Some researchers have made retrospective comparisons of the frequency of exposure to a particular drug in patients who have experienced an unwanted effect with the frequency of exposure to the same drug in a control group of patients who have not experienced the reaction. Others have compared prospectively the occurrence of untoward reactions in those who receive a particular drug with that in a control group. The methods may be applied in hospital-based services, as for example in the Boston Collaborative Drug Surveillance Program (BCDSP; Jick *et al.*, 1970) or in general practices as in 'Prescription Event Monitoring' (Inman *et al.*, 1986). In these methods there is a known denominator which allows for a measure of the frequency of occurrence of the reaction.

The BCDSP has specifically addressed itself to psychiatric reactions, including depression. Danielson *et al.* (1981) investigated such reactions in almost 27 000 intensely monitored in-patients with no history of mental illness in 22 participating hospitals in Boston, Glasgow and Paris. The monitors, mostly nurses, recorded a variety of psychic reactions, including depression which was encountered in 48 patients, giving a prevalence of 1.8 per 1000. The drugs thought to be causally related to at least one case of depression are shown in Table 6.1.

The findings were consistent with previous reports in the literature and this could possibly have influenced the researchers in their judgement of the relationship between reaction and drug. Many of the patients who had drug-related depression were receiving polypharmacy—often combinations of drugs each thought to produce depression. For the group as a whole, there were no important associations between age, sex and type of psychic disturbance, but depression was correlated with cardiovascular disease. Antihypertensive and anxiolytic-sedative agents, which are alleged to cause depression, are frequently used in patients with these illnesses.

DRUGS ALLEGED TO CAUSE DEPRESSION

The evidence for and against depression being caused by the drugs identified in the BCDSP study and others highlighted in the medical literature is as follows.

Table 6.1 Drugs judged to have induced depression [reproduced by kind permission of Springer International (Danielson *et al.*, 1981)]

Drug	Number of cases
Diazepam[a]	3
Diazepam + sedative hypnotics[b]	7
Reserpine[a]	2
Reserpine + other suspect drug(s)	5
Reserpine + steroids	3
Methyldopa[a]	3
Methyldopa + other suspect drug(s)	4
Digoxin[a]	3
Amitriptyline[a]	1
Amitriptyline + other suspect drug(s)	3
Steroids + other suspect drug(s)	4
Phenobarbital + other suspect drug(s)	2
Levodopa[a]	1
Other combinations of two or more drugs	7
Total	**48**

[a] Sole implicated drug.
[b] Flurazepam, nitrazepam, phenobarbital, triclofos.

1. Antihypertensive drugs

Many reports of depression occurring during the course of treatment with the Rauwolfia alkaloids, especially reserpine, appeared during the 1950s (Doyle and Smirk, 1954; Freis, 1954; Wilkins, 1954; Achor *et al.*, 1955; Doyle *et al.*, 1955; Genest *et al.*, 1955; Locket, 1955; Macarthur and Isaacs, 1955; Muller *et al.*, 1955; Schroeder and Perry, 1955; Smirk and McQueen, 1955; Wallace, 1955; Lemieux *et al.*, 1956; Litin *et al.*, 1956; Platt and Sears, 1956; Krogsgaard, 1958; Quetsch *et al.*, 1959; Sturup and Gruener, 1958). The depression was accompanied by a wide variety of other affective symptoms, including psychic and somatic manifestations of anxiety. Descriptions varied from author to author. Many of the symptoms were typical of those seen in depressive illness, while others were atypical. Some patients felt relaxed with a sense of well-being rather than depressed and anxious. The severity of the symptoms varied considerably, with the worst cases requiring admission to hospital and electroconvulsive therapy (ECT). Some patients committed suicide. The depression often developed insidiously after the patient had been on treatment for many months. In some instances it disappeared when the drug was discontinued, but in others it persisted. Many of the investigators noted a positive family and/or past history of depression or a feature in the personality that they thought predisposed the patient to depression.

In the study of Quetsch *et al.* (1959) a comparison was made between patients receiving reserpine and those receiving no specific antihypertensive treatment. Overall, the incidence of depression was higher in the reserpine group, but the proportion of patients who had severe depression was similar in both groups. These findings are of considerable interest, even though the study was retrospective, did not involve random allocation to the two groups and did not specify the factors determining the choice of treatment.

Goodwin and Bunney (1971) reviewed the literature on depression occurring during treatment with reserpine and, after excluding single case reports and studies that did not provide the criteria for the diagnosis of depression or descriptions of the patients' symptoms, analysed data on 286 patients from 16 studies. Nine of these reported the numbers of patients who had depression and the numbers who had received reserpine. From these it was possible to calculate an average incidence of 20 percent but the range was 0–26 percent. On closer analysis of the case material, it appeared that only a quarter of the patients had symptoms compatible with an endogenous-type depression. There was no correlation between the incidence or severity of the depression and the duration and severity of hypertension prior to treatment, the dose of the drug or its antihypertensive effect. The variable that best predicted which patients were most likely to become depressed was a previous history of affective illness and those with such a history developed the more severe depression. Almost a quarter of the patients—about 24 percent of 176 patients in 14 studies—were given ECT (the standard treatment of depression in the 1950s), in most cases after the depression failed to improve when the reserpine was withdrawn. This proportion is consistent with the findings that a quarter of the patients had an endogenous-type depression.

The reviewers concluded that reserpine, alone or in combination with other factors such as stress, precipitates depression in susceptible individuals rather than produces depression de novo. If this is the case, it suggests that theories of the aetiology of depression based on the reserpine-model of depletion of cerebral amines does not have as secure a foundation as is often assumed.

As an alternative to a biochemical explanation, Litin *et al.* (1956) suggested that tranquilization caused by Rauwolfia alkaloids suppresses anger, which leads to a disturbance of relationships and, in turn, depression. Bernstein and Kaufman (1960) suggested that drug-related depression is really a 'pseudo-depression' caused by the way in which the pharmacological effects threaten the patient psychologically. They produce a chemical interference with the patient's defences in which psychomotor activity is used as a means of reassuring himself of his adequacy.

Following the flood of reports of drug-related depression in the 1950s, there was a long period of silence. The reasons for this are unclear. Perhaps it was thought that the reaction was sufficiently well known not to require further reporting or because Rauwolfia drugs were avoided in patients predisposed to depression. It was also suggested that there had been a true decline in the occurrence of reserpine-induced depression (Goodwin and Bunney, 1971). Whatever the case, interest in the relationship between antihypertensive drugs and depression was rekindled following the introduction into clinical practice of methyldopa and other newer drugs.

Bulpitt and Dollery (1973) carried out a self-administered questionnaire study of side effects of these hypotensive agents in 477 patients attending a hypertension clinic. Although their questionnaire had not been evaluated, there was no evidence of an effect of treatment on depression of mood as assessed by the simple question: 'Have you since your last visit been depressed?'. Snaith and McCoubrie (1974) carried out a more sophisticated study using the Wakefield Self-Assessment of Depression Inventory (Snaith *et al.*, 1971) in 264 patients in general practice. They too found no evidence of a relationship between the administration of antihypertensive agents and depressive illness.

The most comprehensive overview of newer antihypertensives was that carried out by Paykel *et al.* (1982). These researchers reviewed the psychiatric side effects of drugs other than reserpine as reported in studies completed by 1977, the date by which most major research on antihypertensives had been carried out. They concluded that over-sedation and sleep disturbance were the commonest unwanted effects, but genuine depression, like toxic confusional states and psychotic reactions, was rare. The incidence of depression in patients receiving methyldopa appeared to be higher than among those receiving the peripheral adrenergic neurone blocking agents, guanethidine, debrisoquine and bethanidine, and also than among those on clonidine, and the β-adrenoceptor blocking drugs, propanolol and oxprenolol—some 3.6 percent in the case of methyldopa compared with 0.3–1.9 percent in the case of the others (see Table 6.2).

Since the appearance of the paper by Paykel and his colleagues, there have been further isolated case reports of depression occurring during treatment with antihypertensives, and two publications focusing on the relationship between propanolol and depression. Griffin and Friedman (1986), recognizing the distinction between true depression and other

Table 6.2 Antihypertensives and depression (after Paykel *et al.*, 1982)

Drug	No. of studies	No. of patients	% with depression
Methyldopa	44	2320	3.6
Clonidine	19	791	1.5
Guanethidine	12	725	1.9
Debrisoquine	9	466	0.4
Bethanidine	4	149	1.3
Propranolol	31	1773	1.1
Oxprenolol	10	367	0.3

symptoms (which they referred to as pseudo-depression), carried out a study in 34 patients receiving propanolol. They used the Hamilton Rating Scale for Depression (Hamilton, 1960). As this is loaded with items measuring somatic symptoms, they also used the Hudson Generalised Contentment Scale (Hudson, 1977), which is loaded with items that rate the type of dysphoria. While accepting that depression cannot be diagnosed by these scales alone, they regarded a high score on the Hamilton scale with a low score on the Hudson scale as being indicative of pseudo-depression and a high score on both scales as being suggestive of a dysphoric state. They found that patients with a past history or family history of depression had significantly higher depression scores than those with a negative history. There was no correlation between the dose of propanolol and the depression scores for the population as a whole, but patients without a previous or family history had a highly significant positive correlation between dosage and depression scores. These findings cannot, however, be accepted as firm evidence that propanolol causes depression, because of the inappropriate use of the rating scales for diagnosing depression, and because of selection bias and the absence of a control group. Also, the population studied was clearly atypical, as the incidence of moderate to severe depression was 47 percent as measured on the Hamilton scale and 50 percent on the Hudson scale.

Avorn *et al.* (1986) reported the prevalence rates of the use of tricyclic antidepressants in a large random sample of 143 250 recipients of Medicaid. They compared the use of tricyclics in patients receiving seven different antihypertensive agents with those on insulin or oral hypoglycaemic drugs. They found that the use of tricyclics in patients taking β-blockers was significantly higher than in those receiving reserpine, hydrallazine, methyldopa and oral hypoglycaemic agents, and they cited this as evidence that propanolol causes depression. This study also can be criticized for a number of reasons. The temporal relationship between the use of propanolol and that of tricyclic antidepressants was not explored and there is therefore the possibility that propanolol was used in many of the patients because other antihypertensives were thought more likely to cause or intensify depression. Patients who became depressed while on other antihypertensive drugs may have been changed to propanolol. It is possible that propanolol was used to treat the somatic symptoms of anxiety, especially tremor and palpitations, that so frequently accompany depression, and it is possible also that propanolol was used to treat tachycardia and/or palpitations caused by tricyclic antidepressants. Antihypertensive drugs with anticholinergic effects, for example methyldopa and clonidine, may have been avoided in patients receiving tricyclics because of concern over summation of these effects, while both propanolol and tricyclics could have been used to treat migraine. The study was based on a single billing claim to Medicaid, and tricyclic antidepressants appear to have been used excessively in the population studied with one patient in four receiving them.

Overall, it appears that antihypertensive agents do not cause depression as often as was previously assumed. Nevertheless, when treating a depressed hypertensive patient or a subject with a past history of affective disorders, it is advisable to 'play it safe' and avoid those drugs that have been thought most liable to depress mood. When depression does occur during treatment, the antihypertensive may need to be changed. Further guidelines for the management of the depressed hypertensive and details concerning relevant drug interactions have been provided by Simpson and Waal-Manning (1971) and Paykel *et al.* (1982).

2. Oral contraceptives

Depression was reported as a possible unwanted effect of oral contraceptives (Kaye, 1963; Wearing, 1963) shortly after they were first used to help control the birth rate in underprivileged women in Puerto Rico (Pincus *et al.*, 1958). Since then there have been numerous reports of depression in individual cases and during uncontrolled or controlled studies of women on the 'pill' (Kane *et al.*, 1967; Nilsson *et al.*, 1967; Moos, 1968; Lewis and Hoghughi, 1969; Herzberg *et al.*, 1970, 1971; Glick and Bennett, 1972; Weissman and Slaby, 1973). In these reports, the depression of mood was accompanied by a variety of other symptoms including anxiety. It was of varying intensity, and in the more severe cases it resulted in women stopping taking the pill and sometimes in suicidal gestures or attempts. In some subjects the depression disappeared on stopping the pill and returned on reintroducing it. Reported incidences have varied widely—from 2.5 to 40 percent.

Problems in relating the depression to the use of the pill arose because similar affective symptoms appear in young women not on oral contraceptives (see Chapter 2) and many subjects who become depressed on the pill have had the same symptoms previously, sometimes as part of the premenstrual syndrome. In fact, women were found to be more liable to depression if they had a past history of affective disorder (Herzberg *et al.*, 1970; Leeton, 1973), although some investigators found that a previous history of depression was not relevant (Kutner and Brown, 1972b). Lewis and Hoghughi (1969) noted that those with a positive previous history developed more severe depression while on the pill than those without such a history. In one study, women who developed depression and irritability as side effects of oral contraceptives had higher neuroticism and extraversion scores than did the pill-taking group as a whole (Hertzberg and Coppen, 1970).

The picture is further complicated by the fact that many women, instead of becoming depressed, have a sense of increased well-being while taking oral contraceptives (Herzberg and Coppen, 1970), while others get relief from the premenstrual syndrome, including its depressive component (Kutner and Brown, 1972a). In keeping with these findings are the results of controlled trials that have failed to show a higher incidence of depression in those taking oral contraceptives than in subjects not on the pill (Goldzieher *et al.*, 1971a,b; Kutner and Brown, 1972a).

There are numerous reasons for the discrepancies in the results of the studies that have been carried out. It is likely that many of the subjects studied were prone to psychiatric symptoms to begin with. They may have been more liable to attend a family planning clinic if already depressed and/or dissatisfied with their current method of contraception—possibly for emotional reasons. It is difficult to allocate subjects randomly to an oral contraceptive or control group, especially if placebo controlled, and equally difficult to conduct a double-blind trial. There are also problems in matching. In most studies, unevaluated instruments or no rating scales at all were used for assessing depression. In view of all these difficulties, it was not surprising that by 1978 34 publications had suggested that depression was an unwanted effect of oral contraceptives while 23 other reports had either failed to confirm this or provided evidence to the contrary (Fleming and Seager, 1978).

During the last decade or so there have been three British publications' worthy of special mention. Fleming and Seager (1978) surveyed 335 women on the contraceptive pill and compared them with a population of 172 women who had previously taken the pill and 179 who had never taken it. The study was carried out in a general practice in a predominantly working class area in South Yorkshire, and depression was rated on a self-administered questionnaire. There was no evidence that women on oral contraceptives were more depressed than those not taking the pill and this applied when the women were matched for age, parity and occupational status.

In keeping with these results are those of Vessey *et al.* (1985) who studied the incidence of serious psychiatric illness, as measured by first referrals to hospital for specialist advice and treatment, in 16 746 women taking part in the Oxford Family Planning contraceptive study. Of these, 9504 were taking oral contraceptives, while the others were using either a diaphragm or an intrauterine device. There were no statistically significant differences between the three groups in the rates per 1000 woman-years of observation for depressive neurosis or affective psychosis.

In the Royal College of General Practitioners oral contraceptive study (Kay, 1984), data were collected by 1400 general practitioners throughout the United Kingdom on 23 000 women on oral contraceptives and 23 000 other women matched for age. At the time the report was published, 19 000 of the total population were still under observation. There were no important differences between these and the women lost to the study. Thirty six percent of those who stopped taking the pill did so because of 'intercurrent morbidity', of which depression was by far the most common diagnosis specified. There was an increased risk of attempted suicide among current pill users, but this was associated with a break-up of relationships rather than the use of the pill. There was not a significantly higher successful suicide rate among those taking oral contraceptives than in the control group. There was a highly significant negative association between depression and the length of time that the women had been on the pill. This reflected 'selection out' at the time of stopping in pill users who became depressed, leaving a residue of users with decreasing susceptibility to depression. This selection out did not occur in relation to attempted suicide and is further evidence that the relationship between depression and attempted suicide is not as clear as supposed.

It was not possible in this general practitioner study to demonstrate a relationship between depression or attempted suicide and the progestogen content of the oral contraceptive, even though such a relationship could not be eliminated with certainty. There was, however, evidence of an effect due to the oestrogen component. By dividing all the brands of oral contraceptives into four oestrogen dose ranges there was a significant trend in relation to depression but not to attempted suicide. There was no correlation between reports of suicide and the duration of use nor the doses of either progestogen or oestrogen. The overall results provided evidence in support of a pharmacogenic depression and were consistent with the clinical impression that depression has ceased to be a common cause of complaint by users of low-dose oestrogen brands (Kay, 1984).

Overall, the balance of evidence suggests that oral contraceptives do not cause depression to the extent that was formerly assumed, although there remains the possibility that the high oestrogen brands used in the past may have produced more affective disturbance than do those in current use. Previous research has suggested a possible mechanism for this. High doses of oestrogens cause deficiency of pyridoxine, which is a coenzyme in many stages of amino-acid metabolism, including decarboxylation and transamination. Pyridoxine deficiency impairs the decarboxylation of 5-hydroxytryptophan to 5-hydroxytryptamine in the brain and elsewhere. The hepatic metabolism of tryptophan is also impaired and this leads to the accumulation of products which inhibit the transport of tryptophan in the brain, further reducing the synthesis of 5-hydroxytryptamine. These changes lead to a corresponding increase in metabolism along the kynurenine–nicotinic acid ribonucleotide pathway (see Fig. 6.1).

These findings are consistent with the cerebral amine theory of depression and they led to the use of pyridoxine in depression occurring in women on the pill (Adams *et al.*, 1973; Drug and Therapeutic Bulletin, 1978; Adams, 1980). The evidence for its effectiveness, however, was not supported by placebo-controlled trials.

3. Neuroleptics

Concern over the long-considered possibility that antipsychotic drugs could cause depression was highlighted when de Alarcon and Carney (1969) reported the occurrence of severe depression in 16 schizophrenic patients treated with fluphenazine enanthate or decanoate, with five of their patients committing suicide. In the same report it was mentioned that

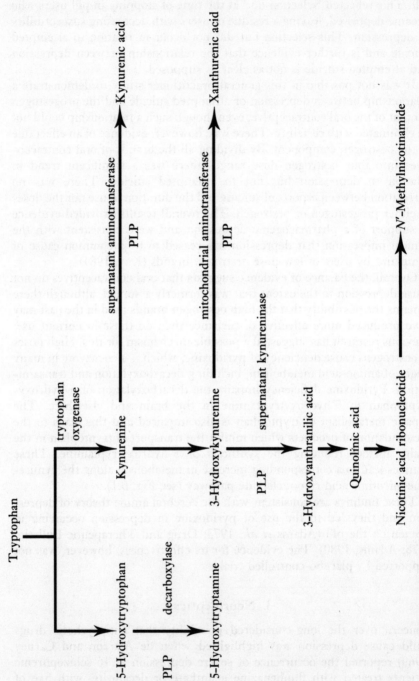

Fig. 6.1 *Major pathways of tryptophan metabolism (PLP = pyridoxal phosphate-dependent enzyme reactions)*

10 (8 percent) of 124 other schizophrenics treated with these drugs developed severe depression. It was suspected that fluphenazine might have been especially prone to cause depression. However, Carney and Sheffield (1975) found that 15 percent of their patients on flupenthixol decanoate also had depression. This was sufficiently severe in some cases for the drug to be withdrawn, and one patient committed suicide. But it is not only depot neuroleptics that have been alleged to cause depression; over the years it has been encountered in patients receiving practically every antipsychotic drug. By 1980, more than 30 publications had drawn attention to the relationship between neuroleptics and depression (Ananth and Ghadirian, 1980), and Galdi *et al.* (1981) presented evidence to suggest that genetically predisposed individuals reacted to neuroleptics with a pharmacogenic depression.

Depression occurring during treatment with neuroleptics is not necessarily due to the drug. Depression was recognized as a symptom of schizophrenia by Kraepelin and Bleuler and it has been referred to in most descriptions of schizophrenia ever since. Post-psychotic depression occurring as a reaction to the illness was described by Meyer-Gross (1920) but depression can occur at any stage of the schizophrenic illness. It may be encountered in untreated first episodes of schizophrenia and in drug-free relapsed chronic schizophrenic patients (Johnson, 1981, 1986). The risk of an episode of depression occurring in a schizophrenic patient was, in fact, found to be more than three times the risk of an acute relapse of the schizophrenia itself and over a 2-year period the duration of morbidity from depression was more than twice that from florid psychotic symptoms (Johnson, 1981).

In a double-blind controlled study, depression was found to occur in the placebo group with a similar frequency to that in the neuroleptic group (Hirsch *et al.*, 1973), while depressive symptoms occurring during acute exacerbations of schizophrenia become less severe during treatment with neuroleptics (Knights and Hirsch, 1981; Möller and von Zerssen, 1981; House *et al.*, 1987; Leff *et al.*, 1988). Such observations lead to the concept of depression being 'revealed' during the course of treatment (Hirsch, 1983). Further evidence against neuroleptics being responsible for depression has been provided by Siris *et al.* (1988), who found no relationship between the severity of depression and either the dose or plasma concentration of fluphenazine decanoate.

Some cases of drug-induced parkinsonism have features similar, if not identical to, severe depressive illness and these respond to anticholinergic agents (Rifkin *et al.*, 1975). Van Putten and May (1978) coined the term 'akinetic depression' to describe this syndrome. The disorder is unlikely to be responsible for a large proportion of cases because depressive symptoms occur in schizophrenic patients receiving antiparkinson agents as often as in those not on these drugs, while anticholinergics are no more effective than placebo in the treatment of depressed schizophrenics (Johnson, 1981).

The risk of suicide in schizophrenic patients is considerably higher than that in the general population (Markowe *et al.*, 1967; Pokorny, 1964;

Evenson *et al.*, 1982; Wilkinson, 1982; Roy, 1986) with 10 percent of patients killing themselves (Miles, 1977). However, no direct causal connection between successful or attempted suicide and treatment with neuroleptics has been demonstrated (Johnson, 1983, 1986; Roy, 1986).

The relationship between neuroleptics and depression is complicated further by the fact that some oral and depot preparations have been found to have a mood-elevating or antidepressant effect in schizophrenia and some have also been found effective in the treatment of depressive illness (Robertson and Trimble, 1982). Other evidence against neuroleptics causing depression is provided by Angst (1987). He carried out a retrospective study of switches from depression to mania and vice versa occurring in patients with manic depressive psychosis between 1920 and 1981. The switches from mania to depression between 1920 and 1970 are shown in Table 6.3, from which it can be seen that there was no significant increase in depression after the introduction of neuroleptics into clinical practice in the 1950s. The length of time from the onset of mania to the switch to depression in the pre-neuroleptic era was 118 days compared with 144 days following the introduction of neuroleptics, a difference that is not statistically significant.

Overall, the evidence suggests that depression is much more likely due to the schizophrenic illness than to antipsychotic medication, although in individual cases distressing extrapyramidal symptoms may well contribute to the patient's low mood.

4. Anxiolytic-sedatives

It is a widely held belief that anxiolytic-sedatives cause depression. The best known and most extensively used antianxiety agent is alcohol and 'boozer's gloom' or 'boozer's remorse' is well known to us all. It is also known that there is a high incidence of suicide among alcoholics, although whether the depression led to the drinking or the alcohol and its attendant problems caused the depression is usually unclear. The use and abuse of barbiturates, and withdrawal from these drugs, have also been cited as causes of depression and suicide.

Benzodiazepines have been similarly incriminated. Depression was noted as a possible side effect during some of the early clinical trials of diazepam (Rao, 1964; McDowell *et al.*, 1966), although some patients who became depressed and suicidal had endogenous psychoses to begin with (Gundlach *et al.*, 1966). Ryan *et al.* (1968) reported seven cases in which

Table 6.3 Switch rates of mania to depression [reproduced by kind permission of Oxford University Press (Angst, 1987)]

	1920–29	1930–49	1950–59	1960–64	1965–70	Total
Sample (*n*)	47	49	55	76	73	300
Switch (percent)	21	22	18	17	25	21

suicidal thoughts and tendencies occurred shortly after starting treatment with diazepam. Two of the patients committed suicide, while two others made serious attempts. Hall and Joffe (1973) reported six further cases of depression occurring during treatment with diazepam. The depression was associated with apprehension, tremulousness, insomnia and suicidal thought.

One question that arises is whether patients who appear to become depressed while taking benzodiazepines were really depressed to begin with. Separate syndromes of an anxiety state and a depressive illness have been demonstrated (Roth *et al.*, 1972; Gurney *et al.*, 1972; Prusoff and Klerman, 1974; Roth and Mountjoy, 1982), but the distinction is not always as clear as we would like to believe (Kendell, 1975) and, if it requires population studies to demonstrate a difference between the two syndromes, it follows that we cannot be sure of the diagnosis in individual cases.

Here too our understanding of the relationship between drug and depression is complicated by the results of trials that have suggested that benzodiazepines have antidepressant properties or at least have a part to play as adjuncts to the treatment of depression (Schatzberg and Cole, 1978; Bellantuono *et al.*, 1980). One of the benzodiazepines, alprazolam, has been said to be as efficaceous as conventional tricyclic antidepressants (Feighner, 1982; Overall *et al.*, 1987; Rickels *et al.*, 1987).

The evidence that has been put forward in support of the belief that benzodiazepines cause depression is largely anecdotal and some of the patients cited in the published case reports had pre-existing physical or major psychiatric illnesses or were on other drugs. There have been no controlled studies showing that benzodiazepines cause depression and we must therefore be sceptical of the claims made. At worst depression occurs as an idiosyncratic reaction in occasional cases (Johnson, 1983).

5. Other drugs

A wide range of other drugs have been reported as causes of depression but, as stated at the outset, it is by no means clear that the authors were referring to depression as understood in psychiatric practice. The depression allegedly caused by these other drugs is often accompanied by psychiatric manifestations of neurotoxicity. Most claims have been based on isolated case reports or 'depression' being noted during a clinical trial— often an uncontrolled trial. Many of the patients who were said to have depression had physical or psychiatric illnesses that could have been responsible. The drugs incriminated include the following.

Antimicrobial agents

Sulphonamides, nalidixic acid, griseofulvin (McClelland, 1973; Whitlock and Evans, 1978) and metronidazole (Voth, 1969; Giannini, 1977), have all been said to cause depression. So has the antituberculous drug, isoniazid

(Goldman and Braman, 1972; Wallach and Gershon, 1972), although this more often causes euphoria. The occurrence of depression during treatment of arthritis with antimalarial drugs (Drew, 1962; Good and Shader, 1977; Schlossberg, 1980) has led to speculation regarding possible links between polyamines and depression (Andrews, 1985).

Corticosteroids

Affective disturbances occurring in Cushing's syndrome have been recognized for many years, with depression being encountered more often than mania (Carpenter *et al.*, 1972). It is not surprising therefore that depression should have been reported during treament with corticosteroids (Borman and Schmallenberg, 1951; Clark *et al.*, 1952, 1953). However, its relationship to the steroids was not confirmed in controlled studies (Lidz *et al.*, 1952; Rees, 1953), although the numbers of patients included in these studies were small. Difficulties also arise in relating the affective disturbance to the corticosteroids, because these drugs are given to patients with serious illnesses, such as leukaemia, lymphoma and systemic lupus erythematosus, that can affect the brain or precipitate depressive reactions.

Cytotoxic drugs

Depression has been noted during treatment with the alkylating agent, dacarbazine, and the vinca alkaloid, vinblastine (Peterson and Popkin, 1980). It is usually unclear if the depression is due to the drug or to the underlying disease, especially when the disease invades the central nervous system. The depression of mood is often part of a more general neurotoxic reaction.

Digoxin

When depression occurs during treatment with digoxin it is usually part and parcel of a more generalized toxic state (Wamboldt *et al.*, 1986; Eisendrath and Sweeney, 1987). It may also be related to the heart disease being treated rather than the drug treatment.

Levodopa

Depression has been reported as an unwanted effect of levodopa by several authors (Barbeau, 1969; Wagshul and Daroff, 1969; Celesia and Barr, 1970; Cherington, 1970; Jenkins and Groh, 1970; McDowell *et al.*, 1970; Cheifetz *et al.*, 1971; Damasio *et al.*, 1971), although not by others. Of the 16 studies reviewed by Goodwin (1971), 10 made no mention of depression or said that it did not occur, while the same number referred to patients who had elation of mood or features compatible with hypomania. This was especially the case when the drug was given in large doses. Subsequent reports have not mentioned depression as a side effect (Hunter *et al.*, 1973; Sweet *et al.*, 1976), and it has been suggested that levodopa might have an antidepressant action in patients with parkinsonism—a suggestion that has not been confirmed in trials of levodopa in depressive illness (Klerman *et al.*, 1963; Goodwin, 1971).

The discrepancies are not surprising when one considers the high prevalence of depression in Parkinson's disease (Mindham, 1970; Celesia and Wanamaker, 1972, Mayeux *et al.*, 1981, 1986). In some cases the depression can be understood as a reaction to the disability, while in others it may result from disappointment at a poor response to treatment. Depression can improve hand in hand with improvement in mobility and increased alertness, providing evidence that, in some cases at least, it is a psychic reaction to the illness rather than a pharmacogenic effect.

Depression may also occur during treament with other antiparkinson agents, for example amantadine (Schwab *et al.*, 1972) but, in this case as with many other drugs, it is part of a more general neuropsychiatric disturbance with confusion, disorientation, anxiety and insomnia.

Nonsteroidal anti-inflammatory analgesics

Depression has been encountered during treatment with phenylbutazone and indomethacin (Thompson and Percy, 1966; Cochrane 1973; Armstrong *et al.*, 1984). It has also been noted during treatment with ibuprofen although no more often than with aspirin (Blechman *et al.*, 1975). As in the case of other drugs, it is difficult to know the extent to which the depression is part of a more general neurotoxic disturbance or whether it is related to the illness being treated, especially as arthritic disorders may be associated with depression.

Stimulants and appetite suppressants

Depression has been observed during treatment with fenfluramine (Gaind, 1969; Imlah, 1970; Steel *et al.*, 1973; Levin, 1975) and while withdrawing from this drug (Oswald *et al.*, 1971; Harding, 1972; Steel and Briggs, 1972). It may occur also during treatment with diethylpropion (Silverstone, 1974) and phentermine (Steel *et al.*, 1973). In some cases at least, depression may be associated with the underlying disorders, including obesity, for which the drugs were prescribed.

Thiazide diuretics

Eight cases of depression in patients receiving thiazide diuretics were described by Okada (1985), but these could possibly have been coincidental and related to the underlying disease or to antihypertensive drugs taken with the diuretics.

Tricyclic antidepressants

Paradoxical though it may sound, depression has been reported as an unwanted effect of tricyclic antidepressants (Oswald *et al.*, 1972; Danielson *et al.*, 1981; Meador-Woodruff and Grunhaus, 1986). This highlights the fact that dysphoria that accompanies other effects on psychomotor function can be mistakenly regarded as a pharmacogenic depression. In some patients at least, the affective disturbance may be due to disillusionment at the slow response to treatment or a psychic reaction to other troublesome side effects.

Miscellaneous drugs

Isolated reports of depression during treatment with many other drugs, including choline (Tamminga *et al.*, 1976), cimetidine (Jefferson, 1979), disulfiram (Liddon and Satran, 1967), and pizotifen (Carrol and Maclay, 1975), have appeared in the literature but the general points made throughout this chapter apply equally to such cases. During the last four years, reports of depression related to metaclopramide (Bottner and Tullio, 1985), flunarazine (Chouza *et al.*, 1986; D'Alessandro *et al.*, 1986; Meyboom *et al.*, 1986), ranitidine (Billings and Stein, 1986), and tizanidine (Nab and Hommes, 1987) have been published; and with 24 cases having been notified to the CSM, there is now suspicion that nifedipine may also be a cause of depression. Many more drugs will undoubtedly be incriminated in the future.

6. Drugs of abuse

Some of the aforementioned drugs, such as anxiolytic-sedatives and psychostimulants, may be abused but special mention should be made of drugs taken illegally. Methadone (Weissman *et al.*, 1976), amphetamines, especially when being withdrawn (Kalant, 1966; Grinspoon and Hedblom, 1979, Grinspoon and Bakalar, 1985) and lysergic acid diethylamide (LSD; Ungerleider *et al.*, 1966) have all been alleged to cause depression. However, in the case of illegal drug abusers, perhaps to a greater extent than with other patients, it is extremely difficult to know the extent to which the depression is related to individual drugs, because most subjects are polydrug abusers. It is equally difficult to know the extent to which personality, social and medical problems account for the affective symptoms.

THE FUTURE

The more critical and authoritative reviews have suggested that the frequency with which drugs cause depression has been exaggerated. A detailed phenomenological assessment shows that drug-related 'depression' is often not depression in the psychiatric sense of the word. A better understanding of the patients affected and of their attitude towards their illness and its treatment, and more sophisticated epidemiological studies often reveal more likely causes of depression than the suspected drug. But this does not mean that we should abandon our search for a pharmacological model of depression.

The history of the pharmacotherapy of depression, from which current theories of its aetiology have been derived, suggests that future discoveries are just as likely to result from chance observations in general medicine or in the laboratory as from ongoing neuropsychiatric research. Classical examples of such observations led to the introduction into psychiatric practice of the phenothiazines, monoamine oxidase inhibitors, tricyclic antidepressants and lithium. Chlorpromazine was synthesized during attempts to create a more sedative analogue of promethazine, which was being investigated as an antihistamine compound, and its tranquillizing properties were noted by chance by the French anaesthetist–surgeon, Laborit (Laborit *et al.*, 1952). This led to trials in psychotic patients by Delay and Deniker (1952). The antidepressant properties of imipramine, which was synthesized by making small structural alterations in the phenothiazine molecule, were found while it was being tested as an antipsychotic drug (Kuhn, 1958). Iproniazid was first used as a treatment for tuberculosis because of its similarity to the antituberculous drug, isoniazid, and it was noted that patients receiving it had an elevation of mood and euphoria. Sedation in guinea pigs receiving lithium urate during the search for an abnormal substance in the urine of manic patients led to the use of lithium in mania (Cade, 1949). The sequence of chance observations continued with the discovery of the butyrophenones from the analgesic, meperidine, and that of the substituted benzamides used in psychiatry from the antiarrhythmic drug, procainamide.

The frequency with which depressive illness occurs in all communities and the great suffering caused to individuals demand that every avenue of research should be explored. If we are to learn from history, this must include the constant search for psychic reactions to new and established drugs and the careful monitoring of drugs to identify any depressive reactions that occur.

REFERENCES

Achor R. W. P., Hanson N. O., Gifford R. W. (1955). Hypertension treated with *Rauwolfia serpentina* (whole root) and with reserpine: controlled study disclosing occasional severe depression. *Journal of the American Medical Association*, 159, 841–5.

Adams P. W. (1980). Pyridoxine, the Pill and depression. *Journal of Pharmacotherapy*, 3, 20–9.

Adams P. W., Wynn V., Rose D. P., *et al.* (1973). Effect of pyridoxine hydrochloride (vitamin B_6) upon depression associated with oral contraception. *Lancet*, 1, 897–904.

Ananth J., Ghadirian A. M. (1980). Drug-induced mood disorders. *International Pharmacopsychiatry*, 15, 59–73.

Andrews R. C. R. (1985). The side effects of antimalarial drugs indicate a polyamine involvement in both schizophrenia and depression. *Medical Hypotheses*, **18**, 11–8.

Angst J. (1987). Switch from depression to mania, or from mania to depression. *Journal of Psychopharmacology*, **1**, 13–9.

Armstrong R. D., Laurent R., Panayi G. S. (1984). A comparison of indoprofen and indomethacin in the treatment of ankylosing spondylitis. *Pharmacotherapeutica*, **3**, 637–41.

Avorn J., Everitt D. E., Weiss S. (1986). Increased antidepressant use in patients prescribed β-blockers. *Journal of the American Medical Association*, **255**, 357–60.

Barbeau A. (1969). L-Dopa therapy in Parkinson's disease: a critical review of nine years' experience. *Canadian Medical Association Journal*, **101**, 791–800.

Barker M. G. (1968). Psychiatric illness after hysterectomy. *British Medical Journal*, **2**, 91–6.

Bellantuono D., Reggi C., Tognoni G., Garattini S. (1980). Benzodiazepines: clinical pharmacology and therapeutic use. *Drugs*, **19**, 195–219.

Bernstein S., Kaufman, M. R. (1960). A psychological analysis of apparent depression following Rauwolfia therapy. *Journal of Mount Sinai Hospital*, **27**, 525–30.

Billings R. F., Stein M. B. (1986). Depression associated with ranitidine. *American Journal of Psychiatry*, **143**, 915–6.

Blechman W. J., Schmid F. R., April P. A., *et al.* (1975). Ibuprofen or aspirin in rheumatoid arthritis therapy. *Journal of the American Medical Association*, **233**, 336–40.

Borman M. C., Schmallenberg H. C. (1951). Suicide following cortisone treatment. *Journal of the American Medical Association*, **146**, 337–8.

Bottner R. K., Tullio C. J. (1985). Metoclopromade and depression. *Annals of Internal medicine*, **103**, 482.

Boyd J. H., Weissman M. M. (1982). Epidemiology. In *Handbook of Affective Disorders* (Paykel E. S., ed.). New York: Churchill Livingstone, pp. 109–25.

Bulpitt C. J., Dollery C. T. (1973). Side effects of hypotensive agents evaluated by a self-administered questionnaire. *British Medical Journal*, **3**, 485–90.

Cade J. F. J. (1949). Lithium salts in the treatment of psychotic excitement. *Medical Journal of Australia*, **2**, 349–52.

Carney M. W. P., Sheffield B. F. (1975). Forty-two months experience of flupenthixol decanoate in the maintenance treatment of schizophrenia. *Current Medical Research and Opinion*, **3**, 447–52.

Carpenter W. T., Strauss J. S., Bunney W. E. (1972). The psychobiology of cortisol metabolism: clinical and theoretical implications. In *Psychiatric Complications of Medical Drugs* (Shader R. I., ed.). New York: Raven Press, pp. 49–72.

Carrol J. D., Maclay W. P. (1975). Pizotifen (BC 105) in migraine prophylaxis. *Current Medical Research and Opinion*, **3**, 68–71.

Celesia G. G., Barr A. N. (1970). Psychosis and other psychiatric manifestations of levodopa therapy. *Archives of Neurology*, **23**, 193–200.

Celesia G. G., Wanamaker W. M. (1972). Psychiatric disturbances in Parkinson's disease. *Diseases of the Nervous System*, **33**, 577–83.

Cheifetz D. I., Garron D. C., Leavitt F., *et al.* (1971). Emotional disturbance accompanying the treatment of parkinsonism with L-dopa. *Clinical Pharmacology and Therapeutics*, **12**, 56–61.

Cherington M. (1970). Parkinsonism, L-Dopa and mental depression. *Journal of the American Geriatrics Society*, **18**, 513–6.

Chouza C., Scaramelli A., Caamano J. L. *et al.* (1986). Parkinsonism, tardive dyskinesia, akathisia and depression induced by flunarizine. *Lancet*, **i**, 1303–4.

Clark L. D., Bauer W., Cobb S. (1952). Preliminary observations on mental disturbances occurring in patients under therapy with cortisone and ACTH therapy. *New England Journal of the Medicine*, **246**, 205–16.

Clark L. D., Quarton G. C., Cobb S., Bauer W. (1953). Further observations on mental disturbances associated with cortisone and ACTH therapy. *New England Journal of Medicine*, **246**, 178–83.

Cochrane G. M. (1973). A double-blind comparison of naproxen with indomethacin in osteoarthritis. *Scandinavian Journal of Rheumatology* (Suppl. 2), 89–93.

D'Alessandro R., Benassi G., Morganti G. (1986). Side-effects of flunarizine *Lancet*, **2**, 463.

Damasio A. R., Lobo-Antunes J., Macedo C. (1971). Psychiatric aspects in Parkinsonism treated with L-dopa. *Journal of Neurology, Neurosurgery and Psychiatry*, **34**, 502–7.

Danielson D. A., Porter J. B., Lawson D. H., *et al.* (1981). Drug-associated psychiatric disturbances in medical inpatients. *Psychopharmacology*, **74**, 105–8.

de Alarcon R., Carney M. W. P. (1969). Severe depressive mood changes following slow-release intramuscular fluphenazine injection. *British Medical Journal*, **2**, 564–7.

Delay J., Deniker P. (1953). Les neuroplegiques en therapeutique psychiatrique. *Thérapie*, **8**, 347–64.

Doyle A. E., McQueen E. G., Smirk F. H. (1955). Treatment of hypertension with reserpine, with reserpine in combination with penta-pyrrolidinium, and with reserpine in combination with varatrum alkaloids. *Circulation*, **11**, 170–81.

Doyle A. E., Smirk F. H. (1954). Hypotensive action of reserpin. *Lancet*, **1**, 1096–97.

Drew J. E. (1962). Concerning the side effects of antimalarial drugs used in the extended treatment of rheumatic disease. *Medical Journal of Australia*, **2**, 618–20.

Drug and Therapeutics Bulletin (1978). Depression and oral contraceptives: the role of pyridoxine. *Drugs and Therapeutics Bulletin*, **16**, 86–7.

Eisendrath S. J., Sweeney M. A. (1987). Toxic neuropsychiatric effects of digoxin in therapeutic serum concentrations. *American Journal of Psychiatry*, **144**, 506–7.

Evenson R. C., Wood J. B., Nuttall E. A., Cho D. W. (1982). Suicide rates among public mental health patients. *Acta Psychiatrica Scandinavica*, **66**, 254–64.

Feighner J. P. (1982). Benzodiazepines as antidepressants. A triazolobenzodiazepine used to treat depression. *Modern Problems of Pharmacopsychiatry*, **18**, 196–212.

Fleming O., Seager C. P. (1978). Incidence of depressive symptoms in users of the oral contraceptive. *British Journal of Psychiatry*, **132**, 431–40.

Freis E. D. (1954). Mental depression in hypertensive patients treated for long periods with large doses of reserpine. *New England Journal of Medicine*, **25**, 1006–8.

Gaind R. (1969). Fenfluramine (Ponderax) in the treatment of obese psychiatric out-patients. *British Journal of Psychiatry*, **115**, 963–4.

Galdi J., Rieder R. O., Silber D., Bonato R. R. (1981). Genetic factors in the response to neuroleptics in schizophrenia: a psychopharmacogenetic study. *Psychological Medicine*, 11, 713–28.

Genest J., Adamkiewicz L., Robillard R., Tremblay G. (1955). Clinical uses of Rauwolfia. *Canadian Medical Association Journal*, 72, 483–9.

Giannini A. J. (1977). Side effects of metronidazole. *American Journal of Psychiatry*, 134, 329–30.

Glick I. D., Bennett S. E. (1972). Side effects of progesterone and oral contraceptives. In *Psychiatric Complications of Medical Drugs* (Shader, R. I., ed.) New York: Raven Press, pp. 295–332.

Goldman A. L. Braman S. S. (1972). Isoniazid: a review with emphasis on adverse effects. *Chest*, 62, 71–7.

Goldzieher J. W., Moses L. E., Averkin E., *et al.* (1971a). A placebo-controlled double-blind crossover investigation of the side effects attributed to oral contraceptives. *Fertility and Sterility*, 22, 609–23.

Goldzieher J. W., Moses L. E., Averkin E., *et al.* (1971b). Nervousness and depression attributed to oral contraceptives: A double-blind placebo-controlled study. *American Journal of Obstetrics and Gynecology*, 111, 1013–20.

Good M. I., Shader R. I. (1977). Behavioral toxicity and equivocal suicide associated with chloroquine and its derivatives. *American Journal of Psychiatry*, 134, 789–801.

Goodwin F. K. (1971). Behavioral effects of L-dopa in man. *Seminars in Psychiatry*, 3, 477–92.

Goodwin F. K., Bunney W. E. (1971). Depressions following reserpine: a re-evaluation. *Seminars in Psychiatry*, 3, 435–48.

Griffin S. J., Friedman M. J. (1986). Depressive symptoms in propanolol users. *Journal of Clinical Psychiatry*, 47, 453–7.

Grinspoon L., Bakalar J. B. (1985). Drug dependence: non narcotic agents. In *Comprehensive Textbook of Psychiatry/IV* vol. 1, 4th edn. (Kaplan H. I., Sadock B. J., eds.). Baltimore: Williams and Wilkins, pp. 1003–15.

Grinspoon L., Hedblom P. (1975). *The Speed Culture: Amphetamine Use and Abuse in America*. Cambridge: Harvard University.

Gundlach R., Engelhardt D. M., Hankoff L., *et al.* (1966). A double-blind outpatient study of diazepam (Valium) and placebo. *Psychopharmacologia*, 9, 81–92.

Gurney C., Roth M., Garside R. F., *et al.* (1972). Studies in the classification of affective disorders. The relationship between anxiety and depressive illness–II. *British Journal of Psychiatry*, 121, 162–6.

Hall R. C. W., Joffe J. R. (1972). Aberrant response to diazepam: a new syndrome. *American Journal of Psychiatry*, 129, 738–42.

Hamilton M. (1960). A rating scale for depression. *Journal of Neurology, Neurosurgery and Psychiatry*, 23, 56–62.

Harding T. (1972). Depression following fenfluramine withdrawal. *British Journal of Psychiatry*, 121, 338–9.

Hertzberg B., Coppen A. (1970). Changes in psychological symptoms in women taking oral contraceptives. *British Journal of Psychiatry*, 116, 161–4.

Hertzberg B. N., Draper K. C., Johnson A. L., Nicol G. C. (1971). Oral contraceptives, depression, and libido. *British Medical Journal*, 2, 495–500.

Herzberg B. N., Johnson A. L., Brown S. (1970). Depressive symptoms and oral contraceptives *British Medical Journal*, 2, 142–5.

Hirsch S. R. (1983). The causality of depression in schizophrenia. *British Journal of Psychiatry*, **142**, 624–5.

Hirsch S. R., Gaind R., Rohde P. D., *et al.* (1973). Outpatient maintenance of chronic schizophrenic patients with long-acting fluphenazine: double-blind placebo trial. Report to the Medical Research Council on clinical trials in psychiatry. *British Medical Journal*, **1**, 633–7.

House A., Bostock J., Cooper J. (1987). Depressive syndromes in the year following onset of a first schizophrenic illness. *British Journal of Psychiatry*, **151**, 773–9.

Hudson W. W., Proctor E. K. (1977). Assessment of depressive affect in clinical practice. *Journal of Consulting and Clinical Psychology*, **45**, 1206–7.

Hunter K. R., Laurence D. R., Shaw K. M., Stern G. M. (1973). Sustained levodopa therapy in parkinsonism. *Lancet* , **2**, 929–31.

Imlah N. W. (1970). Unusual effect of fenfluramine. *British Medical Journal*, **1**, 178–9.

Inman W. H. W., Rawson N. S. B., Wilton L. V. (1986). Prescription-event monitoring. In *Monitoring for Drug Safety* (Inman H. W., Gill E. P., eds.). Lancaster: M T P Press Ltd, pp. 213–35.

Jefferson J. W. (1979). Central nervous system toxicity of cimetidine: a case of depression. *American Journal of Psychiatry*, **136**, 346.

Jenkins R. B., Groh R. H. (1970). Mental symptoms in parkinsonian patients treated with L-dopa. *Lancet*, **2**, 177–80.

Jick H., Mietinen O. S., Shapiro S., *et al.* (1970). Comprehensive drug surveillance. *Journal of the American Medical Association*, **213**, 1455–60.

Johnson D. A. W. (1981). Studies of depressive symptoms in schizophrenia. I. The prevalence of depression and its possible causes; II. A two-year longitudinal study of symptoms; III. A double-blind trial of orphenadrine against placebo; IV. A double-blind trial of nortriptyline for depression in chronic schizophrenia. *British Journal of Psychiatry*, **139**, 89–101.

Johnson D. A. W. (1983). Benzodiazepines in depression. In *Benzodiazepines Divided. A Multidisciplinary Review* (Trimble M. R., ed.). Chichester: John Wiley and Sons, pp. 247–57.

Johnson D. A. W. (1986). Depressive symptoms in schizophrenia: some observations on the frequency, morbidity and possible causes. In *Contemporary Issues in Schizophrenia* (Kerr A., Snaith P., eds.). London: Gaskell, pp. 451–8.

Kalant O.J. (1966). *The Amphetamines, Toxicity and Addiction.* Toronto: University of Toronto Press.

Kane F. J., Daly R. J., Ewing J. A., Keeler M. H. (1967). Mood and behavioural changes with progestational agents. *British Journal of Psychiatry*, **113**, 265–8.

Kay C. R. (1984). The Royal College of General Practitioners' oral contraception study: some recent observations. *Clinics in Obstetrics and Gynaecology*, **11**, 759–86.

Kaye B. M. (1963). Oral contraceptives and depression. *Journal of the American Medical Association*, **186**, 522.

Kendell R. E. (1975). *Role of Diagnosis in Psychiatry.* Oxford: Blackwell, pp. 67–8.

Klerman G. L., Schildkraut J. J., Hasenbush L. L., *et al.* (1963). Clinical experience with dihydroxyphenylanine (DOPA). *Journal of Psychiatric Research*, **1**, 289–97.

Knights A., Hirsch S. R. (1981). Revealed depression and drug treatment for schizophrenia. *Archives of General Psychiatry*, **38**, 806–11.

Krogsgaard A. R. (1958). Side-effects of reserpine in the treatment of essential hypertension with special reference to weight gain and mental depression. *Acta Medica Scandinavica*, **162**, 465–74.

Kuhn R. (1958). The treatment of depressive states with G22355 (imipramine hydrochloride). *American Journal of Psychiatry*, **115**, 459–64.

Kutner S. J., Brown W. L. (1972a). History of depression as a risk factor for depression with oral contraceptives and discontinuance. *Journal of Nervous and Mental Disease*, **155**, 163–9.

Kutner S. J., Brown W. L. (1972b). Types of oral contraceptives, depression, and premenstrual symptoms. *Journal of Nervous and Mental Diseases*, **155**, 153–62.

Laborit H., Hugenenard P., Alluaume R. (1952). Un nouveau stabilisateur vegetatif, le 4560 RP. *Presse Medicale*, **60**, 206–8.

Leeton J. (1973). The relationship of oral contraception to depressive symptoms. *Australian and New Zealand Journal of Obstetrics and Gynaecology*, **13**, 115–20.

Leff J., Tress K., Edwards B. (1988). The clinical course of depressive symptoms in schizophrenia. *Schizophrenia Research*, **1**, 25–30.

Lemieux G., Davignon A., Genest J. (1956). Depressive states during Rauwolfia therapy for arterial hypertension. A report of 30 cases. *Canadian Medical Association Journal*, **74**, 522–6.

Levin A. (1975). The non-medical misuse of fenfluramine by drug-dependent young South Africans. *Postgraduate Medical Journal*, **51** (Suppl. 1), 186–8.

Lewis A., Hoghughi M. (1969). An evaluation of depression as a side effect of oral contraceptives. *British Journal of Psychiatry*, **115**, 697–701.

Liddon S. C., Satran R. (1967). Disulfiram (Antabuse) psychosis. *American Journal of Psychiatry*, **123**, 1284–9.

Lidz T., Carter J. D., Lewis B. I., Surratt C. (1952). Effects of ACTH and cortisone on mood and mentation. *Psychosomatic Medicine*, **14**, 363–77.

Litin E. M., Faucett R. L., Ankor R. W. P. (1956). Depression in hypertensive patients treated with *Rauwolfia serpentina*. *Proceedings of the Staff Meeting of the Mayo Clinic*, **31**, 233–7.

Locket S. (1955). Oral preparations of *Rauwolfia serpentina* in treatment of essential hypertension. *British Medical Journal*, **1**, 809–13.

McClelland H. A. (1973). Psychiatric complications with drug therapy. *Adverse Drug Reactions Bulletin*, **40**, 128–31.

McDowall A., Owen S., Robin A. A. (1966). A controlled comparison of diazepam and amylobarbitone in anxiety states. *British Journal of Psychiatry*, **112**, 629–31.

McDowell F., Lee J. E., Swift T., *et al.* (1970). Treatment of Parkinson's syndrome with L dihydroxyphenylalanine (levodopa). *Annals of Internal Medicine*, **72**, 29–35.

MacArthur J. G., Isaacs B. (1955). Mental effects of reserpine. *Lancet*, **2**, 347.

Maguire G. P., Lee E. G., Bevington D. J., *et al.* (1978). Psychiatric problems in the first year after mastectomy. *British Medical Journal*, **1**, 963–5.

Markowe M., Steinert J., Heyworth-Davis F. (1967). Insulin and chlorpromazine in schizophrenia: a ten year comparative survey. *British Journal of Psychiatry*, **113**, 1101–6.

Mayeux R., Stern Y., Rosen J., Leventhal J. (1981). Depression, intellectual impairment, and Parkinson's disease. *Neurology*, **31**, 645–50.

Mayeux R., Stern Y., Williams J. B. W., *et al.* (1986). Clinical and biochemical features of depression in Parkinson's disease. *American Journal of Psychiatry*, **143**, 756–9.

Meador-Woodruff J. H., Grunhaus L. (1986). Profound behavioral toxicity due to tricyclic antidepressants. *Journal of Nervous and Mental Disease*, **174**, 628–30.

Meyboom R. H. B., Ferrari M. D., Dieleman B. P. (1986). Parkinsonism, tardive dyskinesia, akathisia, and depression induced by flunarizine. *Lancet*, **2**, 292.

Meyer-Gross W. (1920). Über die Stellungsnahme auf abgelaufenen akuten Psychose. *Zeitschrift für die Gesamte Neurologie und Psychiatrie*, **60**, 160–212.

Miles C. P. (1977). Conditions predisposing to suicide: a review. *Journal of Nervous and Mental Disease*, **164**, 231–46.

Mindham R. H. S. (1970). Psychiatric symptoms in Parkinsonism. *Journal of Neurology, Neurosurgery and Psychiatry*, **33**, 188–91.

Möller H. J., von Zerssen D. (1981). Depressive Symptomatik in stationären Behandlungsverlauf von 280 schizophrenen Patienten. *Pharmacopsychiatria*, **14**, 172–9.

Moos R. H. (1968). Psychological aspects of oral contraceptives. *Archives of General Psychiatry*, **19**, 87–94.

Muller J. C., Pryor W. W., Gibbons J. E., Orgain E. S. (1955). Depression and anxiety occurring during Rauwolfia therapy. *Journal of the American Medical Association*, **159**, 836–8.

Nab H. W., Hommes O. R. (1987). Depression associated with tizanidine. *British Medical Journal*, **295**, 612.

Nilsson A., Almgren P-E. (1968). Psychiatric symptoms during the post-partum period as related to use of oral contraceptives. *British Medical Journal*, **1**, 453–5.

Nilsson A., Jacobson L., Ingemanson C-A. (1967). Side-effects of an oral contraceptive with particular attention to mental symptoms and sexual adaptation. *Acta Obstetrica et Gynecologica Scandinavica*, **46**, 537–56.

Okada F. (1985). Depression after treatment with thiazide diuretics for hypertension. *American Journal of Psychiatry*, **142**, 1101–2.

Oswald I., Brezenova V., Dunleavy D. L. F. (1972). On the slowness of action of tricyclic antidepressant drugs. *British Journal of Psychiatry*, **120**, 673–7.

Oswald I., Lewis S. A., Dunleavy D. L. F., *et al.* (1971). Drugs of dependence though not of abuse: fenfluramine and imipramine. *British Medical Journal*, **3**, 70–3.

Overall J. E., Biggs J., Jacobs M., Holden K. (1987). Comparison of alprazolam and imipramine for treatment of outpatient depression. *Journal of Clinical Psychiatry*, **48**, 15–9.

Paykel E. S., Fleminger R., Watson J. P. (1982). Psychiatric side effects of antihypertensive drugs other than reserpine. *Journal of Clinical Psychopharmacology*, **2**, 14–39.

Peterson L. G., Popkin M. K. (1980). Neuropsychiatric effects of chemotherapeutic agents for cancer. *Psychosomatics*, **21**, 141–53.

Pincus G., Rock J., Garcia C-R., *et al.* (1958). Fertility control with oral medication. *American Journal of Obstetrics and Gynecology*, **75**, 1333–46.

Platt R., Sears H. T. N. (1956). Reserpine in severe hypertension. *Lancet*, **1**, 401–3.

Pokorny A. (1964). Suicide rates in various psychiatric disorders. *Journal of Nervous and Mental Diseases*, **139**, 499–506.

Prussoff B., Klerman G. L. (1974). Differentiating depressed from anxious neurotic outpatients. *Archives of General Psychiatry*, **30**, 302–9.

Quetsch R. M., Achor R. W. P., Litin E. M. Faucett R. L. (1959). Depressive reactions in hypertensive patients. A comparison of those treated with Rauwolfia and those receiving no specific antihypertensive treatment. *Circulation*, **19**, 366–75.

Rao A. V. (1964). A controlled trial with 'Valium' in obsessive compulsive state. *Journal of the Indian Medical Association*, **42**, 564–7.

Rees L. (1953). Psychological concomitants of cortisone and ACTH therapy. *Journal of Mental Science*, **99**, 497–504.

Rickels K., Chung H. R., Csanalosi I. B., *et al.* (1987). Alprazolam, diazepam, imipramine, and placebo in outpatients with major depression. *Archives of General Psychiatry*, **44**, 862–6.

Rifkin A., Quitkin F., Klein D. F. (1975). Akinesia. A poorly recognised drug-induced extrapyramidal behavioral disorder. *Archives of General Psychiatry*, **32**, 672–4.

Robertson M. M., Trimble M. R. (1982). Major tranquillisers used as antidepressants. *Journal of Affective Disorders*, **4**, 173–93.

Roth M., Mountjoy C. Q. (1982). The distinction between anxiety states and depressive disorders. In *Handbook of Affective Disorders* (Paykel E. S., ed.). Edinburgh: Churchill Livingstone, pp. 70–92.

Roth M., Gurney C., Garside R. F., Kerr T. A. (1972). Studies in the classification of affective disorders. The relationship between anxiety and depressive illness—I. *British Journal of Psychiatry*, **121**, 147–61.

Roy A. (1986). Suicide in schizophrenia. In *Suicide* (Roy A., ed.). Baltimore: Williams and Wilkins, pp. 97–112.

Ryan H. F., Merrill B., Scott G. E., *et al.* (1968). Increase in suicidal thoughts and tendencies. Association with diazepam therapy. *Journal of the American Medical Association*, **203**, 135–7.

Schatzberg A. F., Cole J. O. (1978). Benzodiazepines in depressive disorders. *Archives of General Psychiatry*, **35**, 1359–65.

Schlossberg D. (1980). Reaction to primaquine. *Annals of Internal Medicine*, **92**, 435.

Schroeder H. A., Perry H. M. (1955). Psychosis apparently produced by reserpine. *Journal of the American Medical Association*, **159**, 839–40.

Schwab R. S., Poskanzer D. C., England A. C., Young R. R. (1972). Amantadine in Parkinson's disease. Review of more than two years' experience. *Journal of the American Medical Association*, **222**, 792–5.

Silverstone T. (1974). Intermittent treatment with anorectic drugs. *Practitioner*, **213**, 245–52.

Simpson F. O., Waal-Manning H. (1971). Hypertension and depression: interrelated problems in therapy. *Journal of the Royal College of Physicians,*, **6**, 14–24.

Siris S. G., Strahan A., Mandeli J., *et al.* (1988). Fluphenazine decanoate dose and severity of depression in patients with post-psychotic depression. *Schizophrenia Research*, **1**, 31–5.

Smirk F. H., McQueen E. G. (1955). Comparison of rescinnamine and reserpine as hypotensive agents. *Lancet*, **2**, 115–6.

Snaith R. P., Ahmed S. N., Mehta S., Hamilton M. (1971). The assessment of the severity of primary depressive illness. *Psychological Medicine*, **1**, 143–9.

Snaith R. P., McCoubrie M. (1974). Antihypertensive drugs and depression. *Psychological Medicine*, **4**, 393–8.

Spitzer R. L., Endicott J. (1978). *Schedule for Affective Disorders and Schizophrenia*. New York: Biometrics Research, Evaluation Section, New York State Psychiatric Institute.

Spitzer R. L., Endicott J., Robins E. (1978a). *Research Diagnostic Criteria*. New York: Biometrics Research, Evaluation Section, New York State Psychiatric Institute.

Spitzer R. L., Endicott J., Robins E. (1978b). Research diagnostic criteria: rationale and reliability. *Archives of General Psychiatry*, **35**, 773–82.

Steel J. M., and Briggs M. (1972). Withdrawal depression in obese patients after fenfluramine treatment. *British Medical Journal*, **2**, 26–7.

Steel J. M., Munro J. F. Duncan L. J. P. (1973). A comparative trial of different regimens of fenfluramine and phentermine in obesity. *Practitioner*, **211**, 232–6.

Sturup H., Gruener A. (1958). Long-term combined drug therapy in non-malignant hypertension. *Acta Medica Scandinavica*, **160**, 251–60.

Sweet R. D., McDowell F. H., Feigenson J. S., *et al.* (1976). Mental symptoms in Parkinson's disease during chronic treatment with levodopa. *Neurology*, **26**, 305–10.

Tamminga C., Smith R. C., Chang S., *et al.* (1976). Depression associated with oral choline. *Lancet*, **2**, 905.

Thompson M., Percy J. S. (1966). Further experience with indomethacin in the treatment of rheumatic disorders. *British Medical Journal*, **1**, 80–3.

Ungerleider J. T., Fisher D. D., Fuller M. (1966). The dangers of LSD. Analysis of seven months' experience in a university hospital's psychiatric service. *Journal of the American Medical Association*, **197**, 389–92.

van Putten T., May P. R. A. (1978). 'Akinetic depression' in schizophrenia. *Archives of General Psychiatry*, **35**, 1101–7.

Vessey M. P., McPherson K., Lawless M., Yeates D. (1985). Oral contraceptives and serious psychiatric illness: absence of an association. *British Journal of Psychiatry*, **146**, 45–9.

Voth A. J. (1969). Possible association between metronidazole and agitated depression. *Canadian Medical Association Journal*, **100**, 1012–3.

Wagshul A. M., Daroff R. B. (1969). Depression during L-Dopa treatment. *Lancet*, **2**, 592.

Wallace D. C. (1955). Treatment of hypertension. Hypotensive drugs and mental changes. *Lancet*, **2**, 116–7.

Wallach M. B., Gershon S. (1972). Psychiatric sequelae to tuberculous therapy. In *Psychiatric Complications of Medical Drugs* (Shader R. I., ed.). New York: Raven Press, pp. 201–12.

Wamboldt F. S., Jefferson J. W., Wamboldt M. Z. (1986). Digitalis intoxication misdiagnosed as depression by primary care physicians. *American Journal of Psychiatry*, **143**, 219–21.

Wearing M. P. (1963). The use of norethindrone (2 mg) with mestranol (0.1 mg) in fertility control. *Canadian Medical Association Journal*, **89**, 239–41.

Weissman M. M., Slaby A. E. (1973). Oral contraceptives and psychiatric disturbance: evidence from research. *British Journal of Psychiatry*, **123**, 513–8.

Weissman M. M., Slobetz F., Prusoff B., *et al.* (1976). Clinical depression among narcotic addicts maintained on methadone in the community. *American Journal of Psychiatry*, **133**, 1434–8.

Whitlock F. A., Evans L. E. J. (1978). Drugs and depression. *Drugs*, **15**, 53–71.

Wilkins R. W. (1954). Clinical usage of Rauwolfia alkaloids, including resperine (Serpasil). *Annals of the New York Academy of Science*, **59**, 36–44.

Wilkinson G. (1982). The suicide rate in schizophrenia *British Journal of Psychiatry*, **140**, 138–41.

Wing J. K., Cooper J. E., Sartorius N. (1974). *Measurement and Classification of Psychiatric Symptoms: An Instructional Manual for the PSE and CATEGO Program*. New York: Cambridge University Press.

SECTION 3.

The Life Cycle and Depression

7 *Depression in adolescence*

WILLIAM Ll. PARRY-JONES

INTRODUCTION

During the last decade, there has been a rapid expansion of clinical and research interest in childhood depression, but the adolescent aspects have received less attention. In general, adolescent health care is a relatively neglected subject, in terms of both awareness of special health needs and service delivery. During medical training, there is only likely to be minimal supervised experience of working with psychiatrically disturbed adolescents. General practitioners often report difficulties in interviewing and establishing rapport with young people and their apprehensions about missed cases of depression. Their task is complicated by a variety of commonly held ideas about adolescent disorders, especially that they are difficult to diagnose precisely because they are atypical forms of adult presentations. It is the case that the clinical presentation of depression in adolescents is often complex and, at first sight, is not clearly part of a familiar 'adult' nosological entity. However, several characteristic patterns of depression in teenagers can be distinguished. At the same time, the similarities and continuities with disorders of both childhood and adulthood should not be overlooked. Psychiatric disorders in adolescents include those present since childhood and those arising for the first time in adolescence. The latter comprise both specific psychiatric syndromes, with increasing resemblance to adult forms, and a variety of reactions to developmental and situational stresses. Although the maturational stresses themselves are unique to this age group and the stage of personality development is different, the kinds of reactions that occur when adults face life crises are essentially the same.

Depression is a normal human emotion—teenagers, like people of all ages, experience depressive feelings and show, in their behaviour, signs of sadness, gloom, despondency and unhappiness, especially after losses, disappointments and frustrations that are felt to be personally important. The stage at which depression becomes abnormal remains a controversial question and the decision must be arbitrary, with criteria concerned with the duration, severity and quality of the symptoms and their dysfunctional effects. Although depressive behaviour may be displayed from early childhood, the capacity to express and articulate feelings of lowered mood does not develop before cognitive maturity begins to emerge in adolescence

(Graham, 1986). Subsequently, although distress may be acknowledged, adolescents are often unwilling to talk spontaneously about their deeper and softer feelings and, instead of lowered mood, they may describe more indirectly a sense of emptiness or absence of feelings. This can make the presence of depressed mood difficult to recognize and, in the late 1960s, the emphasis on the concomitant behavioural abnormalities of states of inconspicuous depression generated the concepts of 'masked' depression and of the expression of depression through a variety of 'depressive equivalents' (Glaser, 1967). Since then, several studies have cast doubt on the clinical validity of these concepts (Kovacs and Beck, 1977; Pearce, 1978).

In recent years, research on childhood depression has expanded considerably, particularly in the USA, and Rutter *et al.* (1986) have provided a comprehensive review of current thinking. The view that adult criteria can be used in the identification of depressive disorder in children and adolescents (Puig-Antich *et al.*, 1978) has been strengthened. A number of systematic interview schedules have been developed (Kazdin and Petti, 1982; Birleson *et al.*, 1987; Kazdin, 1987) and significant progress has been made in establishing more widely accepted criteria for the diagnosis of affective disorders in children and adolescents. Several studies have confirmed the similarity of manifestations of depression during adolescence and adulthood (Strober *et al.*, 1981; Friedman *et al.*, 1983), although it is clear that puberty has significant modifying effects on psychological markers of depressive illness (Puig-Antich, 1986). Nevertheless, there continues to be controversy about the stage at which children begin to experience depressive symptoms of a type found in adults (Shaffer, 1985). The delay is due to supposed emotional, cognitive and neurochemical immaturity, but such a general explanation is unsatisfactory and this constitutes an important field for continuing research.

In this chapter, the general view is taken that depression can occur at any age and is manifested by different symptom patterns from early childhood, through adolescence into adulthood. Reliance on adult-type presentations as the frame of reference for depression in other age groups is to be discouraged, and the clinician's primary task is the recognition of depression at all stages.

PREVALENCE

There is a major lack of empirical data on the prevalence of depressive disorders in adolescents in non-clinic populations, although there is more information about the frequency of depressive symptoms (Kaplan *et al.*, 1984; Kandel and Davies, 1982). Research is complicated by problems of imprecise terminology in definitions and classification. In a study of a community sample of adolescents, Kashani *et al.* (1987) reported a prevalence of 4.7 percent for major depression and 3.3 percent for dysthymic disorder, using DSM-III criteria (Diagnostic and Statistical Manual; American Psychiatric Association, 1980). These rates are significantly higher than those for pre-adolescents (Kashani and Carlson, 1987). The Isle of Wight study revealed a 1-year prevalence of affective disorder of 1.4 per 1000 in 10–11 year olds and a threefold increase in the rate for depression from pre-adolescence to adolescence (Rutter *et al.*, 1976). This study also demonstrated a sharp rise in depressive feelings during the pubescent period. In younger children, the sex ratio for depression is roughly equal, but during the adolescent years the ratio changes progressively so that girls outnumber boys by up to 4:1. Amongst psychiatric populations, some investigators have suggested that depression is rare, whilst others have found that about 25 percent of adolescent psychiatric patients suffer from clinical depression (Robbins *et al.*, 1982).

CHARACTERISTIC PATTERNS OF ADOLESCENT DEPRESSION

Depressive symptoms can occur in many psychiatric syndromes in adolescents, such as anorexia nervosa and schizophrenia, and also in physical illnesses like glandular fever and influenza. In this section, however, attention is confined to disorders in which low mood, of varying severity, is the central feature. The classification of these disorders in adolescence is particularly challenging because, in this age span, typical child and adult presentations can occur or be admixed. Depression in adolescents tends to be influenced by environment more readily than in adults and lowering of mood is less fixed, in keeping with the typically rapid fluctuation of adolescent moods.

Single approaches to classification based on aetiology, symptoms or course are not wholly satisfactory. The most widely used classification is based on the distinction, used in the International Classification of Diseases (ICD-9; World Health Organization, 1978) between 'understandable', situationally determined, depressive disorders and those that are not explicable in terms of the current life situation. In the clinical setting, however, this traditional reactive–endogenous distinction is of limited value because symptom intensity is not necessarily related to exposure to stressful life events. The application to adolescents of diagnostic criteria and classifications that have proved useful with adults is still experimental. For example, Robbins *et al.* (1982) have shown that the use of the Research Diagnostic Criteria (RDC) (Spitzer *et al.*, 1978) is feasible. For everyday clinical purposes, however, especially for general practitioners, the recognition of commonly occurring patterns of disorder is as important as precise classification. Whilst there is much in common between adolescent and adult presentations, there are a number of distinctive features and characteristic patterns of presentation which inform and influence clinical practice with patients of this age.

Depression related to maturational stress

Adolescence is a time of rapid physiological and psychological change, of intensive readjustment to the family, school, work and social life and of preparation for adult roles. The period demands the completion of a number of maturational tasks and their sequential nature makes a useful frame of reference in the clinical assessment and treatment of adolescents. The tasks of coping with the physical changes of puberty, of separating from the family and becoming independent, of developing intimate relationships with others, especially persons of the opposite sex, and of discovering one's capacities or talents for work may all lead adolescents into an unhappy, sad, demoralized state of mind, as the unknown is faced. There is a relinquishment of childhood gratifications and attachments— inevitable losses which have to be mourned. Similarly, the ending of the school years and leaving home, especially when not fully prepared for it, can be disturbing. The sudden realization of the overwhelming problems facing humanity can be another factor which increases the burden on the adolescent, especially when it becomes clear that adults are equally helpless.

For most adolescents, such maturational tasks are achieved comfortably, involving essentially healthy and appropriate periods of lowered mood which, characteristically, are transient and do not interfere with everyday functioning. A small number of adolescents, however, experience a persistent mood of sadness, hopelessness and apathy which interferes with performance and can lead to considerable personal suffering (Albert and Beck, 1975; Rutter *et al.*, 1976). Such adolescents may complain directly of depression or, more commonly, of a lack of feelings and a sense of emptiness. Although these depressive states are usually mild, there may be expressions of worthlessness and self-denigration, and the sense of loneliness and hopelessness about things ever changing for the better may reach the point when suicidal ideas arise. Fears of failure are likely to be prominent—concerned with, for example, never being able to become an effective, worthwhile adult and of never being able to make a sexual relationship. In many instances, there is likely to have been a history of behavioural problems, difficulties in school, episodes of anxiety, difficulties with peers and tenuous family relationships.

Depression related to external causes

The concept of depression related to normal developmental processes and the specific strains of adolescence can be widened to include the provoking effects of environmental stresses and life events. Usually, these involve loss events like bereavement, or other personal setbacks, misfortunes and disappointments, such as the breaking up of a close relationship or an academic failure, resulting in the loss of an important hope or ambition. Problems in the adolescent's social life at home, in school or in the peer group may be the precipitants. The intensity of depression depends on the size of the loss and the individual's susceptibility to the implications of reversal. This type of disorder, which is also called neurotic depression, often arises in individuals who have previously shown evidence of vulnerability, anxiety, phobias, obsessional or hysterical symptoms.

It is possible to recognize tentatively during adolescence, or even before, those features of personality make-up which apparently predispose to the development of depression. In the cognitive theories of depression, developed by Beck (1972), emphasis is placed on the part played by pessimistic thoughts or depressive cognitions. Clinical experience indicates that these can begin to emerge in late childhood. They include negative thoughts about oneself, sets of expectations that result in negative conclusions and distorted thinking that leads to negative ends. The suggested theory is that children and adolescents who habitually adopt these ways of thinking and have low self-esteem are more likely to become depressed when faced with reversals. A rebuff or some derogatory comment is much more likely to lead to depression in a teenager who needs to be 'on top' all the time and liked by everyone. At present, the processes that interact with cognitive development to produce low self-esteem and negative self-evaluation are ill understood (Cicchetti and Schneider-Rosen, 1986) and the significance of these apparent vulnerability factors is uncertain.

Masked depression

In some young people, lowered mood may not be conspicuous or described spontaneously, although the suspicion that the person is depressed is borne out, on detailed inquiry of the adolescent and the parents, by the presence of characteristic depressive symptomatology. Under these circumstances, the term 'masked depression' has been used (Glaser, 1967; Carlson and Cantwell, 1980). Whilst it is accepted that masked depression does not constitute a separate diagnostic entity, retention of the term in adolescent practice draws attention usefully to the fact that depression, whatever the aetiology, can easily go unrecognized. In adolescents, the presenting features that may conceal depression take a variety of forms including, for example, restless boredom and a persistent search for new activities, complaints of fatigue, bodily preoccupations and somatic symptoms like headache, and other aches and pains. Alternatively, there may be uncharacteristic antisocial or delinquent behaviour, risk-taking, such as reckless driving, promiscuity and solvent or drug abuse. Kashani *et al.* (1985) confirmed an association between depression and substance abuse. Several studies have shown that depression and conduct disorder may occur concomitantly (Marriage *et al.*, 1986) and Shaffer (1974) found that antisocial behaviour preceded a high proportion of child suicides.

Affective psychosis

Affective psychoses are rare before puberty but gradually increase in their incidence during mid and late adolescence to reach adult levels (Gammon *et al.*, 1983). The developmental processes that may account for this are ill understood (Rutter, 1986). The clinical features are essentially the same as those occurring in adulthood. They include single or recurrent episodes of moderate or severe depression and depression alternating with episodes of mania or hypomania. Characteristically, these features arise in adolescents who have not been exposed to any obvious external stresses in their current life situation. Although the underlying cause is not understood, the disorder is usually construed in biological terms with a strong genetic element. As in its adult counterpart, the depressive illness has prominent physical or biological features, such as sleep disturbance, loss of appetite and weight, lack of energy and poor concentration. Compared with depression which is more clearly understandable in reactive terms, there is likely to be less changeability in the mood. A family history of bipolar illness is often present (Strober and Carlson, 1982).

Unless the presenting features are acute, the recognition of the first episode of a manic-depressive illness may be difficult, especially in younger adolescents, until second and subsequent attacks have occurred and a recurrent or cyclical pattern has become clear. Instead, attempts tend to be made by clinicians to construe symptoms in terms of personal and interpersonal difficulties. In the differential diagnosis, affective disturbance in early schizophrenia has to be considered as well as depressive psychoses, with symptoms similar to manic-depressive psychoses, but apparently provoked largely or entirely by saddening stresses, such as bereavement. Such psychotic states are diagnostically puzzling and prolonged observation may be needed, although the lack of a working diagnosis compounds the difficulties of coping with ambiguity in the clinical situation.

EXAMINATION OF DEPRESSED ADOLESCENTS AND THEIR FAMILIES

The initial contact

Adolescents are likely to find it difficult to ask for help themselves, so self-referral is infrequent and when help is sought the reasons are likely to reflect an urgent need for reassurance, guidance or protection. In most referrals, the presenting problems are those identified by others. When brought unwillingly to the initial interview with the doctor, however, the depressed adolescent may present in a confused, provocative, volatile or negativistic way, and may be unwilling or unable to identify specific problems. Further, the acknowledgement of difficulties may itself be seen as a capitulation to parental pressures and exacerbates a sense of inadequacy. The stage management of the initial professional contact is important in gaining the confidence and cooperation of those involved (Parry-Jones, 1985). Wherever possible, the approach needs to include consideration of the adolescent's family and, as a general rule, the parents or substitute care-givers of adolescents up to 16 years should be involved routinely. Beyond this age, the procedure may vary as, quite appropriately, some young people may prefer to be seen without parental knowledge or, at least, separately from them. A combination of joint and separate interviews with adolescent and parents is usually the most productive. Particular attention needs to be given to the feelings and attitudes of the parents and a sensitive response made to their predicament, which may include regret and guilt about past actions.

Interviewing and diagnostic assessment

The diagnostic process in adolescent psychiatric disorders need not differ from that used in other age groups, and systematic consideration is given to the clinical history, accurate mental state examination, the adolescent's life circumstances and any associated family, educational, work, social and recreational problems. Similarly, the differential diagnosis of the clinical psychiatric syndrome in adolescents includes all disorders occurring in other age periods. However, the process of history taking and the examination of mental state often needs to be more flexible because some teenagers are likely to find the face-to-face interview daunting.

In the opening interview, particular consideration has to be given to establishing trust and confidence in adolescents who are withdrawn, uncommunicative and fearful of being thought of as 'mad'. The confidence of demoralized and suspicious young people is most likely to be gained by listening without condemning, and any hint of phoneyness or forcing the pace will be detected swiftly. A key step in assessment, therefore, is engaging the adolescent and developing sufficient rapport to make possible further enquiry and discussion about the young person's feelings and life situation. The strength of the alliance is crucial in determining the clinician's effectiveness in providing support and reducing the sense of isolation, in achieving compliance with individual treatment, and in negotiating and facilitating changes within the family.

The central and most challenging task of assessment is disentangling manifestations of abnormal functioning that constitute evidence of depressive disorder, from age appropriate reactions that are likely to settle when stress is reduced or eliminated with further development and the passage of time. Consideration needs to be given, therefore, to evidence of actual change in behaviour and mental state, the extent to which these changes are in keeping with the young person's age and sex, and the frequency, persistence and pervasiveness of the abnormal features. Having established the evidence of abnormality, its effects on the adolescent's development, social life and day-to-day functioning need to be evaluated, as well as the effects on others. Diagnosis is likely to be unreliable without obtaining evidence about the adolescent's behaviour in a variety of settings, and information from the parents about the adolescent, the family, the home background and the extended family and friends. Physical examination is often indicated because depressive symptoms can occur in certain physical diseases and, further, the examination may provide a useful opportunity to discuss issues concerned with self-image and bodily functions and changes. This emphasizes the importance of the clinician having a thorough familiarity with the phenomena of normal adolescence and a sensitive appreciation of the internal and external stresses likely to be experienced.

The suicide rate rises rapidly during early and mid-adolescence and the possibility of suicide and parasuicide always needs to be considered when a teenager presents with depressive symptoms (Hawton *et al.*, 1982; Brooks-bank, 1985). Prevention is difficult, but professionals working with young people should be able to identify the warning signs sufficiently clearly to initiate appropriate action and to ensure the adolescent's safety. Any talk of suicide should be treated seriously. The main pointers to serious risk are persistent, severe depression; previous self-destructive behaviour; unusually stressful events, like school failure, the break-up of a love affair; and poor communication with others, especially parents. The risk is likely to be greater if the suicide attempt was carried out in isolation, if it was timed to make intervention unlikely, if precautions were taken to avoid discovery, if a suicide note was left or if there was evidence of extensive premeditation.

THERAPEUTIC APPROACHES

Before intervention, there has to be a realistic appraisal of objectives, the optimum arrangements for their implementation, and their practical feasibility. Prognostic pointers need to be taken seriously and over-optimism about outcome, on the basis that adolescence is a 'passing phase', may be misplaced. Decisions about intervention can carry the risk of both underestimating the seriousness of the problem, because the adolescent will 'grow out of it', or of overreacting in the belief that something has to be done urgently. The initial objectives of intervention should be the relief of distress for the adolescent and the family, the provision of appropriate support and, if necessary, a place of safety.

Most depressed teenagers will be channelled to a general practitioner, who will a have the main responsibility for decision-making. The majority should be manageable at home by the general practitioner, especially when the disorder is clearly understandable as a reaction to passing developmen-tal strains or to short-term stressful experiences. Despite the considerable literature on the management of depression in general practice, little is known about the diagnostic, decision-making and treatment difficulties experienced by general practitioners with adolescent patients. If mild depression does not respond to treatment within a reasonable time, or if depression is severe and associated with threats or attempts at suicide, referral to a psychiatrist is indicated. Only a very small proportion of depressed adolescents are likely to require hospitalization for intensive psychiatric assessment and treatment.

Therapeutic work with adolescents

Counselling, psychotherapy or some form of social intervention is likely to be successful in most cases of 'understandable' depression. The aim is to help the youngster recover or develop a fresh confidence in coping with difficulties and facing up to unpleasant situations. The clinician has to guard against fostering dependency by taking over too much responsibility. It is important not to overreact to minor, age-appropriate ups and downs when all that may be needed is reassurance of parents and, on occasion, other significant adults such as teachers, that there is no cause for alarm. The most common difficulties in individual work with adolescents are in establishing trust, talking about feelings like rejection, alienation and anger, and coping with defensive or help-rejecting behaviour. In order to progress, the adolescent patient needs to be able to accept the interest that is shown, which inevitably is related to the genuineness of the clinician's responses to the adolescent's feelings. The form of intervention ranges from direct practical help in resolving personal, situational and relationship problems to individual psychotherapy systematically planned to enable the adolescent to develop new ways of feeling more authoritative and confident. This may develop, perhaps for the first time, a sense of self-worth. Engaging the adolescent's interest and commitment in treatment is facilitated if the focus of attention is on clearly relevant issues and on the active steps that can be taken to produce change.

Some young people may have developed such a chronically negative view of themselves that it is difficult to shift the focus on to assets and achievements, and away from losses, regrets and inadequacies. In such cases, the techniques of cognitive behaviour therapy may be particularly effective (McAdam, 1986; Young, 1984), because they are problem-orientated and concerned with the adolescent's current experiences. In general their use with adolescents awaits evaluation. Cognitive restructuring techniques have the added advantage of discouraging dependency and regressive behaviour, which may develop with prolonged psychotherapy. Specialized psychoanalytic approaches emphasize the significance of mourning and depression as part of adolescent development and the importance of being able to experience and bear depression (Baker, 1978).

Although there is a natural reluctance to use psychotropic drugs with young people, the clinician will have to decide whether or not to use antidepressants. The literature on this topic is sparse, with few studies of the effectiveness of drugs in children and adolescents (Strober and Carlson, 1982). Clinical practice suggests that medication is indicated in the small number of patients who have biological symptoms, such as sleep disturbance and psychomotor retardation, or who are displaying psychotic symptoms. The author's preference is for a tricyclic antidepressant administered at night and employed in maximum dosage for several weeks before concluding that it is ineffective. The use of minor tranquillizers is discouraged strongly and hypnotic drugs are best avoided. In general terms, one needs to be cautious in prescribing antidepressants, so as not to run the risk of undermining the attempts being made by the adolescent and the family to cope constructively with painful feelings. The place of lithium in adolescent psychiatric treatment is not wholly clear, but there is evidence to suggest that it is as effective in manic-depressive disorder in this age group as it is in adults (Youngerman and Canino, 1978). Following two or three major affective episodes, it would be appropriate to consider long-term prophylactic treatment with lithium. The main difficulty is the likelihood of poor compliance with an extended regime. Electroconvulsive therapy is used rarely with adolescents, but may be indicated in severe, protracted depression which has proved resistant to other forms of treatment.

Parental and family work

Some form of specific work with the parents or families of depressed adolescents is usually indicated. Little is known about the extent of the burdens borne by the parents and siblings of depressed adolescents. Clinical experience suggests that it can be considerable, but the need for further research investigation is clear. Parents may feel responsible in some way for the adolescent's state and unsure about how to deal with mood disturbance in a young person who seems cut-off, completely alone and not reassured by comfort. Many factors within the family may generate outwardly disturbed behaviour in its adolescent members.

Parental responses to age-appropriate changes may be disorganized or obstructive, complicating the completion of maturational tasks and perceived by adolescents as increasing stress. Such processes, particularly those involving separation from parents, may need to be tackled in family therapy; Guttman (1983) has reviewed the place of this approach in treatment. Elaborate family involvement, however, is not appropriate in all cases, especially with older adolescents, and the objectives need to be identified clearly in the light of the overall diagnostic formulation.

RECURRENT OR CHRONIC DEPRESSION AND THE CONTINUITIES WITH ADULT DISORDERS

Little is known about the natural history of adolescent depressive disorders and it is difficult to predict with any certainty the occurrence of relapses.

There have been few recent studies of the outcome of child and adolescent depression. Welner *et al.* (1979) found that early onset bipolar affective illness had an unfavourable outcome, and it has been reported that a significant proportion of manic–depressive adults commence their disorders in the adolescent years (Carlson, 1983). However, in a systematic study of patients seen as children and adults, Zeitlin (1986) showed that, in many cases, adult depression was not preceded by childhood disorder. There has been considerable clinical and research interest in the relationship between traumatic events in childhood and adolescence, especially the loss of a parent, and adult depression, but the evidence is still difficult to interpret. In this context, it is also necessary to consider the effects of depressed parents on their children. The possibility remains speculative that the negative cognitions of adult depression could have their origins in negative self-schemata developed during childhood and adolescence, as a result of such factors as early loss or parental depression. Consideration of the possible links and continuities between child, adolescent and adult disorders has clinical and research implications. For child and adolescent psychiatric services, it highlights the need for the early, precise identification and the rigorous treatment of young people with potentially recurrent or chronic depressive disorders. The research priorities in this field include both prospective studies to clarify the natural history of adolescent depression and to establish predictors of outcome, and investigation of the antecedents, in childhood and adolescence, of adult affective disorders.

REFERENCES

Albert N., Beck A. (1975). Incidence of depression in early adolescence: a preliminary study. *Journal of Youth and Adolescence*, 4, 301–7.

American Psychiatric Association (1980). *Diagnostic and Statistical Manual of Mental Disorders*, 3rd edn. Washington: American Psychiatric Association.

Baker R. (1978). Adolescent depression: an illness or developmental task? *Journal of Adolescence*,1, 297–307.

Beck A. T. (1972). *Depression: Causes and Treatment*. Philadephia: University of Pennysylvania Press.

Birleson P., Hudson I., Buchanan D.G., Wolff S. (1987). Clinical evaluation of a self-rating scale for depressive disorder in childhood (Depression Self-rating Scale). *Journal of Child Psychology and Psychiatry*, 28, 43–60.

Brooksbank D. J. (1985). Suicide and parasuicide in childhood and early adolescence. *British Journal of Psychiatry*, 146, 459–63.

Carlson B. (1983). Bipolar affective disorders in childhood and adolescence. In *Affective Disorders in Childhood and Adolescence: An Update* (Cantwell D., Carlson G., eds.). Lancaster: MTP Press, pp. 61–83.

Carlson G. A., Cantwell D. P. (1980). Unmasking masked depression in children and adolescents. *American Journal of Psychiatry*, 137, 445–9.

Cicchetti D., Schneider-Rosen D. (1986). An organizational approach to childhood depression. In *Depression in Young People. Developmental and Clinical*

Perspectives (Rutter M., Izard C. E., Read P. B., eds.). New York: The Guildford Press, pp. 71–134.

Friedman R. C., Hurt S. W., Clarkin J. F., *et al.* (1983). Symptoms of depression among adolescents and young adults. *Journal of Affective Disorders*, 5, 37–43.

Gammon G., John K., Rothblum E. *et al.* (1983). Use of a structured diagnostic interview to identify bipolar disorder in adolescent in-patients; frequency and manifestation of the disorder. *American Journal of Psychiatry*, 140, 543–7.

Glaser K. (1967). Masked depression in children and adolescents. *American Journal of Psychotherapy*, 21, 565–74.

Graham P. (1986). *Child Psychiatry. A Developmental Approach.* Oxford: Oxford University Press, pp. 110–5.

Guttman H. A. (1983). Family therapy in the treatment of mood disturbance in adolescence. In *The Adolescent and Mood Disturbance* (Golonbek H., Garfinkel B. D., eds.) New York: International Universities Press, pp. 263–72.

Hawton K., O'Grady J., Osborn M., Cole D. (1982). Adolescents who take overdoses: their characteristics, problems and contracts with helping agencies. *British Journal of Psychiatry*, 140, 118–23.

Kandel D. B., Davies M. (1982). Epidemiology of depressive mood in adolescents. *Archives of General Psychiatry*, 39, 1205–12.

Kaplan S. L., Hong G. K., Weinhold C. (1984). Epidemiology of depressive symptomatology in adolescents. *Journal of the American Academy of Child Psychiatry*, 23, 91–8.

Kashani J. H., Carlson G. A. (1987). Seriously depressed pre-schoolers. *American Journal of Psychiatry*, 144, 348–50.

Kashani J. H., Keller M. B., Solomon N., *et al.* (1985). Double depression in adolescent substance users. *Journal of Affective Disorders*, 8, 153–7.

Kashani J. H., Carlson G. A., Beck N. C., *et al.* (1987). Depression, depressive symptoms, and depressed mood among a community sample of adolescents. *American Journal of Psychiatry*, 144, 931–4.

Kazdin A. E. (1987). Children's depression scale: validation with child psychiatric inpatients. *Journal of Child Psychology and Psychiatry*, 28, 29–41.

Kazdin A. E., Petti T. A. (1982). Self-report and interview measures of childhood and adolescent depression. *Journal of Child Psychology and Psychiatry*, 23, 437–57.

Kovacs M., Beck A. T. (1977). An empirical clinical approach towards a definition of childhood depression. In *Depression in Children: Diagnosis, Treatment and Conceptual Models* (Schulterbrandt J., Raskin A., eds.). New York: Raven Press.

McAdam E. (1986). Cognitive behaviour therapy and its application with adolescents. *Journal of Adolescence*, 9, 1–15.

Marriage K., Fine S., Moretti M., Haley G. (1986). Relationship between depression and conduct disorder in children and adolescents. *Journal of the American Academy of Child Psychiatry*, 25, 687–91.

Parry-Jones W. Ll. (1985). Adolescent disturbance. In *Child and Adolescent Psychiatry. Modern Approaches* (Rutter M., Hersov L., eds.). Oxford: Oxford University Press, pp. 584–5.

Pearce J. (1978). The recognition of depressive disorders in children. *Proceedings of the Royal Society of Medicine*, 71, 494–500.

Puig-Antich J. (1986). Psychobiological markers: effects of age and puberty. In

Depression in Young People: Developmental and Clinical Perspectives (Rutter M., Izard C. E., Read P. B., eds.). New York: The Guilford Press, pp. 341–81.

Puig-Antich J., Blau S., Marx N., *et al.* (1978). Prepubertal major depressive disorder: a pilot study. *Journal of the American Academy of Child Psychiatry*, 17, 695–707.

Robbins D. R., Alessi N. E., Cook S. C., *et al.* (1982). The use of the Research Diagnostic Criteria (RDC) for depression in adolescent psychiatry inpatients. *Journal of the American Academy of Child Psychiatry*, 21, 251–5.

Rutter M. (1986). The developmental psychopathology of depression: issues and perspectives. In *Depression in Young People: Developmental and Clinical Perspectives* (Rutter M., Izard C. E., Read P. B., eds.). New York: The Guilford Press, pp. 3–30.

Rutter M., Graham P., Chadwick O., Yule W. (1976). Adolescent turmoil: fact or fiction? *Journal of Child Psychology and Psychiatry*, 17, 35–56.

Rutter M., Izard C. E., Read P. B., eds. (1986). *Depression in Young People: Developmental and Clinical Perspectives.* New York: The Guilford Press.

Shaffer D. (1974). Suicide in childhood and early adolescence. *Journal of Child Psychology and Psychiatry*, 15, 275–91.

Shaffer D. (1985). Depression, mania and suicidal acts. In *Child and Adolescent Psychiatry: Modern Approaches* (Rutter M., Hersov L., eds.). Oxford: Blackwell Scientific Publications, pp. 698–719.

Spitzer R. L., Endicott J., Robins E. (1978). *Research Diagnostic Criteria (RDC) for a Selected Group of Functional Disorders.* New York: New York State Institute.

Strober M., Carlson G. (1982). Bipolar illness in adolescents with major depression. *Archives of General Psychiatry*, 39, 549–55.

Strober M., Green J., Carlson G. (1981). Phenomenology and subtypes of major depressive disorder in adolescence. *Journal of Affective Disorders*, 3, 281–90.

Welner A., Welner Z., Fishman R. (1979). Psychiatric and adolescent in-patients: 8–10 year follow-up. *Archives of General Psychiatry*, 36, 698–700.

World Health Organization (1978). *Ninth Revision of the International Classification of Diseases: Mental Disorders.* Geneva: World Health Organization.

Young H. S. (1984). Counselling strategies with working class adolescents. *British Journal of Cognitive Psychotherapy*, 2, 21–32.

Youngerman J., Canino I. A. (1978). Lithium carbonate use in children and adolescents. A survey of the literature. *Archives of General Psychiatry*, 35, 216–24.

Zeitlin H. (1986). *The Natural History of Psychiatric Disorder in Children.* Oxford: Oxford University Press.

8 *Depression in the puerperium: a conceptual controversy*

JOHN L. COX

INTRODUCTION

The position of this chapter between 'Depression in Adolescence' and 'Depression in the Elderly' heightens an important and persistent controversy about whether or not there are distinctive characteristics of depression which follows childbirth. From the first descriptions of postnatal mental illness by Hippocrates and the 19th Century clinical observations of Marcé (1858) to those of the present day, post partum mental illness has continued to receive specific attention in the literature; and the debate as to what Marcé actually said about the features of this disorder still continues. Karnosh and Hope (1937), for example, as well as Boyd (1942), have quoted Marcé as asserting that these psychiatric disorders are *not* specific clinical entities and that their symptoms are also found in psychoses which occur at other times. Yet Hamilton (1962) has concluded that Marcé put forward the opposite view—namely that it is the combination of symptoms (i.e. syndromes) which are different from those observed in non-puerperal mental illness. Andrews (1988), in a more recent review, believes that both these interpretations of what Marcé said are also misleading:

Hamilton is right in saying that Marcé thought that there was a condition 'mental illness related to childbirth' but wrong in attributing this to considerations of symptom pattern. Marcé describes a 'caractere speciale' that the post partum period gives to the symptomatology but it is the temporal relationships and co-temporal variations of physiological and psychopathological states that led him to believe that there was such a condition.

Karnosh and Hope, and Boyd, are right in saying that the symptomatology of the condition according to Marcé was not unique to the puerperium but wrong in concluding that Marcé therefore thought that puerperal and non-puerperal conditions were the same.

In addition to this historical debate, which may never fully be resolved, there is the contemporary confusion caused by the aetiological assumptions of the terms 'postnatal depression' and 'puerperal psychoses', which suggest a causal relationship between childbirth and psychiatric disorder when all that may be implied is a temporal association.

Because of this continuing conceptual controversy about the nature of postnatal mental illness, two of the widely used classificatory systems, the International Classification of Diseases (ICD-9; World Health Organization, 1978), and the American Diagnostic and Statistical Manual (DSM-III; American Psychiatric Association, 1987), do not include the category of puerperal psychoses at all. There remains a paradox that at a time when research into the aetiology, prevention and treatment of postnatal mental illness is underway, and when the popular press brings this topic to the attention of the public, these nomenclatures do not reflect this widespread general concern. It would seem that the recognition in English law of the offence of 'infanticide' more accurately reflects public opinion, as well as clinical concern. Thus, although the Infanticide Act dates from 1938, the recent Criminal Law Revision Committee (1980) has retained this special offence. Almost all of the defendants receive a non-custodial sentence, or a treatment order.

It is a purpose of this chapter, therefore, to describe some of the clinical, socio-cultural and research facets of these orders which may explain why the diagnoses of 'puerperal psychosis' and 'postnatal depression' are still used and why our society continues to regard these disorders as of particular importance.

EVIDENCE FOR AN INCREASED FREQUENCY OF MENTAL ILLNESS FOLLOWING CHILDBIRTH

Although the likelihood of a mother with a puerperal psychotic illness requiring admission is small (1–2 per 1000 live births) compared with at least 10–15 percent of women with a post partum depressive disorder in the community, the increased risk of being admitted to a psychiatric hospital in the puerperium is nevertheless substantial. Thus Kendell *et al.* (1987), using linked data from obstetric and psychiatric case registers, showed that over a 12-year period 54 087 births were recorded which resulted in 120 psychiatric admissions within 90 days of parturition. They also showed that in the first 30 days after childbirth there were nearly seven times as many admissions when compared with the average monthly rate before pregnancy (68 versus 10.). They concluded that this dramatic rise in the admission rate post partum suggests that powerful biological factors were involved or that the parapartum weeks were exceptionally stressful, and that such stress *exceeded* that which followed other events such as the loss of a job, or moving house. Their finding that being unmarried, having a first baby, and delivery by Caesarean section were associated with a yet greater likelihood of psychiatric admission does give support to those who believe that psychological stresses make a substantial contribution to this increased risk of psychiatric morbidity post partum.

However, not all women who were admitted to a psychiatric unit had a psychotic illness; in fact a quarter had a minor depressive disorder or a personality disorder only (Dean and Kendell, 1981). In a further analysis carried out by Dean (1989), these mothers with minor depressions were found to have more non-birth-related, long-term difficulties than those admitted with psychoses, and were more likely to have been admitted later in the puerperium. Six of the 16 women with minor depressions were unmarried and a further four had marital problems compared with only nine of the 51 with major depressions who were unmarried and seven with marital problems. These data suggest that there may be at least two subgroups of post partum depression.

The first group is those women with a major affective disorder, predominantly depressive, which occurs in women genetically predisposed towards manic depressive illness, and which usually has an onset within two weeks of childbirth. Their subsequent psychiatric morbidity has been shown by Platz and Kendell (1988) to be similar to the non-puerperal affective psychoses. In a study by Dowlatashi and Paykel (1989), women with puerperal affective psychoses did not have the adverse social, marital and economic factors which generally characterize those with non-psychotic depressions—findings which would suggest that their aetiology may be more closely related to neuroendocrine disturbance.

The second group are women with later onset milder depressions who are mostly at home and rarely consult psychiatrists. Several prospective studies have shown that at least 10–15 percent of women suffer from these depressive disorders within six months of childbirth (Paykel *et al.*, 1980; Cox *et al.*, 1982; Kumar and Robson, 1984; Watson *et al.*, 1984). Nott (1987) found an incidence rate of 18 percent at nine months. Although community studies of depression in women, whether or not childbearing, have shown rather similar rates (Brown and Harris, 1978; Dean *et al.*, 1983), further analysis of the community study carried out by Bebbington *et al.* (1989) has suggested that married and parous women do have particularly high rates of depression. It is possible, therefore, that if the episodes of depression which occurred post partum are excluded from the analysis of general population studies of women, then the frequency of depression, whether or not childbearing, would be considerably lower than that reported in the postnatal studies.

To determine the frequency of postnatal depression in a community sample and to compare the frequency with that found in pregnancy, a prospective study was carried out on a fully representative sample of women in Edinburgh (Cox *et al.*, 1982). The sample comprised 105 mothers, who were first interviewed using the Standardised Psychiatric Interview of Goldberg *et al.* (1970) at the booking-in clinic of the Simpson Memorial Maternity Pavilion. The other three psychiatric interviews took place during the last trimester of pregnancy, within 10 days of delivery, and at 4–5 months after childbirth. The proportion of mothers with a definite depressive illness in the puerperium (13 percent) was a three-fold increase compared with that found in pregnancy; in 9 of these 13, the illness was not preceded by any depression during pregnancy. Such women were similar in most respects to those described by Pitt (1968) as having an 'atypical' (neurotic) depression. There were, however, a further 17 women (16 percent) with milder depressions which, though lasting in 15 patients for at least four weeks, had improved by the time the 5-month postnatal interview was carried out. These women with milder disorders were referred to as having depressive 'symptoms'. If the 13 women with depressive illness are combined with those having depressive 'symptoms' then the research suggests that at least 1 in 4 of the women were depressed at some time after childbirth. Such women were likely to report a deterioration in their marital relationships, and had commonly experienced a marked reduction in sexual satisfaction, usually due to loss of libido.

To determine how accurately a mother recalled postnatal depressions three years later, 11 of these 13 women were interviewed again, and it was found that seven recalled very precisely the previous postnatal depression. There was an 88 percent agreement between depressive ratings made when the mother was depressed and those obtained retrospectively three years later (Cox *et al.*, 1984). Of the four who did not recall these events, three had been pregnant again and two of these three had experienced a second postpartum depression. When these two mothers were asked why they had not recalled their earlier postnatal depression they said that the second postnatal depression had been so bad that it had overshadowed the memory of the previous one. Thus in no less than 7 (50 percent) of the 13 depressed mothers (7 percent of the total sample) the postnatal depressive illness had lasted for at least 12 months. These findings are similar to those of Pitt (1968) and Nott (1987).

The pressing need to answer more definitely the question of whether or not there is an increased frequency of depression in postpartum women compared with non-puerperal women demands further controlled studies. The only such study to be reported is that in the US by O'Hara (1989), who selected friends of the Index subject as controls and found that the difference in the frequency of depression between the childbearing and the control group did not quite reach statistical significance. Thus 10.4 percent of the 182 childbearing women interviewed were depressed compared with 7.8 percent of the controls. In another comprehensive prospective study of postnatal depression using the Present State Examination, Cooper *et al.* (1988) found a point prevalence of non-psychotic psychiatric disorder of 8.8 percent at six months postpartum; a finding which they suggest is no different from what might be expected in a general population sample.

These researchers have therefore drawn attention to several important methodological issues which need to be taken into account by those who attempt to replicate their findings. O'Hara, for example, found a marked practice effect of giving repeated measures of psychiatric morbidity over a limited period of time. The non-childbearing controls showed a reduction in psychiatric morbidity as the study proceeded. This work also demonstrated the need to determine the characteristics of any subject who drops out from a study during its progress and to ensure that the minor depressions, which can be socially disabling, are also identified. In an attempt to clarify these important matters with regard to postnatal depression myself and Dr. Declan Murray are carrying out a study of postnatal depression in Stoke on Trent using individually matched controls obtained from local General Practitioner lists.

CHILDBIRTH: A DISTINCTIVE LIFE EVENT

Although the seminal findings of Brown and Harris (1978) showed that having young children was a vulnerability factor for depression, the *precise* contribution of the childbirth event itself to such depression was not fully established. Nevertheless, the depressed women in their study had twice the rate of pregnancy and birth events than the non-depressed although the research design did not distinguish clearly between the women who were pregnant and those who had recently delivered. However, Brown and Harris showed that it was the contribution of other problems (for example, bad housing and major marital difficulties) which were the main triggers for the onset of depression in many instances. They concluded that childbirth had brought home to a woman the 'disappointment and hopelessness of her position and that aspirations are made distant as she becomes more dependent on an uncertain relationship'.

The method used to rate the 'childbirth event' is therefore very complex and necessitates, for example, the interviewer determining the extent of 'contextual' threat of the birth event to a mother. This interview procedure illustrates how such measures of threat and social disadvantage must initially reflect the changing attitudes of a society towards childbirth. At the present time, a single mother who became pregnant might be regarded as experiencing a less threatening event than formerly because of the increased acceptance of single parent families. Likewise an assumption that a mother who brings up small children in a house with an 'inadequate' number of rooms is experiencing a particularly 'negative' event may be unwarranted. This assessment needs to be set within a socio-cultural context, as not all families would regard this as being such a major disadvantage. Several researchers have therefore attempted to improve the Life Events research methodology by measuring the components of the stress factors associated with childbirth and including an evaluation of those *non-childbearing* related events which could be particularly threatening if they occurred during childbearing. Thus the death of a parent before delivery, for example, is a particularly traumatic experience for a mother, and moving house with three children under five years is also especially stressful. Likewise the stress caused by adverse obstetric factors, such as Caesarean section, may also need to be considered.

In a study by Watson *et al.* (1984), Life Events and Difficulties were recorded using an adaptation of the Brown and Harris interview method; they found that *only* 3 of the 29 women with episodes of affective disorder before or after childbirth had *no* other Life Event which could have brought this about. The depressed mothers were divided into five categories according to the relationship of depression to non-childbirth-related Life Events, as well as to long-term social difficulties. These five categories were:

depression clearly *unrelated* to a pregnancy and childbirth event, such as a bereavement or housing crisis;

depression associated with Life Events which were themselves derived from pregnancy or childbirth, such as serious antenatal complications or a premature birth;

depressive episodes which occurred to a mother who faced continuing life difficulties rather than an acute Life Event;

depression in pregnancy caused by the memory of a sad event during an earlier pregnancy, such as a previous stillbirth;

depression which followed the birth event only and occurring in a mother who had no experience of any previous adverse Life Event or Difficulty, and had no past psychiatric history.

O'Hara *et al.* (1986) have also wrestled with these problems of how to measure the childbirth event. They have divided the stresses of childbirth into three categories:

those which occurred during pregnancy;
those related to the stress of the delivery itself;
those which were related to child care.

They then developed a Peri-Partum Stress Scale with two subscales based on these three aspects of childbirth. Likewise Barnett *et al.* (1983) recognized the need to rethink how the Life Events associated with childbirth were to be recorded. Because they could not identify a Life Event Scale which fully acknowledged the unique aspects of the obstetric stress, they developed a self-report scale of their own.

Kumar and Robson (1984) in their study of postnatal depression used four categories of birth-related Life Events:

marital or occupational changes of the mother or partner;
health considerations;
domestic or social change;
crises such as burglaries, theft or witnessing disturbing events.

The authors found that the most important contribution of events to depression following childbirth was an impaired marital relationship, and antenatal depression from a previous termination. However, they did also conclude that the childbirth event per se had a 'particular and deleterious effect on the mental health of a substantial proportion of first time mothers'. Similarly, Paykel *et al.* (1980) found that although the stress of pregnancy and childbirth were important as additional stresses in tenuous situations, there was a small subgroup of women whose depression appeared to have a primary biological cause and which seemed to be independent of socially determined events.

CHILDBIRTH AS A 'RITE DE PASSAGE'

Medical anthropologists have made a unique and vital contribution to this discussion by their understanding of childbirth as a 'Rite de Passage' which has three phases: (a) the Rite of Separation which includes the cleansing and purifying of the subject; (b) the Liminal Period when the subject has no status, is in limbo and when private humiliation may be inflicted; and (c) the Rite of Incorporation when the subject moves back to a new status which is usually symbolized by new clothing, and followed by much feasting and rejoicing. Seel (1986) has shown how these childbirth-related rituals are important not only for the individual who participates in them but also as expressions of dominant social values.

Thus, in most societies, the change in status from 'childless woman' to 'mother' is a major role change which requires considerable adjustment of her relationships to her mother, her husband and siblings, as well as to the wider society. Such a marked change in social status should be marked appropriately by a public ceremony and by carrying out a complete 'Rite de Passage'. Seel observes, however, that whilst the 'separation' and the 'liminal period' are indeed *highly* elaborated in Western obstetrics (the mother is admitted to hospital and puts on new clothes), the final phase of 'incorporation' and the return to society is *unfinished*. The hypothesis is put forward that because of this *lack* of social structure in the puerperium, parents have to fend for themselves as best they can. A new mother in Western society may, for example, receive conflicting advice as to the amount of domestic activities which can be undertaken, and there is no concensus as to when sexual relationships are to be resumed. The mother's status is thus ambiguous and her role as a provider for her children is perhaps less valued than formerly. It is therefore a most plausible hypothesis that this lack of postnatal structure may threaten self-esteem, result in less social support being available and so may initiate a clinical depression. The husband's role in childbirth is also uncertain, which makes it more difficult to determine the type of practical support to give his wife and child.

FAMILY IMPLICATIONS

The direct observations by Murray (1988) in Cambridge, using a complex video technique, have shown how mothers who are depressed have a less well-timed responsiveness to their children, and how these children look to their mothers less and engage in more self-directed activity. These direct observations support those by Cohn Tronick *et al.* (1983), who observed that babies spent more time protesting, crying and looking away from the mother who was role-playing being 'depressed', compared with a mother who behaved in a more animated and cheerful manner. The impact of maternal depression at such a time of social change and new bonding is therefore likely to be considerable, and these studies have suggested that the depressed affective tone generated at that time in the baby could have an enduring quality, which may even influence subsequent temperamental development.

It is striking that the role of the father in the puerperium is only just beginning to be investigated and that so little information is available on the frequency of depression in this partner. Yet several studies of puerperal depression have shown a clear relationship between depression post partum and marital difficulties (Cox *et al.*, 1982; Kumar and Robson 1984; Watson *et al.*, 1984). This neglect of an aspect of parenting therefore needs to be urgently rectified as fathers assume more multiple roles. Brown and Harris (1978) have shown that a confiding relationship between partners is threatened considerably by childbirth and in some instances is disconti- nued irrevocably. The role of the husband is not only as a supporter, providing instrumental help for the mother and practical care for the baby, but also crucially as a confidant. If the husband becomes depressed secondarily to his wife's difficulties, or as a primary problem, then the likelihood of the childbirth 'Rite de Passage' being optimally completed is substantially diminished.

HEALTH PERSONNEL: THE NEED FOR SPECIFIC TRAINING IN POSTNATAL MENTAL ILLNESS

The implications for the training of health personnel who are already working with these young mothers is considerable. Clinical experience suggests that postnatal depression can, with training, be readily recog- nized by primary care workers and that they have an essential preventative and curative task to undertake. Again, clinical experience, as well as research findings, have shown that principles of non-directive counselling are particularly appropriate for the treatment of puerperal depression and that health visitors are most receptive to acquiring these extra skills.

A controlled study which sought to demonstrate how effective such counselling is when carried out by a health visitor who is already in regular contact with young mothers has been reported (Holden *et al.*, 1989). Health visitors are in a particularly good position to be concerned with the detection and management of postnatal depression as they provide an essential link between a recently delivered mother and her general practitioner, and are routinely involved in the care of puerperal mothers and their children. They can also initiate contact with women and are therefore well placed to detect early symptoms of psychiatric disorder.

In the controlled study of non-directive counselling, health visitors were first given three one and-a-half hour training sessions which included a role play, discussions and observing a video. Fifty women with a depressive illness that fulfilled Research Diagnostic Criteria for depression were included in the study and had been randomly allocated to a counselled group ($n = 26$) and to a control group ($n = 24$). The counselled group received eight weekly half-hour sessions of non-directive counselling by their own health visitor. The women in both groups were then interviewed 13 weeks later by a doctor who did not know to which group the mother had been allocated and had specifically asked the mother not to inform her about this.

The main finding was that over two-thirds (69 percent) of the 26 depressed women in the counselled group showed no evidence at follow-up of having a major or minor depressive illness compared with only 9 (38 percent) of the 24 women in the control group. Other comparisons using psychiatric symptom scores showed a highly significant reduction of symptoms in mothers in the counselled group and no reduction in the controls. These findings therefore would suggest that non-directive counselling by a health visitor can indeed bring about an improvement in such depression—although which component of the counselling was therapeutic could not be determined precisely. It is important to observe, however, that a third of mothers in the control group had *also* improved by 13 weeks, and that a third of the counselled group did *not* improve. Mothers in this latter category may be those who require a combination of antidepressants as well as counselling if their depression is to be fully alleviated.

Other research in Lewisham, outer London (S. Elliott and T. Leverton, work in progress) has found that an intervention during pregnancy to mothers at high risk of depression after childbirth was also effective in bringing about a reduction in postnatal depression. These findings were sufficiently encouraging for a three-centre study in Lewisham, Edinburgh and Keele to be put in progress to determine how this approach can be generalized into the ordinary routine practice of busy health visitors. Experience had already indicated that the majority of health visitors, given encouragement and diagnostic skills, can indeed assist in the treatment of depressed mothers, provided they have good back-up from a mental-health professional such as a community psychiatric nurse or an interested psychiatrist.

There is also a need to encourage family physicians to identify antenatal and postnatal depression, and to collaborate fully with other primary care professionals when planning a management strategy. This need for a more widespread education about the recognition and management of postnatal mental illness, however, is not confined to these personnel. There may be a similar need for hospital-based psychiatrists to obtain information if they are to support and educate the primary health care professionals. Although obstetricians may regard these problems as occurring after they have discontinued their own involvement, it is important that their training should nevertheless include information about the high frequency of psychiatric morbidity associated with childbearing and about the need to identify mothers with mental illness after childbirth. It is understood that the Royal College of Obstetricians and Gynaecologists is presently revising its own examination requirements to include greater emphasis on these psychological and psychiatric aspects of childbearing.

DETECTION OF PARANATAL DEPRESSION: THE NEED FOR NEW MEASURES

During earlier studies, it became clear that the existing Self-Report Scales for measuring anxiety and depression, if administered to childbearing women, lacked the validity and practical usefulness that had been apparent when standardized on other subjects. Thus, the Anxiety and Depression Scale (SAD) of Bedford and Foulds (1978) was found to have marked limitations when administered to pregnant women. Of the 13 women who scored above Fould's threshold for personal illness (6 +) only 3 had any form of psychiatric disorder and 4 had minor psychiatric symptoms only (Cox *et al.*, 1983). The observations of Nott and Cutts (1982) that 89 (45 percent) of 200 puerperal women scored highly on the 30-item General Health Questionnaire (Goldberg *et al.*, 1970) but only 37 (18 percent) were psychiatric cases also suggests there may be difficulties with other widely used questionnaires when employed in the puerperium. Thus O'Hara *et al.* (1983) showed that the Beck Depression Inventory (Beck *et al.*, 1961) also had limitations when used on childbearing women. Measures of self-control that predicted subsequent postnatal depression using the Beck scale were not confirmed when a clinical syndrome diagnosis of depression was made.

There are several possible explanations as to why these scales are unsatisfactory. The somatic symptoms associated with the physiological changes of pregnancy, such as abdominal pain, back ache and palpitations, may cause a high score on psychiatric questionnaires but are not necessarily associated with a mood disturbance. An item used to measure lack of pleasure—'I have enjoyed watching television or reading a good book as much as I usually do'—may lack face validity for use in the puerperium. Likewise, questions about sleep disturbances (which are not linked specifically with an abnormal mood) might give a morbid rating indicating depression when the disturbance may actually be caused by a crying baby or by the need for night feeds. A suitable postnatal depression scale, therefore, must have face validity for the subject and also be able to be completed easily in a short period of time. If the scale is to be completed during a visit by a health professional, such as a health visitor or community psychiatric nurse, then these time constraints are particularly important.

A self-report scale specifically designed to detect those mothers who were depressed following childbirth has therefore been devised; a task helped by the earlier work of Snaith (1981, 1983), who had clearly recognized the need to modify existing scales used to measure depression for use in novel clinical situations and who was also aware of the need to develop a screening questionnaire to detect postnatal depression. This latter need has long been regarded (Kumar, 1982; Cox *et al.*, 1983) as a particularly important research priority.

Details of the development of the Edinburgh Postnatal Depression Scale (EPDS) have been fully documented elsewhere (Cox, 1986, Cox *et al.*, 1987). In summary, a 13-item scale was first validated on a sample of 63 puerperal women living near a Health Centre in Livingston New Town, 20 miles from Edinburgh. This study showed that whilst these 13 items distinguished clearly between depressed and non-depressed mothers, two irritability items (both of which were derived from the Irritability Sub-Scale of the Irritability Depression and Anxiety Scale (Snaith *et al.*, 1978)) and the only item related directly to mothering ('I have enjoyed being a mother') belonged to a separate 'non-depression' factor. Therefore a second validation study of the 10-item scale was conducted, and it was found that a threshold score of 12/13 identified all of the 21 women with major depressive illness and 2 of the 3 women with a probable major depressive illness. Four of the 11 women with definite minor depressions were false negatives. The sensitivity of this 10-item scale was 86 percent and the specificity was 78 percent.

Subsequent clinical study has confirmed that the EPDS is particularly useful in the routine work of community health workers as a screening scale, as well as in confirming the health professionals' opinion that a mother may have a marked psychiatric disorder. The self-report EPDS has proved as effective in detecting postnatal depression as two well-established interview rating scales—the Montgomery–Asberg (1979) Depression rating scale and the Raskin three-area scale (Raskin *et al.*, 1970).

The scale has also now been validated for use during pregnancy on a sample of 100 women attending the antenatal clinic at North Staffs Maternity Hospital. This study showed that a higher threshold (14/15) identified the eight women with a Major Depression in late pregnancy, but that the scale was less satisfactory than in the puerperium for detecting women with minor depression. The EPDS was fully acceptable to the pregnant women and its administration at a busy antenatal clinic seemed to cause little practical difficulty (Murray and Cox, 1988).

THE NEED FOR SPECIFIC CLINICAL FACILITIES

It is apparent from earlier discussion in this chapter that to provide an optimum facility for mothers with postnatal-related mental illness requires staff who have a particular sensitivity for these problems and who are familiar with developmental psychology as well as well trained in counselling techniques. Collaboration between the health visitor and the family physician is also of much importance if an optimum service is to be provided. The base for such a community service requires an appropriately equipped nursery, staffed by nursery nurses.

Reasons why so much puerperal mental illness goes undetected are that such mothers so rarely describe their symptoms in detail to professional workers; and women are reluctant to be separated from their family for treatment. A psychiatric service, therefore, needs to be fully sensitive to these issues and to have a facility to arrange for domiciliary management of disturbed mothers as well as for in-patient treatment. Oates (1988) in Nottingham manages to look after mothers with quite marked puerperal mental illness in their homes with the assistance of community psychiatric nurses and her own substantial commitment of time. At the Parent and Baby Day Unit in Stoke on Trent, it has been feasible to provide a more limited domiciliary service. The main thrust of resources is there linked to the provision of day hospital-based counselling, with the opportunity for assessment by a psychiatrist. The admission to psychiatric hospital of at least six women who would otherwise have required it has proved preventable. The need for nursery nurses recognizes the specific clinical implications of the treatment of depression in the puerperium which are not precisely paralleled in the treatment of depression at other stages of the life cycle.

An in-patient mother and baby unit is also an important clinical facility for mothers with psychoses, such as mania, schizophrenia or a profound depressive psychosis associated with suicidal or infanticidal risk. These mothers will require active treatment and observation by psychiatrists *and* a facility to admit the baby with them into a hospital setting. The development of the large regional Mother and Baby In-Patient Unit in Manchester has been described (Brockington and Margison, 1982), but no systematic study has yet been carried out to evaluate the effectiveness of an in-patient unit in comparison to a day hospital service. Although most Health Districts with a population of 3–400 000 require a 2- or 3-bedded in-patient mother and baby unit, the problems of staffing such units, which may only be full intermittently, are considerable. It is likely that these units will only function optimally if they are closely linked to a day hospital resource which provides a bridge between in-patient management and the reintegration of the mother into the community after discharge from hospital. It is also possible that nursing staff could be moved with greater flexibility between a day hospital and an in-patient unit and so be able to respond to clinical needs, which fluctuate markedly from month to month.

CONCLUSION

This chapter has endeavoured to indicate quite distinctive clinical and academic aspects of post partum depression. When a depressive illness occurs in the setting of such massive role changes for the mother and the family, it may have major consequences for the optimum adoption of these new roles, for the satisfactory development of the baby and for the bonding of the marriage. Thus, although the symptoms of postnatal depression *may* not differ substantially from depression occurring in non-childbearing women, the content of the depressive 'thoughts' usually reflects the preoccupation of the new mother with her baby. Research findings suggest that non-psychotic depression is largely determined by personality and social factors and that the birth of the baby may enhance the negative impact and threat of other adverse events and difficulties.

For some families the birth of a baby is an extremely satisfying and consistently joyous occasion. However, for at least 1 in 10 families the baby represents a long-term difficulty which can threaten the mother's coping skills and, in the absence of consistent family support, provoke a sense of hopelessness and low self-esteem. This may then develop into a more prolonged depressive illness. However, the wider recognition of the extent of postnatal depression, the availability of simple screening tests for this disorder, and the recognition that counselling skills can be readily assimilated by health visitors have enhanced the possibility that these distressed mothers and their families can now be treated.

It is hoped that hospital-based specialists, such as psychiatrists, obstetricians and paediatricians, will continue to raise the profile of these depressions which follow childbirth, and through their influence on Examination Boards and Colleges ensure that the medical profession is better informed about these serious emotional sequelae to childbirth. It is an event which cannot be regarded just as biologically determined and technological but as the beginning of a process of re-adjustment for the woman and her partner. For 1 in 7 parents it is followed by a depressive disorder.

The epidemiological, psychological and clinical aspects of depression associated with childbearing *are* therefore in some ways distinctive and so justify retention of the diagnostic labels 'puerperal psychosis' and 'postnatal depression', even if the symptoms are similar to those occurring in depression at other times, and even if the aetiological contribution of the birth event itself is less important than was at one time believed.

REFERENCES

Andrews H. (1988). *The Diagnosis of the Puerperal Psychoses*. Doctorate Thesis, University of Nottingham.
American Psychiatric Association (1987). *Diagnostic and Statistical Manual of Mental Disorders* 3rd edn. revised. Washington: American Psychiatric Association.
Barnett B. F. W., Hanna B., Parker G. (1983). Life event scales of obstetric groups. *Journal of Psychosomatic Research*, 27, 313–30.
Beck A. T., Ward C. H., Mendelson M., *et al.* (1961). An inventory for measuring depression. *Archives of General Psychiatry*, 4, 53–63.

Bedford A., Foulds G. (1978). *Delusions–Symptoms–States. State of Anxiety and Depression* (manual). Windsor: National Foundation for Educational Research.

Bebbington P. E., Dean C., Der G., *et al.* (1989). Gender, parity and the prevalence of minor affective disorder. Under Review for *British Journal of Psychiatry*.

Boyd D. A. (1942). Mental disorders associated with childbearing. *American Journal of Obstetrics and Gynecology*, 43, 335–49.

Brockington I., Margison F. (1982). Psychiatric Mother and Baby Unit. In *Motherhood and Mental Illness* (Brockington I., Kumar R., eds.). London: Academic Press.

Brown G. W., Harris T. (1978). *Social Origins of Depression*. London: Tavistock Publications.

Cohn J. F., Tronick E. Z. (1983). Three month old infants' reaction to simulated maternal depression. *Child Development*, 54, 185–93.

Cooper P. J., Campbell E. A., Day A., *et al.* (1988). Non-psychotic psychiatric disorder after childbirth: a prospective study of prevalence, incidence, course and nature. *British Journal of Psychiatry*, 152, 799–806.

Cox J. L. (1986). *Postnatal Depression—A Guide for Health Professionals*. Edinburgh: Churchill Livingstone.

Cox J. L., Connor Y., Kendell, R. E., (1982). Prospective study of the psychiatric disorders of childbirth. *British Journal of Psychiatry*, 140, 111–7.

Cox J. L., Connor Y., Henderson I., *et al.* (1983) Prospective study of the psychiatric disorders of childbirth by self report questionnaire. *Journal of Affective Disorders*, 5, 1–7.

Cox J. L., Rooney A., Thomas P. F., Wrate R. W. (1984). How accurately do mothers recall postnatal depression? Further data from a 3 year follow-up study. *Journal of Psychosomatic Obstetrics and Gynaecology*, 3, 185–9.

Cox J. L., Holden J. M., Sagovsky R. (1987). Detection of postnatal depression: development of the 10-item Edinburgh postnatal depression scale (EPDS). *British Journal of Psychiatry*, 150, 782–6.

Criminal Law Revision Committee (1980). 14th Report. *Offences against the Person?* London: HMSO.

Dean C. (1989). *Childbirth as a Life Event* Symposium Proceedings (Cox J. L., Paykel E. S., Page M. L. eds). Southampton: *Duphar Medical Relations Publications*.

Dean C., Kendell R. E. (1981). The symptomatology of puerperal illnesses. *British Journal of Psychiatry*, 139, 128.

Dean C., Surtees P. G., Sashidharan S. P. (1983). Comparison of research diagnostic systems in an Edinburgh community sample. *British Journal of Psychiatry*, 142, 247–56.

Dowlatashi D., Paykel E. S. (1989). *Childbirth as a Life Event* Symposium Proceedings (Cox J. L., Paykel E. S., Page M. L. eds.). Southampton: *Duphar Medical Relations Publications*.

Goldberg D. P., Cooper B., Eastwood M. R., *et al.* (1970). A standardised psychiatric interview for use in community surveys. *British Journal of Preventive and Social Medicine*, 24, 18–23.

Hamilton J. A. (1962). *Post-partum Psychiatric problems*. St. Louis: C. V. Mosby.

Harris B., Huckle P., Johns S., *et al.* (1989). The use of rating scales to identify postnatal depression. *British Journal of Psychiatry* (in press).

Holden J. M., Sagovsky R., Cox J. L. (1989). Counselling in a general practice setting: a controlled study of health visitor intervention in the treatment of postnatal depression. *British Medical Journal*, **298**, 223–6.

Karnosh L. J., Hope J. M. (1937). Puerperal psychoses and their sequelae. *American Journal of Psychiatry*, **84**, 537–50.

Kendell R. E., Chalmers L., Platz C. (1987). The epidemiology of puerperal psychoses. *British Journal of Psychiatry*, **150**, 662–73.

Kumar R. (1982). Neurotic disorders in childbearing women. In *Motherhood and Mental Illness* (Brockington I. F., Kumar R., eds.). London: Academic Press.

Kumar R., Robson K. M. (1984). A prospective study of emotional disorders in childbearing women. *British Journal of Psychiatry*, **144**, 35–47.

Marcé L. V. (1858). *Traite de la fiole des femmes enceintes des nouvelles accouches et des nourrices*. Paris: Bailliere.

Montgomery S. A., Asberg M. (1979). A new depression scale designed to be sensitive to change. *British Journal of Psychiatry*, **134**, 382–9.

Murray L. (1988). Effects of postnatal depression on infant development: Direct studies of early mother-infant intervention. *Motherhood and Mental Illness* 2 (Kumar R., Brockington I. F.,eds.) London: Wright.

Murray D., Cox J. L. (1988). *Detection of antenatal depression. Validation of the Edinburgh Depression Scale (EPDS)*. Paper presented at 4th International Scientific Meeting of the Marcé Society.

Nott P. N., Cutts S. (1982). Validation of the 30-item General Health questionnaire in postpartum women. *Psychological Medicine*, **12**, 409–13.

Nott P. N. (1987). Extent, timing and persistence of emotional disorders following childbirth. *British Journal of Psychiatry*, **151**, 523–7.

Oates M. (1988). The development of an integrated community orientated service for severe postnatal mental illness. In *Motherhood and Mental Illness* (Kumar R., Brockington I. F., eds.). London: Wright.

O'Hara M. W. (1989). Childbirth as a life event: stressful but not negative. In *Childbirth as a Life Event* (Cox J. L., Paykel E. S., Page M. L., eds.). Southampton: *Duphar Medical Relations Publications*.

O'Hara M. W., Rehm L. P., Campbell S. B. (1983). Postpartum depression: a role for social network and life stress variables. *Journal of Nervous and Mental Disease*, **171**, 336–41.

O'Hara M. W., Varner M. W., Johnson S. R. (1986). Assessing stressful life events associated with childbearing: the peripartum events scale. *Journal of Reproductive and Infant Psychology*, **4**, 85–98.

Paykel E. S., Emms E. M., Fletcher J., Rassaby E. S. (1980). Life Events and social support in puerperal depression. *British Journal of Psychiatry*, **136**, 339–46.

Pitt B. (1968). 'Atypical' depression following childbirth. *British Journal of Psychiatry*, **114**, 1325–35.

Platz C., Kendell R. E. (1988). Matched control follow-up and family study of puerperal psychoses. *British Journal of Psychiatry*, **153**, 90–4.

Raskin A., Schulterbrandt J., Reatig N., McKison J. (1970). Differential response to chlorpromazine, imipramine and placebo. A study of subgroups of hospitalised depressed patients. *Archives of General Psychiatry*, **23**, 164–73.

Seel R. M. (1986). Birth rite. *Health Visitor*, **59**, 182–4.

Snaith R. P. (1981). Rating Scales. *British Journal of Psychiatry*, **138**, 512–4.

Snaith R. P. (1983). Pregnancy-related psychiatric disorder. *British Journal of Hospital Medicine*, **29**, 450–6.

Snaith R. P., Constantopoulos A. A., Jardine M. Y., McGuffin P. (1978). A clinical scale for the self-assessment of irritability. *British Journal of Psychiatry*, **132**, 164–71.

Watson J. P., Elliott S. A. M., Rugg A. J., Brough D. I. (1984). Psychiatric disorder in pregnancy and the first postnatal year. *British Journal of Psychiatry*, **144**, 453–62.

World Health Organization (1978). *Ninth Revision of the International Classification of Diseases: Mental Disorders.* Geneva: World Health Organization.

9 *Depression in the elderly*

ELAINE MURPHY

CONCEPTS OF DEPRESSION IN OLD AGE

Old age is commonly regarded as the season of sorrow and despair. Depression in the elderly has frequently been perceived as a predictable, understandable response to the losses and declines in the last period of life and the wintry themes of ageing and sadness have been closely linked in literature. We know now, however, that the majority of elderly people do not feel depressed, unhappy or unfulfilled and that the pessimism with which many young people regard their future old age is mainly the result of stereotyped misconceptions.

It is important not to exaggerate the extent of depression in the elderly population. Nevertheless, the minority of people who develop severe and significant depression impose a substantial demand for treatment and care. Even though health and social service professionals see only the tip of the iceberg in terms of proportions of the total number of depressed people who exist in the community, those who do reach professionals make a heavy demand on their services. Jolley and Arie (1976) reported that 40 per cent of all referrals to a comprehensive district psychiatric service for the elderly were for depression. Patients requiring in-patient treatment are heavy users of psychiatric beds. Over a 4-year period from 1978 to 1982, one quarter of all the acute beds available in one large psychiatric hospital serving an East London catchment area were occupied by elderly patients with depression (Murphy and Grundy, 1984). It is the chronic and recurrent nature of severe depressions in old age which determines the extensive demand on services.

In spite of the impact of depression on the sufferer and their family, the condition is frequently overlooked or dismissed. The symptoms are easily confused with organic physical symptoms or regarded as an understand-able and untreatable response to the inevitable life stresses of later life. The importance of recognizing the symptoms of depression lies in the fact that the condition is treatable by a variety of medical and social measures and, in general, an isolated episode carries a favourable prognosis for recovery.

CHARACTERISTICS OF DEPRESSION IN OLD AGE

The clinical features of major depressive disorder are generally the same as in younger people. However, the mood disturbance sometimes presents features which may lead the diagnostician astray. Depressed mood is frequently not the main presenting symptom and may be overshadowed by somatic complaints, delusional beliefs, bizarre behaviour disturbances or a picture resembling dementia.

Major depressive disorders in the elderly frequently present in florid form, with significant weight loss, characteristic sleep disturbance and early morning waking. Psychomotor agitation and retardation are common, seen as restless pacing, wringing of the hands, clinging, importuning, begging for help, which engenders a feeling of irritation in those around. At the same time, the sufferer often feels slowed up, unable to think as fast as usual and answers questions in a retarded monosyllabic and distracted fashion. Cognitive changes are usual; loss of concentration and muddled thinking give the appearance of confusion. This, together with a lack of energy, prevents the sufferer completing the simplest task effectively, often interpreted by the patient and sometimes by relatives as evidence of 'laziness' or, even more distressing, as signs of senility and dementia. Delusions of guilt, poverty, nihilism, severe illness, venereal disease, punishment and impending death are often accompanied by somatic complaints of inability to swallow, blocked bowels and a feeling that the insides are rotting or diseased.

The classic presentation of an agitated depressive psychosis described here is characteristic of a severe illness seen in a cohort of elderly people born around the turn of the last century. The best description in the psychiatric literature of affective psychosis of this type was written by Aubrey Lewis (1934), describing his young patients in their 20s, 30s and 40s. We are now seeing the same cohort of patients in their old age (Lewis, 1934). The psychopathology of future generations of elderly people may take a different form.

Depressive stupor

Retardation may be so severe that the patient appears stuporose, immobile, silent (akinetic mutism). A clue to the diagnosis is the determined rejection of food and drink, the alert sometimes frightened eyes and lack of neurological signs. The mortality rate of depressive stupor in old age is very high because of the rapid dehydration and risk of subsequent pneumonia. Rehydration and electroconvulsive therapy (ECT) may not only be life-saving but can be curative.

Milder forms of depressive illness

Not all depressions are severe, however, and milder forms of major depressive disorders, presenting with querulous irritability, anxious clinging and apprehensive pessimism may be difficult to spot. Such elderly people are at risk of being labelled as having 'just personality problems' or 'getting crabby in old age'. Mistakes are easy to avoid if a good history is taken. Usually a time of change from previous normal agreeable personality can be clearly established. There is some evidence that in the USA, depressed elderly people are less likely to express ideas of guilt than younger people (Small *et al.*, 1986) but this has yet to be explored in Europe.

Depression may also present as acute phobic anxiety, usually an intense fear of being alone, with complaints of desperate loneliness and fear. Someone who may have adjusted to years of widowhood and living alone will suddenly become determined to stay close to relatives or friends, needing constant reassurance and continuous company.

Minor depression is much commoner than the florid major depressions—up to five times as common in some surveys (Blazer and Williams, 1980; Gurland *et al.*, 1983). Where depressed mood is not accompanied by biological symptoms, it has sometimes been referred to as 'dysphoria' to distinguish the condition from 'real' depressive disorders. There is no clear borderline between normal unhappiness, as a reaction to life's circumstances, and mild depression as an illness, although attempts have been made to distinguish the two (Gillis and Zabow, 1982). It is probably more useful to regard depressions as falling along a spectrum of disorder with a hierarchy of symptomatology which aids definition of the disorder more clearly as the number of symptoms and severity of the disorder increases (Wing *et al.*, 1974; Gurland *et al.*, 1983).

Distinguishing depression from dementia: 'pseudodementia'

The majority of elderly depressed patients show no evidence of impaired intellect or cognitive decline which is not immediately apparent as a direct consequence of concentration difficulties. Depressed old people frequently complain of poor memory and fears of intellectual decline but, on psychometric testing, performance on tests of immediate and delayed recall do not differ significantly from normal elderly people (Popkin *et al.*, 1982). So common is the complaint of memory problems among depressed elderly people that 15 percent of elderly people referred to a memory clinic for the investigation of early dementia were found to have a diagnosis of depression (Philpot and Levy, 1987).

However, a small but important minority of elderly people with depression present a confused, withdrawn picture which is very difficult to distinguish from dementia. Psychological testing reveals numerous patchy gaps and lowered performance scores which are difficult to interpret. Computerized axial tomography (CAT scan) may be equally unhelpful—a finding of mild cortical atrophy being of little significance. The syndrome of 'pseudodementia' is overdiagnosed and tends to feature in referrals from non-specialists who have not taken sufficient trouble to interview the patient at length to draw out the depressive symptoms which are clearly obvious to the trained person. The rare cases which present real difficulty in diagnosis have been studied by a number of authors (Wells, 1979; Rabins *et al.*, 1984; Thielman and Blazer, 1986). Previous history of depression, rapid onset, variable psychometric performance, all point to a diagnosis of depression. It has been suggested that temporary impairment of cognitive functions may indicate some underlying unspecified cerebral organic disorder, consequent upon ageing, which perhaps affects the physiological arousal mechanisms, and further that this impairment predisposes the patient to depression and recurrences of depression in old age. However, the memory and learning impairments found in elderly people with depression have been shown to be qualitatively different from those seen in the dementias of old age (Whitehead, 1974; Miller and Lewis, 1977).

The commonest reason accounting for a puzzling mixed picture is that the patient has both depression and dementia occurring at the same time. This is said to occur more frequently with multi-infarct dementia (Roth, 1983), although a review of the evidence that mood changes occur more frequently in multi-infarct than in Alzheimer's type of dementia did not support this opinion (Liston and La Rue, 1983).

Hypochondriasis and pain

Hypochondriasis affects approximately two-thirds of elderly depressed people (De Alarcon, 1964) and somatic complaints in general are more commonly found than in younger patients (Gurland, 1976; Zemore and Eames, 1979). The predominance of somatic complaints, frequently compounded by the presence of real physical illness, can mislead the diagnostician when mood is not also obviously lowered. Pain of a persistent, unpleasant, unbearable quality which is difficult to pin down to a precise anatomical location is a common symptom of depression which carries a rather poor prognosis for treatment if it has been going on for many months or years. Physical facial pain is a variant which perhaps carries a better prognosis if vigorously treated (Feinmann *et al.*, 1984).

Depression presenting as behaviour disturbance

Behaviour problems of a wide variety of kinds are frequently symptoms of depression in elderly people who are heavily dependent on others for their day-to-day care. This happens, for example, in residential care, long-stay hospitals, or where the elderly person is living with younger members of the family with whom they have a longstanding difficult relationship. Depressive behavioural problems often occur in the setting of mild intellectual impairment and there is a danger then that the sufferer will be regarded as having advanced dementia. Food refusal and wilful starvation, inappropriate urinary and faecal incontinence with faecal smearing of walls and furniture are reminiscent of the young child with a behaviour disorder. Persistent intermittent blood-curdling screaming, especially at night, frequently denied by the elderly person, seems usually to occur in response to anxious panic as a demand for instant help. In Old People's Homes, the person who has recurrent apparently wilful 'falls' of throwing herself on the floor in a theatrical fashion, the person who has recently 'fallen out' with all the other residents, the person who has begun to bite and scratch the caring staff, or become 'a management problem' should all be suspected of having a depressive disorder.

Depression then can be a rather chameleon-like disorder in elderly people, which is easily overlooked when the mood itself is not obviously sad or distressed. The key to diagnosis is a history of change in the person's mental state coming on over some days or weeks or a month or two rather than years. If there is any doubt about the diagnosis and the condition is of a severity to warrant pharmacological intervention, a good trial of anti-depressant medication is justified and frequently rewarded by a remarkable reversal of bizarre symptoms.

EPIDEMIOLOGY OF DEPRESSION IN OLD AGE

The epidemiology of psychiatric disorders in elderly people living at home and in residential institutions has received a good deal of attention over the past 15 years. A comprehensive and perhaps more optimistic picture is emerging of the distribution of depressions among the general population of elderly people. A clinician tends to see as patients people who are not only at the severest end of the spectrum of depressive disorders but also at the height of the disorder. It is difficult for a specialist to gain a broad perspective of the time course of the illness. Even the primary-care physician, who has a better opportunity to observe the waxing and waning of a disorder over some years, may only have regular contact with a patient during the 'down' periods. Populations of elderly people must be studied systematically to gain a clear picture of the prevalence and natural history of disorders of differing severities.

The major problem which has beset psychiatric epidemiologists has been the definition of what constitutes a 'case' of depression. As depressed mood is an entirely appropriate response to unhappy circumstances and older people may carry a large burden of losses, social difficulties and health problems likely to cause sadness and unhappiness, studies in which a case has been identified merely by depressed mood may be expected to give a higher prevalence of the disorder among elderly people than younger people. This has indeed been the result of studies with these low-threshold criteria, using self-rating scales or standard questionnaires (Zung, 1967; Srole and Fischer, 1980). Clinically this does not have much meaning because the majority of dysphoric elderly people would not be considered appropriate for medical and/or social intervention. However, society at large should perhaps be concerned that elderly people are often dissatisfied and unhappy.

Clinical epidemiologists concerned to seek out cases similar in severity to those seen in clinical practice have used different approaches to psychiatric case definition. This has given rise to problems in comparing results between studies. On the one hand, a quantitative symptom threshold assigns caseness on the basis of a predefined arbitrary cut off level. Most community-based surveys of elderly populations have used global rating scales of psychiatric impairment (For example, the OARS community survey; Blazer, 1978) and the US/UK community survey (Gurland *et al.*, 1983).

The alternative approach is to have clearly defined operational criteria for specified case diagnosis. In this method, signs and symptoms are elicited by interviewers who are highly trained to rate reliably the answers to questions on a structured interview schedule. The ratings are then used to generate diagnoses for specific classification systems. For example the Diagnostic Interview Schedule (DIS) designed by Robins *et al.* (1981) has been extensively used in the United States in a number of studies sponsored by the National Institute of Mental Health, the Epidemiological Catchment Area (ECA) programme. It generates diagnoses using DSM III criteria (American Psychiatric Association, 1980).

These two approaches both have the advantage that studies using these methods can be compared with one another. Urban/rural and international comparisons can be made, allowing us for the first time to examine and test aetiological risk theories between different populations.

What have we learnt so far from studies using these standardized methods? The most surprising finding of all studies, contrasting with stereotyped views of old age, has been that the prevalence rates amongst elderly people for most non-organic mental disorders are in fact similar to, or even slightly lower than other stages of the life cycle (Gurland, 1976; Myers *et al.*, 1984). Recent work in Nottingham suggests a steady prevalence of significant depression of about 10 percent of all age groups among elderly people living at home (Morgan *et al.*, 1987).

Epidemiological surveys of elderly people are made more difficult by the fact that psychiatric morbidity is an important reason for entering permanent residential care, so it is important to include an appropriate sample of those living in institutions—hospitals, nursing homes and retirement homes. This is not always straightforward because of geographical mobility at the time of entering residential care. Some surveys have included those in residential care, others have specifically excluded them and results should be interpreted accordingly.

Table 9.1 shows the prevalence rates of depressive disorders in some recent community surveys. The sex difference in prevalence between men and women is maintained throughout life, women having rates approxi-

Table 9.1 Prevalence rates of depressive disorders in community surveys

Author	Population	Diagnostic method	Findings
Bollerup (1975)	70-year-old cohort study, Copenhagen	Psychiatric interview	1.1% severe depressions requiring psychiatric treatment
Weissman and Myers (1978)	66 + years New Haven, Connecticut	SADS–L structured interview to elicit Research Diagnostic Criteria	5.4% 'major depression': 2.7% 'minor depression'
Blazer and Williams (1980)	65 + years South Eastern US county	OARS depression scale	14.7% 'significant dysphoria'
Gurland et al. (1983)	65 + years, community sample, London and New York	Structured interview; CARE	'Pervasive depression'— 13% New York: 12.4% London
Myers et al. (1984)	65 + years ECA program, community + institutions; 6-month prevalence; New Haven, Baltimore, St. Louis, North Carolina	DIS interview, DSM III criteria	'Major depression' 1.9–3.5%: 'Dysthymia 2.1–3.8%
Morgan et al. (1987)	65 + years, home sample Nottingham	SAD scale, cut-off—6, depression subscale—4: validation by clinical interview	'Depression' 65–74 yrs. 10% 75–79 yrs. 8.9% 80 + yrs. 10.2%

mately 50 percent above that for men. However, the peak prevalence for women falls in the middle years whereas studies suggest that rates for men rise throughout life.

Depression in institutions

Only a small minority of elderly people are permanently resident in hospitals and homes. The proportion of elderly people in institutional care varies from 6 percent in the UK to 12 percent in The Netherlands. It is increasingly recognized that mentally alert residents and those with mild dementias have a markedly higher rate of depression than those living at home in the community. A survey of residents in old people's homes in one London borough found 38 percent had the kind of pervasive depression that was found in only 13 percent of the community-dwelling elderly in the same city (Mann *et al.*, 1984a). The rate in London homes was significantly higher than in similar institutions in New York and Mannheim, Germany but even in those cities the rate was higher than might be expected (Mann *et al.*, 1984b). It is possible that the drab quality of life provided in many residential homes is one reason for the high prevalence, but it is also possible that chronically depressed elderly people are preferentially selected into residential care as a result of their dependence on others and failure to cope adequately alone at home. This hypothesis is currently under investigation in residential homes in Mannheim and London.

The picture overall in the general population of elderly is that moderate severities of depressive disorder are common, but no more common than in any other age group. First-admission rates to psychiatric hospitals for more severe depressions are also not markedly different in the older age groups (Murphy and Grundy, 1984). Recurrent admissions are more common in elderly people, however. Furthermore, there is a good deal of general unhappiness and 'low spirits' amongst elderly people in Western countries which though not reaching a level of clinical significance, nevertheless draws attention to the less than ideal circumstances of many elderly people.

BIOLOGICAL FACTORS IN CAUSATION

It has long been postulated that cerebral ageing may play a part in the aetiology of depression arising for the first time in old age.

Neurotransmitter changes

Studies have focused mainly on noradrenaline and serotonin, the transmitters known to be implicated in depression. Robinson *et al.* (1972) demonstrated that normal people have an age-related decreased concentration of these two neurotransmitters in the hindbrain but 5-HIAA (5-hydroxyindole acetic acid) and MAO (monoamine oxidase) increased with age, the increase in MAO being greater in women. It is tempting to suggest that these changes might predispose elderly people to depression or perhaps attenuate the healing effects of antidepressants and promote chronic illness.

Post mortem studies of the brains of depressed people have not revealed consistent changes in brain noradrenaline or of metabolites. However, decreased levels of serotonin and 5-HIAA have been found in the raphe nuclei of suicide victims (Lloyd *et al.*, 1974) and many studies have reported a lowered cerebrospinal fluid level of 5-HIAA in depressed patients. It has been proposed (Janowsky *et al.*, 1972) that affective disorders result from an imbalance between the noradrenergic and the cholinergic systems, depression occurring when the cholinergic system is dominant and the noradrenergic system depleted.

Neuroendocrine changes—the dexamethasone suppression test (DST)

High circulating levels of cortisol in depressed patients usually return to normal when the patient recovers and thus the high levels of cortisol are linked to the episode of depression itself.

Dexamethasone is a synthetic steroid which results in the suppression of cortisol in the normal subject for up to 24 hours. A positive or abnormal test is one in which the serum cortisol fails to suppress. Several factors interfere with the DST and give false positive results—for example, serious medical illness (especially diabetes), severe infections, significant weight loss, some drugs such as benzodiazepines, and withdrawal from alcohol and other psychotropic drugs. Perhaps most unfortunately for the specialist working with the elderly, 50 percent of dementia sufferers also have a positive test (Raskind *et al.*, 1982; Coppen *et al.*, 1983). Carroll (1982) has claimed that the DST provides a specific laboratory test for melancholia but others are less sanguine about its specificity or indeed whether it will prove to be useful at all as a diagnostic or prognostic aid.

Dexamethasone suppression is influenced by age, depressed elderly people being rather more likely to have abnormal results than younger people. However dexamethasone may not be fully absorbed during the test in elderly people, leading to spuriously high results (Rosenbaum *et al.*, 1984). The uses of the DST in elderly people are few. Certainly it will not help in distinguishing depression from dementia. However, it may be helpful in monitoring the progress of treatment. Although most patients with DST-positive depression return to having a normal DST after treatment, a few do not. These 'continuing non-suppressors' are said to have a worse prognosis even when they do make a clinical recovery (Georgotas *et al.*, 1984).

Neuroradiological changes

The advent of CAT has brought a safe and non-invasive method of imaging the brain. There are changes in the brain with age in 15 percent of elderly people who have no evidence of psychiatric disorder; cortical atrophy and ventricular enlargement are the most common changes reported (Laffey *et al.*, 1984). A longitudinal study of the normal elderly population found 16 percent had increased ventricular size at first assessment and a further 10 percent had enlarged ventricles at follow-up at an average 2.5 years later. Ventricular enlargement was correlated with reduced scores on cognitive tests, as one might expect. However, there was also a higher than expected number of subjects with enlarged ventricles in the 9 percent of the total sample who developed depression during the follow-up study (Bird *et al.*, 1986). However, this contrasts with the findings of Jacoby and Levy (1980), who found no difference in the proportion of depressed elderly patients with enlarged ventricles when compared with age-matched controls. However, the 9 out of 41 depressed elderly people who did have enlarged ventricles were described as clinically dissimilar from other depressed patients, being on the whole older, and having more features of endogenous, retarded depression. At follow-up two years later, 5 of the 9 with the enlarged ventricles were dead compared with only 4 of the 31 depressed with normal ventricles, suggesting that ventricular enlargement may influence the course of depression.

The same investigators found that regional brain densities recorded on CAT scan of depressed elderly patients were intermediate between that of normals and those with dementia (Jacoby *et al.*, 1983), although at present the significance of this finding is unknown. It may be linked to the presence of cerebrovascular disease. The nature of the relationship between vascular disease generally and depression is unclear but many authors have suspected a close link. Kay (1962) found a higher than expected rate of cerebrovascular disease as the attributed cause on death certificates in a mental hospital population diagnosed as having 'functional psychosis'. There is further evidence from the very high incidence of depression after stroke. Up to 60 percent of patients may develop some form of depression following stroke (Robinson *et al.*, 1984). Robinson claimed that depression was commoner in patients with lesions in the left frontal pole compared with right-sided lesions. However, further studies of stroke patients admitted to hospitals (Ebrahim *et al.*, 1987) have not repeated these findings on side of lesion although they do support the very high rate of depression following stroke.

There is further support of the link between cerebrovascular disease and depression from cerebral blood-flow studies. Cerebral blood flow falls during depression in young healthy subjects (Mathew *et al.*, 1980) and glucose metabolism has also been reported as decreased in some regions, on Positron Emission Tomography (PET) scan (Phelps *et al.*, 1984). Whether these findings are linked to the chronicity and high recurrence rate of depression in elderly people is as yet unexplored.

Neurophysiology studies

Both visual- and auditory-evoked potentials have been demonstrated to be delayed in elderly depressed subjects (Hendrickson *et al.*, 1979; Litzelman *et al.*, 1980). These changes do not return to normal after clinical recovery, suggesting an enduring cerebral organic defect.

There are many biological parameters which have been demonstrated to be abnormal in depressed elderly people. Ageing per se produces some of these changes and it appears that ageing may itself produce changes to explain the onset of depression in old age in some individuals. We do not yet know, however, which individuals are at risk because of cerebral biological factors or indeed if these changes are merely a reflection of changes which are a consequence of depression rather than a cause.

PHYSICAL ILLNESS AND DEPRESSION

Many authors have commented on the close association between physical ill health and depression in old age.

The implications of the high physical morbidity in patients with depression

The majority of elderly people presenting to their family doctors or referred on to psychiatrists with depression have substantial physical health problems. These problems are often chronic, degenerative disorders where the symptoms may be improved or controlled by the right medical treatment, but will continue to be a major long-term problem for the patient to cope with. Vigilance is needed to spot depression accompanying chronic ill health but also vigilance is needed on the part of the psychiatrist to detect and treat relevant physical health problems. Close working of psychiatrists and physicians with a special interest in the elderly is essential and joint assessment units staffed by both specialists teams can make the treatment of patients with a complex mix of physical and psychiatric disorder considerably easier.

PSYCHOSOCIAL FACTORS IN CAUSATION

Health, vigour and the well-being of the elderly have more to do with economics and social organization than with the biological inevitability of the laws of nature. Many of the problems of the elderly are susceptible to change by social evolution and political intervention. The exploration of how and to what degree social factors are responsible for mental disorder in old age, especially depression, is therefore of great importance as it has implications for prevention.

Few concepts in psychiatry have been pursued with such enthusiasm over the last 20 years as the notion that adverse factors in the social environment lead to mental illness and to depression in particular. To the lay public, a causal relationship is a foregone conclusion especially for the elderly. It is certainly true that in Western societies, older people do form a socially underprivileged group. They are in general poorer, more likely to live alone and to occupy the worst housing. They have more physical illness and are consequently less mobile, more likely to have poor sight and impaired hearing. Reduction of income, loss of status and sometimes of a useful role are commonplace events in old age. All this is not in doubt. But what empirical evidence is there that low social class, poverty, isolation or the loss events of old age really contribute to the onset of serious depressive illness?

Social models of depression use psychological constructs to explain the origin of depressive disorder. The models postulate that interpersonal and social events external to the individual have an impact on the individual's emotions sufficient to lead to depression. The experience of depression can be traced to the perception of these events, often reflecting the emotional and cognitive reactions of the individual to events in the remote past, usually in early childhood. This model in no way excludes the biological perspective and a comprehensive understanding of the aetiology of depression will need to incorporate both dimensions.

Life events

There are major methodological problems in life-event research which cannot be gone into in great detail here. Recent methods devised by Brown and Harris (1978) provide a sophisticated way of overcoming the major problems (see Chapter 2). Murphy (1982) used this method to examine the recent life events, chronic difficulties and quality of confiding relationships in a study of two groups of depressed subjects who had experienced an onset of depression in the last year. The patients were compared with a group of normal elderly subjects in the general population. The depressed subjects were from two groups: the first consisted of 100 elderly patients referred to psychiatric services for the elderly in east London, a relatively socially-deprived area of the inner city and its adjacent suburbs. In addition to the 100 patients there were 19 subjects in a general population sample who had experienced an onset of depression in the past year. The comparison group was 168 elderly subjects interviewed in the general population who were found to be free of psychiatric disorder at interview.

The findings of this study were very similar to those of Brown and Harris (1978) for younger subjects. Forty-eight percent of depressed patients and 68 percent of depressed community subjects had experienced a severe life event in the year preceding onset compared with only 23 percent of the normal group. The types of severe event which were commoner in depressed subjects were the death of a spouse or child, serious personal physical illness, life-threatening illness to someone close, severe financial loss and enforced change of residence as a result of a demolition programme. Major social difficulties, lasting two years or more, were also significantly associated with depression.

A notable difference between Brown's findings for younger subjects and Murphy's findings was the predicted conspicuous role of chronic poor physical health problems and grave personal health events in older depressed subjects. The overall risk of developing an onset of depression in the year for the total general population sample was approximately 10 percent. For those in good health with no major social problems and no recent severe events, the risk was only 2.5 percent, while the risk in the presence of one of these factors was 16 percent.

Social circumstances and the events of a person's life do then seem to play an important role in depression. However, caution must be used in applying these research findings to individual clinical cases. Almost a quarter of the normal elderly population experienced an event which did not lead to depression, so in a given clinical case it is impossible to be sure that a reported event is causal or not or whether it has occurred coincidentally.

Critics of life-events research have pointed out that the magnitude of the effect of events on the causation of depression may be quite small. Paykel (1982) attempted a hypothetical calculation of the risk of developing depression after a severe event and estimated that the risk was similar in order to the risk of developing clinical tuberculosis after exposure to the bacillus. Just as tuberculosis affects a vulnerable group among those who have contact with the bacillus, we must look for vulnerability factors which predispose individuals to depressive breakdown following life stress.

Social isolation

In Murphy's study (see above), vulnerability to adverse life events, and poor health and major social problems were three times as high in those elderly who reported having no intimate confiding relationship. The question of how the quantity and quality of social relationships predisposes or protects from depression is a complex one in which research is fraught with methodological problems. Most authors are now agreed that simply living alone, or having relatively few daily contacts is not especially disadvantageous for risk of developing depression. Furthermore, depressed people of all ages are more likely to report feeling lonely and unsupported, but elderly people do not report more loneliness than younger age groups. The evidence is that the perceived quality of relationships and their perceived adequacy are the key factors emerging from most studies. It is likely that life-long personality adjustment and the capacity to form good social relationships are very important variables affecting vulnerability.

Social factors and biological factors tend to be studied separately by clinicians, psychologists and social scientists pursuing their own particular area of interest in isolation. The time has come to combine these two approaches if we are to make headway in developing a more comprehensive model of the aetiology of depression.

PHYSICAL METHODS OF TREATMENT

Drug therapy

Recent reviews by Veith (1982) and Busse and Simpson (1983) have concluded that there is little evidence to recommend any single drug as being more effective than any other in the elderly. The choice of medication is usually made on the basis of the physician's experience of a particular drug, the individual patient's ability to tolerate side effects of the traditional tricyclic antidepressants, and the physical health of the patient.

In elderly patients it may well be possible to achieve a therapeutic response with lower doses of the traditional drugs but further studies of other tricyclics are required before any general guidelines can be formulated.

Anticholinergic effects of tricyclic antidepressants are usually the most troublesome in elderly people. Postural hypertension leading to dizziness and falls is possibly the major adverse risk. The risk of cardiotoxicity of these drugs has, however, probably been overstressed. Glassman and Bigger (1981) concluded from a review of the evidence that tricyclic antidepressants are not cardiotoxic at therapeutic levels but that certain patients with abnormalities of intraventricular conduction are at increased risk because tricyclics prolong the PR interval and QRS complexes seen on the electrocardiograph. Veith (1982) found tricyclics to have no significant adverse effect on ventricular function in a group of patients with atherosclerotic or hypertensive heart disease.

The treatment of elderly patients with severe delusional depression presents special problems. The question arises whether to treat with antidepressants alone or whether to add neuroleptic medication. Spiker *et al.* (1985) found a combination of amitryptiline and neuroleptic superior to amitryptiline alone. Monoamineoxidase inhibitors (MAOI) are useful ancillary weapons to have ready in the armoury for a few intractable cases.

The newer antidepressants such as trazodone have been shown to be equally efficacious as imipramine in the elderly and to be well tolerated (Gerner *et al.*, 1980). Similarly, mianserin, a tetracyclic antidepressant, has been shown to be of equal efficacy as amitryptiline in a study of elderly patients by Branconnier *et al.* (1982).

Benzodiazepines have long been used to treat mild depressions and nonspecific neurotic symptoms in primary care. The sedative anxiolytic effects are temporarily comforting, but the long-term disadvantages far outweigh the advantages. The rapidly acquired tolerance leads to increasing doses and marked physical dependence. Psychiatric services for the elderly are seeing increasing numbers of elderly people who have developed serious dependence on diazepam, lorazepam and the shorter-acting hypnotics—temazepam and triazolam. These drugs are not antidepressant and should only be used sparingly in very short courses as an adjunct to antidepressant therapy where severe anxiety and insomnia are not alleviated by a sedative antidepressant.

The use of lithium as a prophylactic against recurrent unipolar depression has not been explored specifically for elderly people but those studies that have included some elderly suggest that it may be useful (Coppen *et al.*, 1983). It is of proven value in the prophylaxis of bipolar manic depressive illness and there is no evidence of a fall-off of efficacy of lithium with age (Murray *et al.*, 1983). However, elderly people are more liable to lithium toxicity and plasma levels should probably be maintained at between 0.4 percent to 0.7 meg/l to avoid toxicity (Jefferson, 1983).

Electroconvulsive therapy (ECT)

Elderly people with severe depressions have long been regarded as good candidates for ECT. ECT can undoubtedly be dramatically effective treatment for a severely retarded depressed person who may be gradually starving to death and refusing fluid. The relapse rate of such illnesses is high but with good prophylaxis established with antidepressants or lithium, the risk of relapse may be diminished.

PSYCHOLOGICAL APPROACHES TO TREATMENT

The provision of emotional support by professionals and relatives during treatment for depression is essential. Depressed elderly patients feel a burden to others, a failure, a nuisance, highly self-critical and selfish. The continued interest of a doctor or a specially trained nurse helps to counteract the feelings of low self-esteem, if the support is given regularly and predictably at a time convenient to the patient. The patient's family also need support. They need to be told what depression is, why their relative appears to be so anxious, irritable, clinging, 'impossible'. Relatives need to learn that depression is treatable and that recovery will eventually take place. Unhelpful responses from relatives are sometimes amenable to education and regular reassurance.

Psychotherapies with the elderly have not yet been subjected to the same research evaluation as the drug therapies and are likely to find little general favour until there is better evidence of their efficacy.

PROGNOSIS, COURSE AND OUTCOME

The introduction of ECT and specific antidepressant drugs have undoubtedly had a major impact on the short-term outcome of major depressive disorders in old age. In spite of the difficulties encountered in treatment, the majority of patients will respond well to treatment within a month (Jarvik *et al.*, 1982), although a third will not respond very satisfactorily. However, the long-term course of depression in old age seems rather less optimistic than for younger people and there has been remarkably little improvement in long-term outcome over the past 15 years.

Mortality

The mortality of patients with depression has been consistently found to be higher than expected when compared with the general population. Kay

(1962) followed a cohort of elderly depressed patients admitted to the Stockholm Psychiatric Clinic between 1931 and 1937 until death or until mid-1956. He found that they had had a mortality rate of twice the expected rate. The increased mortality rate was particularly marked in males (Kay and Bergmann, 1966). The straightforward explanation for this excess mortality is that elderly depressed patients have very poor physical health. However, recently, it has been demonstrated that physical health problems alone do not satisfactorily explain the excess mortality (Murphy *et al.*, in press).

Quality of long-term outcome

There are difficulties in comparing studies of long-term outcome because of differences in judging what constitutes satisfactory outcome, problems in classifying residual symptoms and the choice of subjects studied. The quality of long-term outcome can be most clearly defined and compared in those patients in which recovery is described as a complete return to mental health. Post (1962) recorded a lasting recovery in 27 percent of in-patients admitted around 1950 and followed up to death or up to six years after index admission. In a later study (Post, 1972), 26 percent of a series of patients admitted in 1966 and followed for three years were similarly described as well and lastingly recovered. This similarity in outcome between the two periods of study was interesting because of the introduction of antidepressant drugs between the two series. Fourteen years later, in Murphy's 1979–80 series (Murphy, 1983), 43 percent had made a recovery in a 1-year follow-up and, at four years, this proportion had fallen to 25 percent, a figure very similar to Post's findings. Baldwin and Jolley (1986) reported a rather more optimistic outcome of 58 percent recovered at one year but a similar result over the longer term, using a rather different method of investigation.

The other group it is fairly easy to compare are those who remain chronically, unremittingly ill with depression. Again, the proportions appear to have changed little over the years—17 percent in 1950, 12 percent in 1966 (Post 1962, 1972) and 14 percent in 1979–80 (Murphy, 1983). Modern treatment does not appear to have reduced the hard core of persistently ill patients who make a very heavy demand on social and health services and pose a severe burden on the family.

There is a middle group of between a quarter and a third of patients who, while not remaining severely depressed, do not return to their former good mental health. The biological symptoms remit but the person retains the cognitive and emotional changes of depressed mood. Post (1972) referred to this unsatisfactory outcome as 'residual depressed invalidism', a distressing, fluctuating condition which predisposes to further attacks of the full-blown disorder and which creates enormous social difficulties for the patient and family.

In conclusion, specific treatments appear to have shortened attacks of severe depression and far fewer patients now remain long-term in hospital than in the earlier years of this century. However, a proportion remain seriously depressed for many years, many more have residual problems and only a third have the kind of good recovery which we would like all our patients to achieve.

The clinical importance of these studies in prognosis is that the practice of treating and managing patients and their families should be seen as a potential long-term commitment. Prophylactic medication to prevent relapse may be even more important in older than in younger subjects but, of course, will need close monitoring and supervision. Perhaps more importantly, the after-care arrangements to support those with residual disabilities need very careful thought. Surprisingly little is known about the best way to support such an individual to diminish the chances of relapse. Living accommodation, available social support, day care and respite care for families, and specific case work may all be of importance for certain individuals but evaluation of these various styles of management has so far been poor.

REFERENCES

American Psychiatric Association (1980). *Diagnostic and Statistical Manual of Mental Disorders* 3rd edn. Washington: American Psychiatric Association.
Baldwin R. C., Jolley D. J. (1986). The prognosis of depression in old age. *British Journal of Psychiatry*, **149**, 574–83.
Bird J. M., Levy R., Jacoby R. J. (1986). Computed tomography in the elderly: change over time in the normal population. *British Journal of Psychiatry*, **148**, 80–6.
Blazer D. G. (1978). The OARS Durham Surveys: description and application. In *Multidimensional Functional Assessment: The OARS Methodology* 2nd edn. The Centre for the Study of Ageing and Human Development. Durham: Duke University.
Blazer D. G., Williams C. D. (1980). The epidemiology of dysphoria and depression in an elderly population. *American Journal of Psychiatry*, **137**, 439–44.
Bollerup T. R. (1975). Prevalence of mental illness among 70-year-olds domiciled in nine Copenhagen suburbs: The Glostrup survey. *Acta psychiatrica Scandinavica*, **57**, 327–39.
Branconnier R. J., Cole J. O., Ghazvinian S., Rosenthal S. (1982). Treating the depressed elderly patient: the comparative behavioural pharmacology of mianserin and amitryptiline. *Advances in Biochemistry and Psychopharmacology*, **32**, 195–212.
Brown G. W., Harris T. O. (1978). *Social Origins of Depression*. London: Tavistock.
Busse E., Simpson D. (1983). Depression and antidepressants and the elderly. *Journal of Clinical Psychiatry*, **44**, 35–9.
Carroll B. J. (1982). The dexamethasone suppression test for melancholia. *British Journal of Psychiatry*, **140**, 292–304.

Coppen A., Abou–Saleh M., Miller P., *et al.* (1983). (A) Lithium continuation therapy following ECT. *British Journal of Psychiatry*, **142**, 247–87.

De Alarcon R.D. (1964). Hypochondriasis and depression in the aged. *Gerontologia Clinica*, **6**, 266–77.

Ebrahim S., Barer D., Nouri F. (1987). Affective illness after stroke. *British Journal of Psychiatry*, **151**, 52–6.

Feinmann C., Harris M., Cawley R. (1984). Psychogenic facial pain: presentation and treatment. *British Medical Journal*, **288**, 436–8.

Georgotas A., Stokes P., Krakowski M., *et al.* (1984). Hypothalamic–pituitary–adrenocortical function in geriatric depression. *Biological Psychiatry*, **19**, 685–93.

Gerner R., Estabrook W., Stener J., Jarvik L. (1980). Treatment of geriatric depression with trazodone, imipramine and placebo: a double blind study. *Journal of Chemical Psychiatry*, **41**, 216–20.

Gillis L. S., Zabow A. (1982). Dysphoria in the elderly. *South African Medical Journal*, **62**, 410–3.

Glassman A. H., Bigger J. T. (1981). Cardiovascular effects of therapeutic doses of tricyclic antidepressants. *Archives of General Psychiatry*, **38**, 815–20.

Gurland B. (1976). The comparative frequency of depression in various adult age groups. *Journal of Gerontology*, **31**, 283–92.

Gurland B., Copeland J., Kuriansky J., *et al.* (1983). *The Mind and Mood of Ageing*. London: Croom Helm.

Hendrickson E., Levy R., Post F. (1979). Average evoked responses in relation to cognitive and affective states in elderly psychiatric patients. *British Journal of Psychiatry*, **134**, 494–501.

Jacoby R. J., Levy R. (1980). Computed tomography in the elderly: 3. Affective disorder. *British Journal of Psychiatry*, **136**, 270–5.

Jacoby R. J., Dolan R., Levy R., Baldy J. (1983). Quantitative computed tomography in elderly depressed patients. *British Journal of Psychiatry*, **143**, 124–7.

Janowsky D. S., El–Youset M., Davis J., Serkeske H. (1972). A cholinergic-adrenergic hypothesis of mania and depression. *Lancet*, **2**, 632–5.

Jefferson J. W. (1983). Lithium and affective disorders in the elderly. *Comprehensive Psychiatry*, **24**, 166–78.

Jolley D., Arie T. (1976). Psychiatric services for the elderly: how many beds. *British Journal of Psychiatry*, **129**, 15–28.

Jarvik L. F., Mintz J., Stener J., Geruer R. (1982). Treating geriatric depression: a 26 weeks interim analysis. *Journal of the American Geriatrics Society*, **30**, 713–7.

Kay D. W. K. (1962). Outcome and cause of death in mental disorders of old age: a long term follow up of functional and organic psychoses. *Acta psychiatrica Scandinavica*, **38**, 249–76.

Kay D. W. K., Bergmann K. (1966). Physical disability and mental health in old age. *Journal of Psychosomatic Research*, **10**, 3–12.

Laffey P., Peyster R., Nathan R., *et al.* (1984). Computed tomography and ageing: results in a normal elderly population. *Neuroradiology*, **26**, 2773–8.

Lewis A. (1934). Melancholia; a clinical survey of depressive states. *Journal of Mental Science*, **80**, 277–93.

Liston E. H., LaRue A. (1983). Clinical differentiation of primary degenerative and multi-infarct dementia. *Biological Psychiatry*, **18**, 1451–84.

Litzelman D. K., Thompson L. W., Michaelewski H., *et al.* (1980). Visual event related potentials and depression in the elderly. *Neurobiology of Ageing*, 1, 111–8.

Lloyd K. G., Varley I. J., Deck J., Hornykiewicz O. (1974). Serotonin and 5-HIAA in discrete areas of the brainstem of suicide victims and control patients. In *Serotonin: New Vistas* (Costa, E., Gersa, G., Sandler, M., eds.). New York: Raven Press.

Mann A. H., Graham N., Ashby D. (1984a). Psychiatric illness in residential homes for the elderly: a survey in one London borough. *Age and Ageing*, 13, 257–65.

Mann A. H., Wood K., Cross P., *et al.* (1984b). Institutional care of the elderly: a comparison of the cities of New York, London and Mannheim. *Social Psychiatry*, 19, 97–102.

Mathew L., Meyer J., Semchuk K., *et al.* (1980). Cerebral blood flow in depression. *Lancet*, 1, 1308.

Miller E., Lewis, P. (1977). Recognition memory in elderly patients with dementia and depression: a signal detection analysis. *Journal of Abnormal Psychology*, 86, 84–6.

Morgan K., Dallosso H. M., Arie T., *et al.* (1987). Mental health and psychological well-being among the very old living at home. *British Journal of Psychiatry*, 150, 801–7.

Murphy E. (1982). Social origins of depressions in old age. *British Journal of Psychiatry*, 144, 135–42.

Murphy E. (1983). The prognosis of depression in the elderly. *British Journal of Psychiatry*, 142, 111–9.

Murphy E., Grundy E. (1984). A comparative study of bed usage by younger and older patients with depression. *Psychological Medicine*, 14, 445–50.

Murphy E., Smith E. A. R., Lindesay J. A. B., Slattery J. (1988). Increased mortality rates in late life depression. *British Journal of Psychiatry*, 152, 347–53.

Murray N., Hopwood S., Balfour D., *et al.* (1983). The influence of age on lithium efficacy and side effects in out-patients. *Psychological Medicine*, 13, 53–60.

Myers J. K., Weissman M. M., Tischler G. L., *et al.* (1984). Six month prevalence of psychiatric disorders in three communities. *Archives of General Psychiatry*, 41, 959–67.

Paykel E. S. (1982). Life events and early environment. In *Handbook of Affective Disorders* (Paykel E. S., ed.). London: Churchill Livingstone.

Phelps M. E., Mazziotta J. C., Bastel L., Gernes R. (1984). Positron emission tomography study of affective disorders. *Annals of Neurology*, 15 (suppl.), S149–56.

Philpot M. P., Levy R. (1987). A memory clinic for the early diagnosis of dementia. *International Journal of Geriatric Psychiatry*, 2, 195–200.

Popkin S. J., Gallagher D., Thompson L., Moore M. (1982). Memory complaint and performance in normal and depressed older adults. *Experimental Ageing and Research*, 8, 141–5.

Post F. (1962). *The Significance of Affective Symptoms in Old Age*. Maudsley Monographs 10. London: Oxford University Press.

Post F. (1972). The management and nature of depressive illness in late life: a follow through study. *British Journal of Psychiatry*, 121, 393–404.

Rabins P., Merchant A., Nestradt G. (1984). Criteria for diagnosing reversible dementia caused by depression: validation by two year follow-up. *British Journal of Psychiatry*, **144**, 488–92.

Raskind M., Peskind E., Rivard M., *et al.* (1982). DST and cortisol circadian rhythm in primary degenerative dementia. *American Journal of Psychiatry*, **179**, 1468–71.

Robins L. N., Helzer J., Croughan J., Ratcliff K. S. (1981). National Institute of Mental Health Diagnostic Interview Schedule: its history, characteristics and validity. *Archives of General Psychiatry*, **38**, 381–9.

Robinson D. S., Davies J. M., Nies A. (1972). Ageing monoamines and monoamine oxidase levels. *Lancet*, **1**, 1290.

Robinson R. G., BookStarr L., Price T. R. (1984). A two year longitudinal study of mood disorders following stroke: a six month follow up. *British Journal of Psychiatry*, **144**, 256–62.

Rosenbaum A., Schatzberg A., MacLaughlin M., *et al.* (1984). The DST in normal control subjects: comparison of 2 assays and the effects of age. *American Journal of Psychiatry*, **141**, 1550–5.

Roth M. 1983. Depression and affective disorders in later life. In *The Origins of Depression: Current Concepts and Approaches* (Angst J., ed.). New York: Springer–Verlag.

Small G. W., Komanduri R., Gitlin M., Jarvik, L. F. (1986). The influence of age on guilt expression in major depression. *International Journal of Geriatric Psychiatry*, **1**, 121–6.

Spiker D. G., Weiss J. C., Dealy R. S., *et al.* (1985). The pharmacological treatment of delusional depression. *American Journal of Psychiatry*, **142**, 430–6.

Srole L., Fischer A. K. (1980). The Midtown Manhatten longitudinal study versus the 'Paradise Lost' doctrine. *Archives of General Psychiatry*, **37**, 209–21.

Thielman S., Blazer D. G. (1986). Depression and dementia. In *Dementia in Old Age* (Pitt B., ed.). London: Churchill Livingstone.

Veith R. C. (1982). Depression in the elderly: pharmacological considerations in treatment. *Journal of the American Geriatrics Society*, **30**, 581–6.

Weissman M. M., Myers J. K. (1978). Rates and risks of depressive symptoms in a U.S. urban community. *Acta psychiatrica Scandinavica*, **57**, 219–31.

Wells E. C. (1979). Pseudodementia. *American Journal of Psychiatry*, **131**, 895–900.

Whitehead A. (1974). Factors in the learning defect of elderly depressives. *British Journal of Social and Clinical Psychology*, **13**, 201–8.

Wing J., Cooper J. E., Sartorius N. (1974). *The Measurement and Classification of Psychiatric Symptoms*. London: Oxford University Press.

Zemore R., Eames N. (1979). Psychic and somatic symptoms of depression among young adults, institutionalised aged and non-institutionalised aged. *Journal of Gerontology*, **31**, 283–92.

Zung W. W. K. (1967). Depression in the normal aged. *Psychosomatics*, **8**, 287–92.

SECTION 4

The Management of Depression

10 *Cognitive treatment for depression*

J. MARK G. WILLIAMS

INTRODUCTION

Consider the following statements:

'I haven't the energy to do anything.'
'I know what I ought to do but I can't face doing it.'
'I don't get any pleasure out of being with my friends, they don't want me around.'
'I'm a failure.'
'Everything I do seems to turn out badly.'
'There's nothing to look forward to.'
'I'm useless at everything.'
'I can't concentrate on anything any more.'
'I hate myself.'

These are familiar ideas expressed by depressed people—but what is their causal status in depression? Are they merely symptoms? Recently, several clinical researchers have suggested that although they may indeed arise as symptoms of underlying biological disturbance, they can also play a causal role in depression. If this is true, then therapy directed at changing such thoughts appears plausible. Before going into detail about such treatment, however, let us first describe the ways in which such cognitive factors are ascribed a causal role.

According to Beck's model (1976), for example, these cognitive events (thoughts and images of loss, negative interpretations of ambiguous situations) arise when a stressor activates a long-lasting underlying cognitive structure (a belief, attitude or assumption). These assumptions, such as 'to be happy one must succeed in everything' or 'people who don't work hard at everything are lazy' are not themselves depressive, but in combination with certain situations (for example, a failed exam in the first case; awareness of having not worked at something in the second case) allow a depressive inference to be drawn ('I can't be happy'; 'I am lazy, good for nothing').

According to this cognitive model, the greater the number of these underlying assumptions, the more vulnerable the person will be to becoming depressed as there will be a wider range of stressful situations which will activate one of them. Second, once activated, the underlying depressive structures cause biases in perception and interpretation of current ambiguous situations. Such ambiguity may arise from sources which are external or internal to the person. An example of an external event is when someone does not notice you in the street; the depressed person concludes that this person must not like them. Ambiguity arises from internal sources where, for example, one finds one can't concentrate or can't remember something. The depressed person may conclude that they are dementing. Thoughts and images of loss and rejection predominate.

Finally, by whatever means such negative thoughts, images and interpretations arise, they have subsequent effects on mood and behaviour. Thus, even in cases where such cognitive phenomena are secondary symptoms, they can still play a causal role in *maintaining* the depression once it has started. There is increasing evidence that the length of episode and the probability of relapse is partly a function of how much a mild affective disturbance activates such negative trains of thought (Teasdale, 1988).

In summary, the cognitive model suggests that cognitive structures (beliefs, assumptions) may render a person more *vulnerable* to depression in the face of a stressor; that the combination of assumption and stressor cause a number of cognitive events (ideas of loss) to occur with increased frequency and intensity, which helps to *precipitate* a depressive episode; that whether or not this causal sequence occurs, cognitive factors (depressive interpretations of ambiguous social situations or ambiguous symptoms) may act to *maintain* depression. Note that this model does not suggest that cognitive factors are the sole cause in depression. Rather it sees them as being part of the vicious circle which affects the vulnerability, onset and maintenance of depressive mood and depressive behaviour. Depressed mood can affect cognitions. Cognitions can affect mood. Both cognitive and affective factors can affect behaviour. Each component influences each other. Cognitive therapy brings together a range of techniques which attempt to drive a wedge into this vicious circle by dealing with the cognitive aspect. In this chaper I shall attempt to give a flavour of how this is achieved. Readers who wish to know more may read the work of Beck *et al.* (1979) or Williams (1984).

GENERAL APPROACHES WITHIN THERAPY

If one wishes to intervene at the cognitive level, how should one proceed? Although the therapist may feel that the depressed person is being unduly pessimistic when they say: 'I've got no friends; no one loves me; I'm a failure', simply telling them it is not true, or arguing with them will be of little use. Family, friends and colleagues will have tried to persuade the person that things aren't so black, often to no avail. The problem is that, as far as the person is concerned, they are true. Cognitive therapy therefore tries gradually to loosen the hold such ideas have without making such direct argumentative challenges to the patient. It does so first by systematically assessing and recording the person's thoughts, images and interpretations. Second, it involves forming a collaborative alliance with the person against the 'common enemy' depression, so that, together, patient and therapist can examine the evidence for and against the negative interpretations. Third, patients are taught techniques to help them stand back and evaluate their negative thoughts by themselves, and to come up with some alternative interpretations to situations they are seeing in such a negative way. The keynote atmosphere is collaboration against a background of empathy and warmth. Therapy sessions (and there are usually between 12 and 20 of them, 50 minutes each, over a 3-month period) are structured, and an active coping style is encouraged.

ASSESSMENT

Clearly, at the outset, the therapist will wish to make a thorough assessment of current mental state, family history, current severity of symptoms, and so on. In preparing for cognitive therapy, however, the focus of assessment is then narrowed to examine the interrelationship of thought, affect and behaviour (see Table 10.1). It is useful to supplement this within-session assessment with a daily diary which the patient can complete between sessions. Such a diary can be used to fulfil a number of objectives. First, it can be useful just to record what the patient is doing — and when, in between sessions, they are feeling at their worst. Second, it can be used as evidence that the patient and therapist can look at, within the session, to help evaluate such global negative thoughts as 'I never achieve anything'; 'All I do is sit around all day'. For most people these are inaccurate overgeneralizations, and although they clearly feel they are not achieving as much as they should be achieving, their conclusion that they are actually doing 'nothing' is serving only to exacerbate their mood. A third use of a diary is for the patient, together with the therapist, to assign activities for the next few days or next 24 hours so that they do not have to make a decision in the morning (when the mood is often at its worst) what they are going to do that day. If they have already scheduled some activities the night (or the session) before, this can take the burden of decision away from the periods of time when decisions are most difficult.

Finally, the diary may be used to keep a record of which activities the person finds most pleasurable, and which activities give them a sense of accomplishment. This may be done by asking the patient to put an M or a P against any activity that gave them any sense of mastery (achievement) or pleasure, respectively. For patients who are able to use rating scales they may, in addition, rate each of them on a 0–5 scale. Not all activities that are

Table 10.1 Assessment schedule: this schedule may form the basis of a structured interview which aims to clarify the links between thoughts, feelings and behaviour

Affect	What moods?
	In what situations?
	Other somatic symptoms?
Behaviour	Activities given up or being actively avoided (e.g., social activities, hobbies)?
	Activities which have increased (e.g., lying in bed)?
	Amounts of satisfaction with ongoing activities?
	Concentration or memory failures?
Cognition	Frequency and intensity of:
	negative thoughts and images
	negative interpretation of ambiguous situations
	negative memories of past
	negative predictions for future
	negative underlying assumptions (often later in therapy)

pleasurable give the person a sense of achievement and control over their environment. For example, watching television or listening to music may give the patient some pleasure, but they do not necessarily give the patient a sense of accomplishment (unless they have mended their stereo equipment before listening to the music!). On the other hand, there are some tasks which do not, in themselves, give much pleasure (doing the dishes, mowing the lawn, cleaning a cupboard) but which nevertheless may give a sense that something has been achieved. It is important if patients are to make progress in therapy, for them gradually to increase the number of activities so that there is a balance between activities which give a sense of mastery and a sense of pleasure.

ASSESSING THOUGHTS AND IMAGES

It is sometimes not easy for a patient to grasp exactly what the therapist means by a 'thought' or 'image'. If a depressed person believes that they are a failure or that they have nothing to live for, then as far as they are concerned, this is true. It can take patience and skill for the therapist gradually to begin to enable the patient to see these ideas as merely 'ideas', which may or may not be true. The assessment of thoughts and images has an important role to play, not only in giving vital information about the frequency and intensity of the negative thoughts, but also in allowing the person to begin to distance themselves from them. One method of assessment consists of giving a list of negative thoughts (Williams, 1984; pp. 167–8). The person rates how frequently he or she experiences each of these thoughts, and how intense it is. The therapist can personalize the items, going through the total list with the patient, asking which they have experienced and which they have not. The thoughts they have experienced may then be written on a piece of paper or on cards, which the patient can take home and mark whenever that thought or image occurs. When the patient shows that they are able to identify specific thoughts and images, then they can be encouraged to write them down whenever they occur (*thought catching*).

EVALUATION OF THOUGHTS AS IF THEY WERE HYPOTHESES

This cannot be done until the patient has begun, through *thought catching* within and between sessions, to see the ideas that come into their mind when depressed as just that—ideas, rather than reality. This general notion will have been helped by the assessment diaries in which the person will have noted down the situations in which they have felt depressed, and what ideas ran through their mind at that time. It may have been: 'I'm useless; all I do all day is sit' (in the situation of having sat down for ten minutes after a meal). Or it may be: 'I have no one I can really talk to' (in the situation of having seen two people going down the street laughing with each other). The therapist may then ask the patient what they would have thought if they had not been so depressed. The patient's reply can then be used to help show that their ideas mostly occur when depressed. When the mood is low, not only are these ideas most frequent, but they also feel most valid. They are accepted as true by the patient without stopping to think. The depression produces all these ideas like propaganda—persuading the person they are worthless, stupid, and so forth. One way of dealing with propaganda is to ask every time: 'What is the evidence?' The patient is invited to try it out with their own depressive ideas, for example:

Therapist: Let us start with what you said you felt when you saw those people going along the street. It seemed as if your depressed mood caused you to think: 'I've no one to talk to'. What if you had wanted to argue with your depression? What might you have said to argue back?

(Or alternatively):

Therapist: Let's try and write down the evidence for and against the idea of 'I've no-one to talk to'. In doing this we are trying to look at how things really are rather than what your depression wants you to believe.

The therapist and patient can then collaborate in writing down the following:

Idea to be evaluated ....'I've no one to talk to'

Evidence for

It's a long time since anyone invited me to their house.

My mum lives 100 miles away. I can't keep phoning her.
John (husband) just sits and watches TV in the evening.

Evidence against

I haven't been out for a long time so no one has even *seen* me to invite me round. Dorothy did ask me to call, but I felt too tired.

I *can* talk to mum; if I decided to call each week it may help.
John may talk to me if I talk to him, but I don't really feel like it these days.

The conclusion that this patient reached was that she supposed there were some people (not many) that she could talk to, but that she had been feeling 'too rotten' to make the effort. The importance of going through this procedure is not just to persuade the patient of the therapist's point of view. After all, if it were to be the case that there was really no one that the person could talk to, then therapy might have to focus on increasing the social contacts of this person. However, the exercise may show that the problem is that the person lacks the energy to make the effort to contact people. If so, then the therapist and patient can discuss how, step by step, progress can be made towards that goal. En route, many other depressive ideas may have to be faced—for example: 'Even if I talk to them, they won't want to see me'. The patient can be asked to look out, specifically, for such undermining ideas. After practice in the clinic, the patient might try themselves to evaluate the evidence for and against such a thought.

DEALING WITH UNDERLYING ASSUMPTIONS AND BELIEFS

In most patients, dealing with underlying beliefs will become the focus of therapy towards the end, when they are relatively skilful at thinking objectively about their ideas and feelings. There are two sorts of underlying ideas which can fuel depression, underlying fears and underlying beliefs.

Underlying fears

There may be basic fears of abandonment or fears of failure which are at the root of the other ideas that come to light in therapy. Similarly, people may have basic fears that they are going crazy, that they are dementing, or that they are going to die. Patients may not be aware (or only barely aware) of these fears. How can they be brought to light? First, the therapist needs to notice when there may be an underlying fear that is fuelling the depressed mood. It sometimes becomes clear if the patient feels a severity of mood which does not seem plausibly related to the thought or image that they are aware of and have reported. For example, a young man said he had felt a deep apprehension following the previous session. When the therapist asked whether he was aware of any idea running through his mind, he said he'd been aware of the idea: 'I might not like what I find out about myself in therapy'. The therapist's intuition was that this thought was not sufficient to explain his obviously disturbed mood. He decided to take the patient through a *consequential analysis* of the thoughts:

Therapist: What do you think is the worst that could happen if you find out things about yourself?
Patient: I could break down completely.
Therapist: What would happen then?
Patient: I would have to leave college. My parents would be really disappointed.
Therapist: Anything else?
Patient: I would have to go and live back home. I would have to change careers. There would be nothing left of my life.

We can begin to understand why this man should have felt apprehensive. Although he was conscious of unease about the therapy unearthing things, he was only barely conscious of the inference that this would lead eventually to there being 'nothing left' to his life. Once the underlying fear has been made explicit, the patient and therapist together can analyse the inferences more clearly, examining alternative possibilities. Further, the patient can be asked to imagine the very worst happening, and then to consider what he would do to cope with such a situation. Once the patient is able to imagine coping with the very worst that might happen, much of the lesser negative possibilities can begin to feel more manageable.

Underlying assumptions

Underlying assumptions can also fuel depression by combining with situations to allow the patient to assume the worst. Table 10.2 gives examples of some basic beliefs which have been found characteristic of depressed people. Most of these beliefs are not by themselves likely to produce depression. For example, if I believe that in order to be happy I have to succeed in everything I do, that in itself does not make me depressed. But as soon as I fail something, then that failure combines with the underlying assumption to produce the conclusion: 'I cannot be happy'.

As with other aspects of cognitive therapy, the first way of dealing with these underlying assumptions is to make them explicit, and make the patient aware that they exist. This may be done by asking the patient to complete a questionnaire such as the Dysfunctional Attitude Scale (Weissman and Beck, 1978). The results of this questionnaire can then be discussed with the patient, who can begin to look for evidence of these depressive assumptions between sessions. A useful hint here is for the

Table 10.2 Examples of underlying dysfunction attitudes

It is shameful for people to display their weaknesses
I should be able to please everybody
People should prepare for the worst or they will be disappointed
If people are indifferent to me, it means they don't like me

---

patient to listen for the occurrence of certain words they may use: 'should', 'must', 'ought', 'always', 'never'. Very often when the patient uses these words there is an assumption lying below the surface. For example, one patient became upset when she was describing how little she did around the house. She said: 'I ought to be able to get it all done, it is not a very big house.' When investigated, it became clear that she felt that: 'Unless you keep your house immaculate people will think you are a good-for-nothing lazy-bones.' She also believed: 'If I don't *make* myself do it, it won't get done.'

TECHNIQUES

In achieving the aspects of therapy outlined here, there are many techniques (described by Beck *et al.*, 1979) which the cognitive therapist uses to help assess, clarify, evaluate and change thoughts, feelings and behaviours. Of these, there are some core techniques which are particularly helpful. Note again that the aims of therapy are a) to elicit the patients thoughts, self-talk and interpretation of events; b) gathering, with the patient, evidence for or against the interpretation; and c) setting up experiments (homework assignments) to test out the validity of the interpretations and gather more data for discussion.

Task assignment

This is used to encourage the patient to put themselves into situations they have avoided because of their negative thoughts about it. For example, the patient may not have contacted friends because they feel their friends won't want to hear from them. The task of phoning a friend may therefore be assigned, not simply because the outcome itself may be beneficial, but in order to monitor additional negative thoughts and interpretations which may arise while anticipating or performing the task. These then form the basis for discussion within therapy.

Cognitive rehearsal

This technique is used within a therapy session, in which the patient describes in great detail the stages of engaging in an activity. It is especially useful if a patient has had, or is anticipating having difficulty in carrying out an activity. The patient rehearses the situation, and tells the therapist at each point what thoughts and feelings are occurring. It is a procedure which is useful in two main ways. First, it helps to identify problematical aspects of situations which might not have readily become apparent to either patient or therapist when the activities have been described in more general terms. Each item on the list of difficulties generated during the cognitive rehearsal can become the focus of a behavioural assignment for the patient to do as 'homework'. Second, by imagining that a task is eventually completed the patient can be encouraged to imagine the feelings of satisfaction and accomplishment which accompanies successful completion. For many depressed patients it may have been a long time since they have had a success experience and they may have lost the capacity to remember or imagine what it was like. Cognitive rehearsal offers the opportunity for patients to re-experience at least a little of what is used to be like to feel that they had accomplished a task.

Alternative therapy

Like cognitive rehearsal, this is a forced fantasy technique. In this case, however, the patient is instructed to think of a situation similar to an upsetting situation they have experienced. They are instructed to imagine all the negative thoughts and feelings that would result. In this state (somewhat similar to 'flooding' treatment for phobic patients) the patient attempts to generate very detailed courses of action which could be followed should that situation recur. For example, a patient who is invited by a friend for the weekend could not go for various reasons, but felt sure that her friend would forget her if she refused. She was asked to imagine not taking up the offer and seeing her friends afterwards, and to imagine all the things that could go wrong and how she might cope. Note that the therapist may encourage the patient to confront the worst possible situation. There is no minimalization by the therapist of the scale of the patient's difficulties. The emphasis is not on the advice given by the therapist, but on the patient's solutions. Each solution is then explored in detail using cognitive rehearsal techniques to identify potential 'road blocks' for that action.

EVALUATING THE EFFECTIVENESS OF COGNITIVE THERAPY

There are two aspects to this question. The first is: Does it work in the acute phase of depression? The second is: Does it help to prevent future relapse?

Acute treatment

There are now several controlled trials which have found cognitive therapy to be as effective as antidepressant medication. Early studies appeared to show a better response to cognitive therapy than tricyclic antidepressants, but when the drugs are more carefully controlled (as happened in a trial by Murphy *et al.*, 1984, in which regular blood tests were taken to ensure that blood levels of the drug were within the therapeutic range), the apparent difference between tricyclic antidepressant and cognitive therapy disappeared. The studies using depressed patients (rather than volunteers solicited by advertisement), and using individual rather than group cognitive therapy, are shown in Table 10.3. This gives the degree of change on the Beck Depression Inventory (Beck *et al.*, 1961).

Note that most of these studies have not matched the number of hours of therapist contact between cognitive therapy and drugs. Cognitive therapy patients see their therapist more often for longer. But one important study (McLean and Hakstian, 1979) did control this variable. They had a relaxation and psychotherapy control group in which the patients saw the therapists for just as long as those in the cognitive therapy group. It is important therefore to note that they found results which exactly parallelled the other studies.

It is also worth noting that although one study (Blackburn *et al.*, 1981) appeared to show that cognitive therapy and drug therapy in combination actually did better than either alone (in out-patient depressives at least), this result has not been confirmed by other studies (Murphy *et al.*, 1984; Beck *et al.*, 1985). On the other hand, *no* study has found that drugs and cognitive therapy mutually inhibit each other.

Finally, taking the studies together, one can see that cognitive therapy appears to be effective in a large range of people. The early studies used educated middle- to upper-class patients from University Mental Health Clinics. However, patients treated in later studies (Blackburn *et al.*, 1981; Murphy *et al.*, 1984; Teasdale *et al.*, 1984) were much more evenly spread across the social class range. These factors did not affect the effectiveness of treatment.

These results raise an important issue of cost effectiveness. Cognitive therapy and antidepressant medication are virtually indistinguishable in their effectiveness, so are not antidepressants the treatment of choice on grounds of cost of therapist time alone? For many, if not most patients, this may remain true. But some patients cannot tolerate the side effects of drugs, and others insist that they do not want to take drugs for other reasons. In some patients there is the risk of overdose. For others with heart problems, there may be a problem with the cardiotoxicity of the drugs (especially in overdose). We need a way of managing these patients too.

A second point can also be made with regard to cost. So far, outcome studies have concentrated on delivering the maximum 'dosage' of cognitive

Table 10.3 Studies using Beck Depression Inventory—changes with treatment

Study	Treatment	Subjects	BDI Score		
			Pre	Post	Proportionate change
Rush et al. (1977)	CBT[a]	Out-patients	30.3	5.9	0.81
	Drug[c]	Out-patients	30.8	13.0	0.58
McLean and Hakstian (1979)	CBT	Out-patients	26.8	9.7	0.64
	Drug[d]	Out-patients	27.2	14.1	0.48
	Relaxation	Out-patients	26.8	15.0	0.44
	Psychotherapy	Out-patients	27.0	16.8	0.38
Blackburn et al. (1981)	CBT	GP patients	—	—	0.84
	CBT + Drug[b]	Out-patients	—	—	0.79
	CBT + Drug[b]	GP patients	—	—	0.72
	Drugs[a] alone	Out-patients	—	—	0.60
	CBT	Out-patients	—	—	0.48
	Drugs[b] alone	GP patients	—	—	0.14
Murphy et al. (1984)	CBT	Out-patients	28.7	9.5	0.67
	Drug[e]	Out-patients	29.2	8.9	0.69
	CBT + Drug	Out-patients	29.1	8.8	0.70
	CBT + Placebo	Out-patients	30.3	8.2	0.73
Teasdale et al. (1984)	CBT + Routine treatment	GP patients	30.0	8.0	0.73
	Routine treatment	GP patients	29.0	18.5	0.36
Beck et al. (1985)	CBT	Out-patients	31.0	8.6	0.72
	CBT + Drug[d]	Out-patients	30.0	10.0	0.67

[a]CBT = cognitive behaviour therapy; [b]Amitriptyline and clomipramine; [c]Imipramine; [d]Amitriptyline; [e]Nortriptyline; GP = general practitioner.

therapy. This usually involves at least 12 weeks of 50-minute sessions weekly using the whole range of techniques. My own hope is that further research will concentrate on identifying a small number of 'active ingredients' of therapy that might form the basis of strategies which a person might work through by themselves or under the direction of a general practitioner, health visitor or community psychiatric nurse. This package may become the treatment of choice for some relatively mild but fairly chronic depressives who do not respond to antidepressants, but who nevertheless remain a problem for a physician to manage.

Thirdly, the cost of psychotherapy such as cognitive therapy depends on how long-lasting its effects are. Can it prevent relapse? If so, the long-term cost may be equivalent or less than apparently 'cheaper' therapies which have to be applied again and again. It is evidence on this point that is now considered.

Relapse prevention

It is becoming clear that depression is a chronic relapsing condition. Following one episode, the risk of relapse is especially great in the first months after recovery but remains high thereafter. The estimate of the proportion of people who relapse following the initial response to treatment varies depending on the severity of patients in the sample, the length of the follow-up period and the definition of relapse. Klerman *et al.* (1974) found that 36 percent of their predominantly neurotically depressed out-patients relapsed within eight months following initial response to four to six weeks of amitriptyline, 100–200 mg per day (if given no further treatment). The UK Medical Research Council (MRC) multi-centre trial (Mindham *et al.*, 1973) involved more severely depressed out-patients and found that 50 percent relapsed within six months following initial treatment response if given no further treatment. The US National Institute of Mental Health (NIMH) study (Prien *et al.*, 1974) examined more severely depressed patients and found that 92 percent of a placebo group relapsed within the two years following successful response to initial active treatment. This pattern of results has been replicated in a further MRC trial of maintenance amitriptyline or lithium treatment (Glen *et al.*, 1984): six months after good response to initial treatment, 56 percent of patients given no further treatment had relapsed; this figure had increased to 67 percent after 12 months and 78 percent after 24 months.

Each of these cited studies have also examined to what extent maintenance dosage of antidepressant or lithium can reduce the probability of relapse. Although absolute levels have differed depending on severity of condition, most have found that relapse rates can be (at least) halved by maintenance medication [from 36 percent to 12 percent after eight months (Klerman *et al.*, 1974); from 50 percent to 22 percent after six months (Mindham *et al.*, 1983); from 92 percent to 48 percent after 24 months (Prien *et al.*, 1974]. The most recent estimate from the MRC trial (Glen *et al.*, 1984) is more pessimistic, however. They found that relapse rates at 6 months were reduced from 56 percent to 34 percent; but at 12 months, 45 percent, and at 24 months, 59 percent of patients who remained on maintenance medication had relapsed. It seems that we have a major challenge to find a method of keeping patients well after they have responded during the acute treatment phase. Relying solely on mainten-ance medication for such prophylaxis has the disadvantage associated with long-term drug usage. It depends on patients' compliance with the drugs regimen, carries the risk of overdose, may be contraindicated with patients with heart complaints, and may involve unpleasant side effects over prolonged periods. Has cognitive therapy a role to play here?

There have been three outcome studies which, having compared tricyclic antidepressants with cognitive therapy in the initial treatment, have taken patients who initially responded and examined their outcome over the subsequent 12 or 24 months (Hollon *et al.*, 1984; Blackburn *et al.*, 1986; Simons *et al.*, 1986). Each of these studies has found that patients who have responded to tricyclic antidepressants have a probability of relapse equivalent to that seen in the groups who received no maintenance treatment in the drug trials with moderately to severe depression cited above (Hollon *et al.*, 67 percent at 6 months; Simons *et al.*, 66 percent at 12 months; Blackburn *et al.*, 78 percent at 24 months). Each of these studies has also found, however, that the proportion of patients relapsing was substantially reduced if cognitive therapy had been added to tricyclic antidepressant medication during the acute treatment—Hollon *et al.*, from 67 percent to 18 percent at 6 months (cognitive therapy alone, 25 percent); Simons *et al.*, from 66 percent to 43 percent (cognitive therapy alone, 20 percent); Blackburn *et al.*, from 78 percent to 21 percent at 24 months (cognitive therapy alone, 23 percent).

The results of these studies conducted at different centres in both the US and the UK appear consistent. They are particularly interesting in that two of them (Hollon *et al.*, Simons *et al.*) found differences in relapse rates despite having found no difference between tricyclic antidepressant and cognitive therapy or the combination of the two in the acute phase of treatment. If these results are reliable, it will indicate an important advance in the management of chronically relapsing depressive illness.

FOR WHOM IS COGNITIVE THERAPY MOST SUITABLE?

All the outcome studies have used ambulatory depressed patients who satisfy research diagnostic criteria for unipolar major depressive disorder. They have not examined bipolar patients. Additionally, most therapists would maintain that patients who are too retarded or agitated, or who are extremely suicidal, would not be suitable at that time for any psychother-apy, including cognitive therapy. However, no study has found that the presence of typically 'endogenous' symptoms (e.g., early morning wakening, weight loss, mood worse in the morning) reduces the probability of a good outcome with cognitive therapy. Blackburn *et al.* (1981) found that the longer the duration of the current episode, the worse the outcome. Hollon (cited in Fennell and Teasdale, 1987) analysed the study of Rush *et al.* (1977) and found that four or more of the following items predicted a worse outcome:

Severity—Beck Inventory $\geqslant$ 30 (Beck *et al.*, 1961)
Duration current episode $\geqslant$ 6 months
Inadequate response to previous treatment
Previous episodes $\geqslant$ 2
Associated psychopathology
Overall impairment estimated by clinician as moderate or severe
Poor estimated tolerance for life stress

However, these patients *also* did worse with antidepressants. It appears that further research is needed to find the best methods of managing patients who do not appear to respond to either physical or psychotherapeutic treatments.

In addition to clinical variables, there are hints emerging from several studies about the type of patient who is most likely to do well with cognitive therapy. Murphy *et al.* (1984) found that patients who scored high on a questionnaire measure of 'self-control' (which indicated how much they typically use their own resources in dealing with problems) do better with cognitive therapy. People scoring low (who tend to show a relatively passive style of coping with stress) do better with drugs.

Similarly, Fennell and Teasdale (1987) found that people who responded more favourably at the beginning of therapy to a booklet, '*Coping with Depression*', which described cognitive therapy, did better in therapy than those who failed to find much in the description to which they could relate. The supposition arising from both studies is that those people who tend naturally to have an active coping style, but who find themselves temporarily immobilized by depression, take to the therapy very well, because it suits their natural style. Others have more difficulty. These are only hints, however, and more research is necessary.

Perhaps the surest way of assessing suitability is to try cognitive therapy for three or four weeks. Those studies that have examined the progress of therapy week by week, report that, although the path towards recovery is very variable, one can nevertheless begin to see changes in depression after such time in those who will ultimately benefit most.

WHICH ASPECTS ARE LIKELY TO TRANSFER MOST READILY TO OTHER SETTINGS?

It has already been mentioned that there has not been a systematic investigation of which aspects of cognitive therapy are most suitably used in, for example, a general practitioner's clinic. At this stage, one can therefore only make educated guesses. Ideally, whatever techniques are used should be able to fit into a self-help scheme that a therapist need only supervise in a relatively general way. A common core of those psychotherapies for depression that work well is that they are structured and built around the assignment of activities with encourage the patient gradually to engage in activities they have been avoiding. This suggests that a useful self-help technique would involve the patient in moving gradually towards targets which they have set themselves. They would need to learn how to grade these targets into small chunks, each of which would not be too difficult to achieve. They would also need to learn how to give due reward to themselves when they had achieved a subgoal.

It is relatively easy to imagine how a patient could be encouraged to keep an activity diary and easy to imagine how one might explain, in a booklet form, the importance of including activities which give a sense of accomplishment/mastery and which give a sense of pleasure.

Another important component might be to encourage the patient to keep a diary of their thoughts. One would have to provide examples, such as are included on the Automatic Thoughts questionnaire (Williams, 1984; p. 167), and encourage the patient to rate the frequency and intensity before moving on to evaluate the evidence for and against the thought. Several self-help manuals now exist and it is time that their use was systematically evaluated. Two good examples of such self-help manuals are that of Lewinsohn *et al.* (1978) and of Blackburn (1987).

Other chapters in this book describe how common depression is. Indeed depression has been referred to as the common cold of psychopathology. Common it certainly is, but the psychiatric equivalent of a common cold it is not. In many ways it remains a bewildering condition and no one can afford to be doctrinaire in advocating any single approach to understanding and managing it. The cognitive component of emotional disorders is only one aspect of them, but the evidence is that the range of techniques included in cognitive therapy will continue to provide a useful entry point into the vicious circle of mood, thought and behaviour which characterizes depression.

REFERENCES

Beck A. T., Ward C. H., Mendelson M., *et al.* (1961). An inventory for measuring depression. *Archives of General Psychiatry*, **4**, 561–71.

Beck A. T. (1976). *Cognitive Therapy and the Emotional Disorders*. New York: International Universities Press.

Beck A. T., Shaw A. J., Rush B. F., Emery G. (1979). *Cognitive Theory of Depression*. New York: Wiley.

Beck A. T., Hollan S. D., Young J. E., *et al.* (1985). Treatment of depression with cognitive therapy and amitriptyline. *Archives of General Psychiatry*, **42**, 142–8.

Blackburn I. M. (1987). *Coping with Depression*. Edinburgh: W.R. Chambers.

Blackburn I. M., Bishop S., Glen I. M., *et al.* (1981). The efficacy of cognitive therapy in depression: A treatment trial using cognitive therapy and pharmaco-therapy, each alone and in combination. *British Journal of Psychiatry*, 139, 181–9.

Blackburn I. M., Eunson K. M., Bishop S. (1986). A two year naturalistic follow up of depressed patients treated with cognitive therapy, pharmacotherapy and a combination of both. *Journal of Affective Disorders*, 10, 67–75.

Fennell M. J. V., Teasdale J. D. (1987). Cognitive therapy for depression: Individual differences and the process of change. *Cognitive Therapy and Research*, 11, 253–72.

Glen A. M., Johnson A. L., Shepherd M. (1984). Continuation therapy with lithium and amitriptyline in unipolar depressive illness: a randomized double-blind, controlled trial. *Psychological Medicine*, 14, 37–50.

Hollon S. D., Yuason V. B., Weiner M. J., *et al.* (1984). Combined cognitive-pharmacotherapy vs cognitive therapy alone and pharmacotherapy alone in the treatment of depressed outpatients. Differential treatment outcome in the CPT project (*unpublished ms.*). University of Minnesota and St. Paul Ramsey Medical Center, Minneapolis.

Klerman G. L., DiMascio A., Weissman M., *et al.* (1974). Treatment of depression by drugs and psychotherapy. *American Journal of Psychiatry*, 131, 186–91.

Lewinsohn P. M., Munoz R .F., Youngren M. A., Zeiss A. M. (1978). *Control Your Depression*. London: Prentice Hall International.

McLean, P. D., Hakstian, A. R. (1979). Clinical depression: Comparative efficacy of out-patient treatments. *Journal of Consulting and Clinical Psychology*, 47, 818–36.

Mindham R. H. J., Howland C., Shepherd M. (1973). An evaluation of continuation therapy with tricyclic antidepressants in depressive illness. *Psychological Medicine*, 3, 5–17.

Murphy G. E., Simons K. D., Wetzel R. D., Lustman, P. J. (1984). Cognitive therapy and pharmacotherapy; singly and together in the treatment of depression. *Archives of General Psychiatry*, 41, 33–41.

Prien R. F., Klett C. J., Caffey E. M. (1974). Lithium prophylaxis in recurrent affective illness. *American Journal of Psychiatry*, 131, 198–203.

Rush A. J., Beck A. T., Kovacs M., Hollon S. (1977). Comparative efficacy of cognitive therapy and pharmocotherapy in the treatment of depressed out-patients. *Cognitive Therapy and Research*, 1, 17–37.

Simons A. D., Murphy G. E., Levine J. L., Wetzel R. D. (1986). Cognitive therapy and pharmacotherapy for depression. *Archives of General Psychiatry*, 43, 43–50.

Teasale J. D. (1988) Cognitive vulnerability to persistent depression. *Cognition and Emotion*, 2, 247–740.

Teasdale J. D., Fennell M. J. V., Hibbert G. A., Amies P. L. (1984). Cognitive therapy for major depressive disorders in primary care. *British Journal of Psychiatry*, 144, 400–6.

Weissman A. N., Beck A. T. (1978). *Development and validation of the Dysfunction-al Attitude Scale*. Paper presented at American Educational Research Associa-tion Annual Convention, Toronto, Canada.

Williams J. M. G. (1984). *The Psychological Treatment of Depression: A Guide to the Theory and Practice of Cognitive-Behaviour Therapy*. London: Croom Helm; New York: Free Press.

11 *Developments in antidepressants*

STUART A. MONTGOMERY

INTRODUCTION

The tricyclic antidepressants which were introduced more than a generation ago made an impressive contribution towards improving the quality of life of patients suffering from depressive illness. The efficacy both of these drugs and the so-called second generation antidepressants, which were developed as possible improved treatments, has been quite thoroughly investigated and reviewed, and they are well established in clinical practice in the treatment of depression.

In this chapter, the changes in the way antidepressants are used will be considered, as will the recognition of the patients who will benefit from antidepressant treatment, the dangers of current treatments, the possible advantages of the newer treatments, the need for long-term treatment, and the direction of the future development of antidepressants.

ANTIDEPRESSANTS IN THE TREATMENT OF ANXIETY

One of the problems in psychiatry about which there has been least agreement among clinicians is the separation of anxiety states and depression. There would probably be closer agreement about this categorization if its relevance could be demonstrated, for example, in terms of specific treatments for the separate illnesses. However, the most recent evidence points to a wider spectrum of efficacy of antidepressants than was previously thought and suggests that antidepressants are significantly more effective than benzodiazepines in treating anxiety states. This adds important support for the hypothesis that anxiety states are part of depression and should come within the wider orbit of depressive illness. The recognition of a common basis for the treatment of depression and anxiety is reflected in the approach to the development of new treatments which is emerging. The perception of an antidepressant as having a broad spectrum of effect is leading to compounds with probable antidepressant action being developed as anxiolytics.

Two large, formal studies have recently addressed the issue of the use of antidepressants in the treatment of anxiety. A direct test of the efficacy of antidepressants in anxiety was reported by Kahn *et al.* (1986). In this study, imipramine, chlordiazepoxide and placebo were compared in a large group of patients diagnosed as suffering from anxiety states. The patients treated with imipramine had a significantly better response than those treated with the benzodiazepine or placebo. Although the benzodiazepine was found to be more effective than placebo, it is clear that the antidepressant provided the most effective treatment. The earlier UK Medical Research Council (MRC) study (Johnstone *et al.*, 1980) found that in a large group of patients with anxiety, anxiety/depression, or depression treated with an antidepressant, a benzodiazepine or placebo, the antidepressant, amitritpyline, was effective in the entire group. The benzodiazepine, diazepam, was only effective in a very small group of patients with severe anxiety symptoms. For the majority of patients diazepam was no different to placebo. Both of these studies thus find that the antidepressant acts outside strictly defined depression and appears to be more effective than benzodiazepines in the majority of anxiety states and equally effective in the rest.

The usefulness of antidepressants has also been reported in the more specific categories of anxiety states—for example, in phobic anxiety (Sheehan *et al.*, 1980; McNair and Kahn, 1981; Mavissakalian and Michelson, 1982; Zitrin *et al.*, 1983). There is considerable overlap between the diagnosis of depression/anxiety and the diagnosis of depression/phobias as Angst and Dobler-Mikola (1985) reported in a community survey. Attempts to create separate subdivisions of anxiety for panic states and generalized anxiety disorder are subject to similar problems. The phenomenon of panic has been recognized for some time as being part of the wider symptomatology of depression. In the study of depressive symptomatology which led to the creation of a sensitive instrument for rating depression (Montgomery and Asberg, 1979), the item 'inner tension', which has an element of panic within it, was found to be the most commonly occurring symptom of depression. Furthermore this item was found to be sensitive to change with treatment with antidepressants. There is little doubt that antidepressants are effective in patients diagnosed as suffering from panic states.

The implication of the overlap between the syndromes and the wide spectrum of effect of antidepressants is that the classical division into depression, anxiety states, phobic states and panic disorders is questionable. It seems likely that there is a single underlying disorder of which these different syndromes are manifestations. This may explain why it is possible to treat them all with antidepressant drugs.

BENZODIAZEPINES IN THE TREATMENT OF ANXIETY AND DEPRESSION

Benzodiazepines, which have traditionally been used to treat anxiety states, were originally thought to be safe and the indications for their use were drawn rather broadly. There is, however, increasing awareness of the problems associated with their use. They appear to have a rather narrow spectrum of action compared with antidepressants and it is now well recognized that they are associated with tolerance, dependence and problems on withdrawal.

The risk of dependence appears to increase if the benzodiazepines are used for longer treatment courses. Dependence has been reported to develop in courses as short as four weeks and it is probably wise to avoid using them for periods longer than two to four weeks. Dependence is also more likely in those individuals treated with high doses of benzodiazepines or with benzodiazepines that are particularly potent. It is obviously better to use the lowest possible effective dose, which in some cases may be lower than the minimum strength available. The wide indications for the use of benzodiazepines are misleading. There now seems little justification for their use in mild transient anxiety or sleep disturbance because the risk of dependence will outweigh the benefit of the immediate relief of symptoms, which are likely in any case to resolve naturally. Nor is there evidence of a specific advantage for benzodiazepines in obsessive compulsive disorder for which they have in the past been suggested. This is a long-standing illness where the risk of dependence is rather high. The wide use of benzodiazepines in treating the anxiety associated with personality disorders is also unwise as there is now good evidence of increased disinhibition, aggression and suicidal behaviour associated with benzodiazepines (Gardner and Cowdry, 1985).

The ability of the benzodiazepines to produce immediate short-term relief in severe anxiety states is valuable and it would be a pity if this real advantage were obscured by our concern over their inappropriate long-term use. The recommendation of the Committee of Review of Medicines in the UK that they should only be used for short courses of treatment has regrettably been largely ignored until recently. Some three-quarters of the prescriptions are repeats, many of them for long-term usage.

To avoid dependence, it is wise to encourage patients to take intermittent treatment with a 'drug holiday' every two or three days. Sudden withdrawal may precipitate an acute reaction and a stepwise reduction of dosage is helpful. Withdrawing benzodiazepines from the long-term dependent group is sometimes difficult. It is often helpful to pretreat patients with antidepressants for a month before beginning withdrawal. The withdrawal process may be prolonged and the reduction of dosage should be flexible and responsive to the difficulties encountered by the patient (Montgomery and Tyrer, 1988).

Increasing concern about dependence and withdrawal problems have led to restrictions on the use of all benzodiazepines. The Royal College of Psychiatrists consensus meeting on benzodiazepines and dependence made recommendations for a tightening of the indications for their use (Priest and Montgomery, 1988), which have been supported by the restrictions advised by the Committee on Safety of Medicines (CSM; 1988).

If dependence develops rapidly in many patients treated with benzodiazepines, it seems questionable to embark on treatment of any condition where the symptoms are likely to persist for more than four weeks. The development of benzodiazepines for use as antidepressants seems misguided because antidepressants should be used for a minimum of six months. Antidepressants should not be used simply for the relief of immediate symptomatology but for the longer maintenance phase of treatment until the present episode has completely resolved. It is therefore difficult to envisage a useful role for any new class of benzodiazepines intended for the treatment of depression. To reduce the risk of dependence the drug would need to be withdrawn once the symptoms are resolved and an established antidepressant substituted.

Evidence for the effectiveness of the group of benzodiazepines being developed as antidepressants, such as alprazolam and adinazolam, is in any case questionable, and there is little evidence for their long-term efficacy. To be convincing as antidepressants these benzodiazepines must establish their effectiveness in treating the core symptoms in endogenous depression. The use of the Hamilton Rating Scale (Hamilton, 1967) for depression, which has a high loading of anxiety items, is unwise in pivotal studies. Any sedative or anxiolytic drug may alleviate the anxiety symptoms of depression without treating the underlying illness. It is probably fair to insist on evidence of long-term efficacy in this particular class of compounds.

ANTIDEPRESSANTS AND ADVERSE REACTIONS

We now have a greater concern for safety than before, and require antidepressants with a proven record of safety. Many potential antidepressants are rejected very early in development because of anticholinergic and other unwanted side effects. The higher standards of safety now imposed would probably have the effect of eliminating many of the commonly used older tricyclic antidepressants (TCA) if they were to be discovered now.

Clinicians are conditioned to expect the unpleasant anticholinergic and sedative effects associated with the older TCAs. Indeed, dosage is often titrated against the appearance of side effects although the rationale for this practice has been criticized. The common unwanted side effects should be distinguished from the rarer serious adverse drug reactions. Most of the medicines in use are associated with some risk. With antidepressants these risks include cardiotoxicity, liver reactions, convulsions, blood dyscrasias, hypersensitivity and immunoallergic reactions. If these events occur rarely it is difficult to arrive at an estimate of their incidence until a drug is in wide use. Careful prospective monitoring is obviously necessary in the development stage but a post-marketing surveillance system in the early stage of release into usage is more likely to identify serious but rare adverse drug reactions. There is a tendency for physicians to drop their guard with older drugs and not recognize or report the reactions which occur with them. The true incidence of these side effects is undoubtedly higher with the older drugs than the official statistics suggest. A better measure of the incidence may be seen in formal comparative post-marketing surveillance studies of a new drug compared with an established one. These prospective cohort studies should have a clear end-point which is independent of reporting bias.

Toxicity of antidepressants in overdose

One relatively independent measure of the toxicity of antidepressants is seen in the deaths from overdose. Antidepressants account for some 15 percent of the total deaths resulting from overdosage. The drugs that are named on the death certificate give an indication of the toxicity of those drugs. Often the death certificate names several drugs and the most accurate measure of toxicity would be provided where only one drug is cited, with or without alcohol. The Coroners' reports in England and Wales of deaths from overdose have been used to calculate the relative risks of different antidepressants. When these deaths are related to the usage of antidepressants, as calculated either by the number of patients treated or by the number of prescriptions issued, a consistent picture of toxicity of the older TCAs emerges.

An analysis of the figures (see Table 11.1) from 1977–84 showed that the mean number of fatalities with the TCAs was 106 per million patients

Table 11.1 Comparison of estimated incidences of fatal poisonings with anti-depressants in the UK

Drug	Fatal poisonings per million prescriptions[a] 1975–84	Fatal poisonings per million patients[b] 1977–84
Dothiepin	50.0	143
Amitriptyline	46.5	166
Maprotiline	37.6	103
Doxepin	31.3	106
Imipramine	28.4	106
Trimipramine	27.6	87
Clomipramine	11.1	32
Mianserin	5.6	13

[a]Cassidy and Henry (1987)—England, Scotland and Wales.
[b]Montgomery and Pinder (1987)—England and Wales.

treated (Montgomery and Pinder, 1987). A similar picture (Table 11.1) is seen from the calculations made by Cassidy and Henry (1987), who took all deaths from overdose in the UK and the National Health Service prescription figures as their data base. The most dangerous TCAs appear to be amitriptyline and dothiepin, with 166 and 143 deaths per million patients treated, or approximately 46 and 50 deaths per million prescriptions. This death rate from overdose with the older TCAs is unacceptable. Maprotiline, a bridged tricyclic, is clearly associated with the same risk seen with the older TCAs.

The deaths from the older TCAs are significantly higher than the mean for all antidepressants and the deaths associated with newer antidepressants significantly lower. The safest of the newer antidepressants appear to be mianserin, with six deaths per million prescriptions, and lofepramine. No deaths from overdose with lofepramine alone have been recorded in the first 1.5 million prescriptions. Of the other new antidepressants, trazadone and viloxazine also appear relatively safe.

Clomipramine appears to be the exception among the older TCAs and seems to be relatively safe. On the surface, this is surprising because clomipramine is known to have rather unpleasant anticholinergic side effects and dangerous interactions. There are two possible explanations for the relatively low number of deaths from overdose with clomipramine. One is that clomipramine may be selectively prescribed to obsessional patients with a low risk of suicide. However it is also used in categories of patients with a higher than normal risk of suicide, such as in severe depression, and another explanation should be sought. A second possibility is that clomipramine, by virtue of its ability to inhibit uptake of serotonin (5-hydroxytryptamine; 5-HT), may reduce suicidal thoughts or acts. There is some evidence with other 5-HT uptake inhibitors to support this intriguing possibility. An early reduction in suicidal thoughts was seen during treatment with zimelidine (Montgomery *et al.*, 1981), and similar results have been reported with two other 5-HT uptake inhibitors, fluvoxamine (Muijen, *et al.*, 1988) and fluoxetine (Wakelin and Coleman, 1985).

It seems surprising that the level of deaths directly attributable to the toxicity of a drug is permitted. Zimelidine was withdrawn when deaths from hypersensitivity and Guillain–Barré syndrome were reported an an estimated level of 50 deaths per million prescriptions. This is very much on a par with the rate of deaths from overdose seen with amitriptyline and dothiepin. Nomifensine was withdrawn when only seven deaths per million prescriptions from immunoallergic syndrome were reported (Committee on the Safety of Medicine, 1986).

Reducing the risk of death from overdose

Suicidal thoughts are integral to depression and it is rather difficult to predict which individual patient will make a suicidal attempt. A case can be made for using safer antidepressants in all patients treated at home. If unsafe antidepressants are prescribed, they should be given only in small amounts and preferably in the care of relatives and friends who should be mobilized to support the patient. Certain groups of patients are known to be at a higher risk, in particular those with a history of a previous attempt, the elderly living alone, and those with alcohol problems. A high index of suspicion is needed in these groups where it is particularly important to prescribe safer antidepressants.

DIRECTIONS IN THE DEVELOPMENT OF NEW ANTIDEPRESSANTS

The discovery of imipramine was a chance finding. The range of TCAs developed subsequently are all very similar and have only minor differences in terms of side effects. With the possible exception of clomipramine, there is no evidence of a selective effect on particular subgroups of depression. The TCAs were found to have many different pharmacological effects. It was natural to develop more specific compounds in the hope that one or other of these specific pharmacological properties would prove to have a superior antidepressant effect or faster onset of action. Unfortunately it took many years before selective compounds were available for testing in the clinic. The hope that new selective antidepressants would be more effective, or act on particular subgroups of depressed patients, has not been realized.

A specific test of the relevance of the selectivity of pharmacological action is to compare the clinical effect of relatively specific uptake inhibitors. Both 5-HT uptake inhibitors and noradrenaline uptake inhibitors have been shown to be effective in the same proportion of patients. However, 5-HT uptake inhibitors have not been found to be a specific treatment for the subgroup of depressed patients with low levels of 5-hydroxyindole acetic acid (5-HIAA) in the cerebrospinal fluid (Montgomery *et al.*, 1981). Non-responders on one treatment do not respond selectively to the alternative treatment (Montgomery *et al.*, 1987). The antidepressants with the more selective pharmacological action appear to be just as effective as reference antidepressants and to have the same broad spectrum of antidepressant effect.

5-HT uptake inhibitors

A series of selective 5-HT uptake inhibitors have been developed as antidepressants; their properties are outlined in Table 11.2. Where their efficacy has been established—for example, zimelidine, fluoxetine, fluvoxamine, paroxetine—they appear to have a similar order of efficacy to that of reference antidepressants. In general, they lack anticholinergic effects and therefore do not have the classical side effects seen with the TCAs. By and large, these compounds have been developed without histaminic effects

Table 11.2 Some properties of 5-HT reuptake inhibitors

Where their efficacy has been established it appears to be of the same order as standard antidepressants

Lack of anticholinergic effects, lack of sedation, some gastrointestinal upset, occasional agitation

Selectivity of general antidepressant effect not established

Possible selectivity of action on obsessions, suicidal thoughts, eating disorders, and personality disorders needs investigating

---

and are non-sedative. The rare adverse drug reaction seen with zimelidine is not apparently found with other compounds of this class. This has been tested in a small number of patients who developed the 'zimelidine syndrome' but who did not produce this syndrome during treatment with another 5-HT uptake inhibitor. (Chouinard and Jones 1984; Montgomery *et al.*, 1989). Nausea and nervousness appear to be characteristic side effects with 5-HT uptake inhibitors. The severity of the nausea, which may lead to vomiting, appears to be dose-related and is more prominent with some compounds, for example, fluvoxamine, than with others. Fluvoxamine is also associated with a higher incidence of convulsions, which may be related to dose.

Many of these compounds were developed under the mistaken belief that high levels of uptake inhibition were more effective than moderate levels. Unfortunately, the dosage chosen was often based on open dose-ranging studies, which are notoriously biased towards attributing efficacy to the maximum dose tolerated. Early studies with norzimelidine showed that optimum therapeutic efficacy was seen with lower plasma levels rather than higher levels, indicating that the dose chosen for zimelidine was too high (Montgomery *et al.*, 1981). Almost identical findings have been reported with norfluoxetine, the active metabolite of fluoxetine, again indicating that the dose chosen for the early clinical studies was too high (Montgomery *et al.*, 1986). A comprehensive series of studies of different fixed doses of fluoxetine has shown that the most effective dose is about one-third of that chosen originally on the basis of the early open dose-ranging studies (Wernicke *et al.*, 1987). In these studies, nausea was less frequent at the lower doses and it is possible that the high levels of nausea and vomiting seen with some other 5-HT uptake inhibitors may also be related to too high a dose.

This class of compounds appears to be effective in other groups of psychiatric patients both with and without depression. Clomipramine has an established role in treating obsessive compulsive disorder. Clomipramine itself has strong 5-HT uptake inhibiting properties although its active metabolite is noradrenergic. Placebo-controlled trials (see Table 11.3) have demonstrated the efficacy of clomipramine in obsessive compulsive dis-

Table 11.3 Placebo controlled studies of clomipramine (CMI) in OCD (with and without concomitant depression)

Study	n	Design	Improvement in obsessional symptoms
Depression not excluded			
Thoren *et al.* (1980)	35	Parallel CMI (150 mg) vs placebo	CMI > placebo (5 weeks)
Marks *et al.* (1980)	40	Parallel CMI (136–183 mg) vs placebo	CMI > placebo (4 weeks; self rating only)
Insel *et al.* (1983)	12 11 13	Crossover CMI (236 mg) vs Clorgyline (28 mg) vc placebo	CMI > Clorgyline CMI > placebo (4 + 6 weeks)
Flament *et al.* (1985)	19	Crossover CMI (141 mg) vs placebo	CMI > placebo (5 + 5 weeks)
Marks *et al.* (1988)	25 12	Parallel CMI (127–157 mg) vs placebo (plus identical exposure conditions)	CMI > placebo (8 weeks)
1° + 2° depression excluded			
Montgomery 1980	14	Crossover CMI (75 mg) vs placebo	CMI > placebo (4 weeks)

order both in patients without concomitant depression (Montgomery, 1980) and in patients with variable concomitant depression (Thoren *et al.*, 1980; Marks *et al.*, 1980; Insel *et al.*, 1983; Flament *et al.*, 1985). Open treatment studies suggest that the new 5-HT uptake inhibitors are also effective in this group and this is supported by a recent placebo-controlled study with fluvoxamine (Cottraux *et al.*, 1987). There is also a suggestion that 5-HT uptake inhibitors may have a specific effect in treating bulimia nervosa. Serotonin uptake inhibitors might well have some specific and selective effects in personality disorders and in obsessional illness. There is a considerable body of work examining impulsivity and suicidal behaviour in personality disorders in which the serotonin system appears to be involved, and it would seem reasonable to investigate drugs with 5-HT effects in these groups.

Specific 5-HT antagonists and agonists

Mianserin and trazadone are established atypical antidepressants. Both have some effects on 5-HT receptors but it has not been possible to say if these actions are principal to their antidepressant effects because both have other pharmacological actions. Trazadone selectively inhibits reuptake of 5-HT but is paradoxically a central and peripheral serotonergic antagonist. It has an active metabolite, *m*-chlorophenylpiperazine (*m*CPP), which is a postsynaptic agonist at 5-HT_1 receptors. Apart from its α-adrenergic blocking properties, mianserin has 5-HT_2 antagonist effects as well as $α_2$-adrenoceptor antagonism.

The recognition of different 5-HT receptor types (5-HT_1-like, 5-HT_2 or 5-HT_3) has allowed a new range of agonists and antagonists to be developed. How many of these approaches will turn out to be useful in depression or anxiety remains to be tested.

Buspirone, a 5-HT_1 antagonist, has been developed as an anxiolytic and appears to be effective in alleviating anxiety (Goldberg and Finnerty, 1979; Rickels, 1981; Schweizer *et al.*, 1986). It is interesting that the onset of anxiolytic effect is subject to a delay similar to conventional antidepressants (Feighner *et al.*, 1982). Although it is probably an antidepressant this has not been adequately tested. Gepirone, a 5-HT_2 antagonist, has possible antidepressant efficacy although the evidence is based at the moment only on open studies (Amsterdam *et al.*, 1987). Clinical studies on ritanserin, a 5-HT_2 antagonist, indicate some potential efficacy in dysphoric states. Unfortunately, these studies are hard to evaluate and until they have been adequately reported and replicated it is not possible to generalize from the results. The relation between 5-HT_1- and 5-HT_2-receptors is particularly intriguing. The 5-HT_3 antagonists appear to have a role in inhibiting vomiting associated with whole-body treatment of carcinoma with radio-therapy or drugs. Whether they are effective in anxiety or depression remains to be tested.

Alpha$_2$-adrenoceptor antagonism

The rationale behind the development of $α_2$ antagonists is that it is necessary to enhance noradrenergic synaptic activity for antidepressant effect. Blocking presynaptic $α_2$-adrenergic receptors would interrupt the negative feedback system and increase the available noradrenaline. The antidepressant effect of mianserin, which has α-adrenergic antagonistic effects, is thought to be mediated by this mechanism. More potent and specific centrally acting $α_2$ antagonists are necessary to test the relevance of this theory.

A number of compounds with more specific $α_2$ antagonist effects are now in development, some of which have reached clinical testing. One of the earliest of these was idazoxan for which there is some evidence of antidepressant efficacy in major depression. Unfortunately idazoxan also has $α_2$ agonist effects so that more precise testing of the theory awaits a more selective compound.

Phosphodiesterase inhibitors

The effect of noradrenaline centrally may be enhanced by focusing on the adenylate cyclase system, which acts as a second messenger to the β-adrenergic receptors. A phosphodiesterase inhibitor might allow cyclic adenosine monophosphate (cAMP) to accumulate and to increase the noradrenergic effects in the brain. Rolipram is the only example to reach clinical practice. Unfortunately, the results on antidepressant efficacy are mixed and although there have been positive results in small active-comparator studies in Europe, a large multicentre placebo–controlled study in the USA could not confirm efficacy (Feighner, 1987).

Antidepressants with important dopaminergic effects

Nomifensine has effects on noradrenaline and 5-HT, as well as inhibition of dopamine reuptake. Its undoubted efficacy as an antidepressant has led to the development of a series of new antidepressants with principal effects on the dopamine system.

Minaprine was introduced in France in 1980 for 'inhibitory states'. It blocks the reuptake of dopamine in vivo although not in vitro, and it also has effects on 5-HT (Biziere *et al.*, 1985). The concept of inhibitory states is peculiar to France and it is not clear how closely patients suffering from this condition resemble depressives. Preliminary studies, however, suggest there is efficacy in major depression. Bupropion, with undoubted antidepressant efficacy (Preskorn and Othmer, 1984), has relatively weak dopamine reuptake-inhibiting properties. In the high doses used in the large pivotal studies on depression in the USA, the dopaminergic effects may, however, have been important. At these high doses, bruproprion had little in the way of anticholinergic, histaminic or cardiotoxic effects. Agitation, insomnia, dizziness and nausea were, however, common. The initial reports suggest a rather wide spectrum of action with some effects on depression associated with personality disorders. The high incidence of convulsions has held back the release of this interesting drug until further testing has been completed. A far more selective dopamine reuptake inhibitor (GBR 12909) is currently being tested clinically as an antidepressant. Because of its more potent and selective action, the results with this compound may elucidate the clinical importance of the facilitation of dopamine transmission in the treatment of depression.

Monoamine oxidase inhibitors (MAOI)

The monoamines 5-HT and noradrenaline, which have been thought to have an important involvement in depression, are metabolized predominantly by the A form of monamine oxidase (MAO), so the development of new MAOIs has focused on compounds which are selective for this form. It is, of course, possible that inhibitors of either form would have antidepressant efficacy, as irreversible inhibition at the rates needed to change brain concentrations of one form would, over time, affect both forms. The selectivity for one form is less marked in vivo than in vitro. One problem with existing MAOIs is that they are associated with the tyramine pressor response, the so-called cheese effect. The development of new MAOIs has been concentrated on reversible selective monoamine oxidase A (MOA-A) inhibitors in an attempt to produce compounds which would be free of this effect.

Perlindole, a short-acting reversible MAO-A inhibitor, has been shown to have reasonable efficacy in placebo-controlled trials. Moclobemide, similarly, has short-acting reversible MAO-A inhibition but inhibition of platelet MAO-B is also observed—possibly because there are active metabolites with an effect on MAO-B (da Prada *et al.*, 1986). The clinical studies suggest there is probable antidepressant efficacy. The early results with moclobemide are promising in that they suggest efficacy in a dose where the cheese effect is not seen (Tiller *et al.*, 1986). The irreversible inhibitor of MAO-B, L-deprenyl, has been available in many countries as an adjunct for treatment in parkinsonism. There was interest in its possible usefulness in depression because of its lack of the cheese effect. Clinical trials have given mixed results in depression and the exact role of MAO-B inhibition in antidepressant effects remains to be established.

LONG-TERM TREATMENT WITH ANTIDEPRESSANTS

Antidepressant efficacy is normally evaluated only in acute depression studies. The risk of adverse effects is calculated from large groups of patients exposed to the drugs. It is on this basis that a risk-benefit calculation is usually made. These acute depression studies are usually conducted for a period of four to six weeks and the response is defined by the appropriate reduction in severity of depressive symptoms registered on observer rating scales. Longer term studies are required by regulatory authorities to establish the safety of a drug in long-term usage, often in 100 patients treated for a year. Evidence of the efficacy of antidepressants in the long term has not been required by regulatory authorities until recently.

Most antidepressants were introduced before the concept of long-term treatment had been properly formulated. All the evidence now points to the need to continue antidepressant treatment well beyond the acute period until the episode has completely resolved. If antidepressants are withdrawn before four to six months there is an increased chance of the return of symptoms which would register inadequate treatment of the current episode. This phase of treatment of the acute episode is referred to as the continuation phase and should be clearly distinguished from the prophylactic phase which follows. The exact length of the continuation phase has been the matter of some debate. Prien and Kupfer (1986), in a retrospective analysis of the relapse rates on placebo in an earlier study (Prien *et al.*,

1973), found a relatively high overall relapse rate (44 percent) in the first 16 weeks, with the highest chance of relapse occurring in the first 8 weeks. Their results argue for the maintenance phase being continued for at least four months after the acute symptoms have resolved; other investigations have suggested that at least six months is needed.

There is relatively strong evidence for antidepressants, particularly amitriptyline, being effective over this continuation phase of acute treatment. However, the evidence for many, widely used standard antidepressants is based on open observation without formal testing. The ability of an antidepressant to maintain response over this continuation phase is an important aspect of efficacy. It is simply not sufficient to claim efficacy on the basis of an acute study lasting six weeks when it is clear that antidepressants need to be used for the continuation phase of four to six months following response.

For patients with recurrent depression, antidepressants are used to prevent the development of new episodes. Very few studies have examined the role of antidepressants in the true prophylaxis of recurrent depression. Some of the studies which have been carried out were so poorly designed (Medical Research Council, 1981) that it was clear from the start they would contribute little to our knowledge. Many failed to calculate the number of patients that would be needed to test the hypothesis and were thus far too small. Some studies made the quite obvious mistake of confusing the continuation phase with the prophylactic phase of treatment. Only those studies which have included a defined symptom-free period are able to provide us with an estimate of the usefulness of antidepressants in true prophylaxis.

Lithium is of course established for the prophylaxis of bipolar depression but the studies using lithium as a prophylactic agent in unipolar depression are less clear. Schou (1979), in a metanalysis of 76 unipolar depressives treated with lithium and 77 treated with placebo in several different studies concluded that lithium was effective. Prien *et al.* (1984), on the other hand, suggest that there is insufficient evidence on which to recommend lithium for prophylaxis in unipolar depression.

In unipolar depression, there are not enough studies on any compound to establish a reference by which other prophylatic agents might be judged. There are only five studies which included a defined symptom-free period and one of these is too small to permit valid conclusions. There is only one positive study of amitriptyline (Coppen *et al.*, 1978), which had a rather short symptom-free period of six weeks. There are two studies examining the prophylactic ability of imipramine, lithium and placebo. The largest of these (Prien *et al.*, 1984) again used a rather short symptom-free period of two months and found that lithium was no better than placebo over a 2-year period whereas imipramine was. The second very small study (Kane *et al.*, 1982) unfortunately included too few patients to be sure of the results. There have been two studies on 5-HT uptake inhibitors; Bjork (1983) used a 4-month symptom-free period and found zimelidine was better than placebo over a 1.5-year period; a recent large multicentre study (Montgomery *et al.*, in press) which used a 4.5-month symptom-free period found that fluoxetine was better than placebo over a 1-year period. This last study is the only one large enough to unequivocally demonstrate prophylactic efficacy.

Many of the antidepressants currently in wide usage, both new and old, do not appear to have been adequately tested for their ability to prevent new episodes of depression arising. The draft guidelines for the European Economic Community on the testing of antidepressants make the point that long-term efficacy must be tested separately from efficacy in acute treatment. Although such studies are time consuming, it is possible to get a closer measure of the long-term efficacy of antidepressants. It will not be long before we require evidence of efficacy of all antidepressants in prophylaxis separately from acute treatment.

RECURRENT TRANSIENT MOOD CHANGES IN PERSONALITY DISORDERS

There is increasing concern that classificatory systems like the Diagnostic and Statistical Manual (DSM III; American Psychiatric Association, 1980) might miss mood changes which are transient yet disabling. This is a difficult group to investigate and one approach has been to examine the associated behavioural disturbance such as suicidal behaviour.

Transient mood states are found in personality disorders suffering from recurrent suicidal acts. In a series of studies on multiple suicide attempters where DSM III depression was excluded, it was clear that the occurrence of transient mood disturbance predicted subsequent suicidal acts (Montgomery *et al.*, 1983). These mood disturbances were accompanied by rateable depressive symptomatology. On the Montgomery–Asberg Depression Rating Scale (MADRS; Montgomery and Asberg, 1979) the symptoms which predicted a subsequent suicide attempt after one month on placebo were suicidal thoughts, reduced appetite, reduced sleep, apparent sadness, and lassitude. The MADRS score itself also predicted subsequent suicidal attempts. It is interesting that this series of symptoms does not include reported sadness. In other words, in this group the condition may not be perceived as depression by the patient.

The recurrent brief depression group that Angst and Dobler–Mikola (1985) have reported in their epidemiological survey in the normal population has a similar pattern of symptomatology. The psychopathological symptoms which showed a highly significant difference from normals ($p < 0.001$) were anxiety, sleep disturbance, exhaustion and weakness, appetite loss and suicidal thoughts. They found that a large number of symptoms traditionally rated as depressive were present and that, apart from the brevity of the episodes, the condition satisfied DSM III criteria for major depression. These findings are very similar to those in the studies on the prevention of suicidal behaviour in personality disorders. Angst and

Dobler–Mikola also found that recurrent brief depression occurred in about 5 percent of the general population, that some 80 percent had a spontaneous resolution in a few days, and that the occurrence seriously impaired their social functioning.

These controlled investigations on the prevention of suicidal behaviour are the only ones to have examined prophylactic treatment effects prospectively in this group. A positive effect would not be expected in an acute treatment study. It is necessary to use a prophylactic design in a condition which recurs for a few days every so often for a year or more. The antidepressant, mianserin, was not significantly different from placebo (Montgomery *et al.*, 1983) and this result supports the general clinical view that antidepressants are not particularly effective in treating transient lowered mood associated with personality disorders. In the parallel study of the depot neuroleptic, flupenthixol, given in a low dose (Montgomery and Montgomery, 1982), there was a highly significant reduction in suicide attempts when compared with placebo. These results are supported by a further study of low-dose neuroleptics in which low-dose thiothixene appeared to be effective in reducing the characteristic features of borderline personality disorder (Goldberg *et al.*, 1986).

These studies imply that antidepressants which are effective in such a wide range of anxiety and depression may not be effective in this group of personality disorders. The usefulness of low-dose neuroleptics in this group suggests that the condition may need a different pharmacological approach. It is possible that drugs which affect the dopamine system have a selective effect on this form of illness. There are some indications of this in the evolution of potential antidepressants that affect the dopamine system. The wide use of low-dose neuroleptics in France as antidepressants is interesting in this context. The development of potential antidepressants with principal effects on the dopamine and serotonin systems may provide the opportunity to investigate this area further.

CONCLUSION

There are a large number of very interesting compounds being developed as antidepressants or anxiolytics. Selective compounds have a particular value in investigating the underlying mechanisms of psychiatric illness. They are already pointing to some of the inconsistencies and deficiencies of existing classificatory systems. The definition of depression in the DSM III and Research Diagnostic Criteria (Spitzer *et al.*, 1975) reflects the experience of which patients are likely to respond to conventional antidepressants. Some of the patients who do not fulfil these diagnostic criteria may suffer from conditions allied to depression and could benefit from treatment. It is possible that new psychoactive compounds may be effective in conditions that are not yet clearly defined. We must be careful not to let rigid classificatory systems obstruct the progress of knowledge.

194 *Depression: An integrative approach*

REFERENCES

American Psychiatric Association (1980). *Diagnostic and Statistical Manual of Mental Disorders.* Washington: American Psychiatric Association.

Amsterdam J. D., Berwish N., Potter L., Rickels K. (1987). Open trial of gepirone in the treatment of major depressive disorder. *Current Therapeutic Research*, **41**, 185–93.

Angst J., Dobler–Mikola A. (1985). The Zurich Study—a prospective epidemiological study of depressive neurotic and psychosomatic syndromes. *European Archives of Psychiatry and Neurological Sciences*, **234**, 408–16.

Biziere K., Worms P., Kan J.-P. *et al.* (1985). Minaprine, a new drug with antidepressant properties. *Drugs Experimental and Clinical Research*, **11**, 831–40.

Bjork K. (1983). The efficacy of zimelidine in preventing depressive episodes in recurrent major depressive orders—a double blind placebo controlled study. *Acta psychiatrica Scandinavica*, **68**, 182–9.

Cassidy S., Henry J. (1987). Fatal toxicity of antidepressant drugs in overdose. *British Medical Journal*, **295**, 1021–4.

Chouinard G., Jones B. (1984). No crossover of hypersensitivity between zimelidine and fluoxetine. *Canadian Medical Association Journal*, **131**, 1190.

Committee on Safety of Medicines (1986). Update—withdrawal of nomifensine. *British Medical Journal*, **293**, 41.

Committee on Safety of Medicines (1988). Benzodiazepines, dependence and withdrawal symptoms. *Current Problems*, **21**.

Coppen A., Ghose K., Montgomery S., *et al.* (1978). Continuation therapy with amitriptyline in depression. *British Journal of Psychiatry*, **133**, 28–33.

Cottraux J., Nury A. M., Mollard E. (1987). *Fluvoxamine and exposure in obsessive-compulsive disorders.* Presented at Royal College of Psychiatrists, London.

da Prada M., Kettler R., Keller H. H., Bonetti E. P. (1986). *Moclobemide, a new antidepressant inhibiting platelet monoamine oxidase type-B activity in man.* Paper presented at 3rd World Conference Clinical Pharmacology and Therapeutics, Stockholm.

Feighner J. P. (1987). Paper presented at International Symposium on New Directions in Depressive Disorders, Jerusalem.

Feighner J. P., Merideth C. H., Hendrickson G. A. (1982). A double-blind comparison of buspirone and diazepam in outpatients with generalized anxiety disorder. *Journal of Clinical Psychiatry*, **43**, 103–7.

Flament M. F., Rapoport J. L., Berg C. F., *et al.* (1985). Clomipramine treatment of childhood obsessive-compulsive disorder. *Archives of General Psychiatry*, **42**, 977–83.

Gardner D. L., Cowdry R. W. (1985). Alprazolam-induced dyscontrol in borderline personality disorder. *American Journal of Psychiatry*, **141**, 98–100.

Goldberg H. L. K., Finnerty R. J. (1979). The comparative efficacy of buspirone and diazepam in the treatment of anxiety. *American Journal of Psychiatry*, **136**, 1184–7.

Goldberg S. C., Schulz S. C., Schulz P. M., *et al.* (1986). Borderline and schizotypal personality disorders treated with low-dose thiothixene vs placebo. *Archives of General Psychiatry*, **43**, 680–6.

Hamilton M (1967). Development of a rating scale for primary depressive illness. *British Journal of Social and Clinical Psychology*, 6, 278–96.

Insel T. R., Murphy D. L., Cohen R. M., *et al.* (1983). Clomipramine and clorgyline in OCD. *Archives of General Psychiatry*, 40, 605–12.

Johnstone E. C., Cunningham Owens D. G., Frith C. D., *et al.* (1980). Neurotic illness and its response to anxiolytic and antidepressant treatment. *Psychological Medicine*, 10, 321–8.

Kahn R. J., McNair D. M., Lipman R. S., *et al.* (1986). Imipramine and chlordiazepoxide in depressive and anxiety disorders. *Archives of General Psychiatry*, 43, 79–85.

Kane J. M., Quitkin F. M., Rifkin A., *et al.* (1982). Lithium carbonate and imipramine in the prophylaxis of unipolar and bipolar II illness. *Archives of General Psychiatry*, 39, 1065–9.

McNair D. M., Kahn R. J. (1981). Imipramine and chlordiazepoxide for agoraphobia. In *Anxiety: New Research and Changing Concepts* (Klein D. F., Rabkin J. G., eds.). New York: Raven Press, pp. 169–80.

Marks I. M., Stern R. S., Mawson D., *et al.* (1980). Clomipramine and exposure for obsessive compulsive rituals. *British Journal of Psychiatry*, 136, 1–25.

Mavissakalian M., Michelson L. (1982). Agoraphobia: behavioural and pharmacological treatments. *Psychopharmacology Bulletin*, 18, 91–103.

Medical Research Council Drug Trials Subcommittee (1981). Continuation therapy with lithium and amitriptyline in unipolar depressive illness: a controlled clinical trial. *Psychological Medicine*, 3, 5–17.

Montgomery S. A. (1980). Clomipramine in obsessional illness: a placebo controlled trial. *Pharmaceutical Medicine*, 1, 189–92.

Montgomery S., Asberg M. (1979). A new depression scale designed to be more sensitive to change. *British Journal of Psychiatry*, 134, 382–9.

Montgomery S., Montgomery D. (1982). Pharmacological prevention of suicidal behaviour. *Journal of Affective Disorders*, 4, 291–8.

Montgomery S. A., Pinder R. (1987). Do some antidepressants promote suicide? *Psychopharmacology*, 92, 265–6.

Montgomery S. A., Tyrer P. J. (1988). Benzodiazepines: time to withdraw. *Journal of the Royal College of General Practitioners*, April 146–147.

Montgomery S. A., McAuley R., Rani S. J., *et al.* (1981). A double blind comparison of zimelidine and amitriptyline in endogenous depression. *Acta Psychiatrica Scandinavica*, suppl. 290, 63, 314–27.

Montgomery S. A., Roy D., Montgomery D. B. (1983). The prevention of recurrent suicidal acts. *British Journal of Clinical Pharmacology*, 15, 183S–8S.

Montgomery S. A., James D., de Ruiter M., *et al.* (1986). *Weekly oral fluoxetine treatment of major depressive disorder*. Paper presented at 15th CINP Congress, Puerto Rico.

Montgomery S. A., James D., Montgomery D. (1987). Pharmacological specificity is not the same as clinical selectivity. In *Clinical Pharmacology in Psychiatry* (Dahl L., Gram L., eds.). Berlin: Springer Verlag.

Montgomery S. A., Dufour H., Brion S., *et al.* The prophylactic efficacy of fluoxetine in unipolar depression. *British Journal of Psychiatry Supplement* (in press).

Montgomery S. A., Gabriel R., James D., *et al* (1989). The specificy of the zimelidine reaction. *International Clinical Psychopharmacology*, 4, suppl. 1, 27–9.

Muijen M. (1988). A comparative clinical trial of fluoxetine, mianserin and placebo with depressed outpatients. *Acta Psychiatrica Scandinavica*, **78**, 384–90.

Preskorn S. H., Othmer S. C. (1984). Evaluation of bupropion hydrochloride: the first of a new class of atypical antidepressants. *Pharmacotherapy*, **4**, 21–34.

Prien R. F., Klett C. J., Caffey E. M. (1973). Lithium carbonate and imipramine in the prevention of affective episodes. *Archives of General Psychiatry*, **29**, 420–5.

Prien R. F., Kupfer D. J., Mansky P. A., *et al.* (1984). Drug therapy in the prevention of recurrences in unipolar and bipolar affective disorders. *Archives of General Psychiatry*, **41**, 1096–104.

Prien R., Kupfer D. J. (1986). Continuation drug therapy for major depressive episodes: how long should it be maintained? *American Journal of Psychiatry*, **143**, 18–23.

Priest R. G., Montgomery S. A. (1988). Benzodiazepines and dependence. *Royal College of Psychiatrists Bulletin*, **12**, 107–9.

Rickels K. (1981). Recent advances in anxiolytic therapy. *Journal of Clinical Psychiatry*, **42**, 40–4.

Schou M. (1979). Lithium as a prophylactic agent in unipolar affective illness. *Archives of General Psychiatry*, **36**, 849–51.

Sheehan D. V., Ballenger J., Jacobsen G. (1980). Treatment of endogenous anxiety with phobic, hysterical, and hypochondriacal symptoms. *Archives of General Psychiatry*, **37**, 51–9.

Spitzer R., Endicott J., Robins E. (1975). *Research Diagnostic Criteria* Instrument No. 58. New York: New York State Psychiatric Institute.

Thoren P., Asberg M., Cronholm B., *et al.* (1980). Clomipramine treatment of obsessive compulsive disorder. *Archives of General Psychiatry*, **37**, 1281–5.

Tiller J. W. G., Schweitzer I, Maguire K. P., *et al.* (1986). *A controlled study of moclobemide in atypical depression.* Paper presented at 3rd World Conference on Clinical Pharmacology and Therapeutics, Stockholm.

Wakelin J. S., Coleman B. S. (1985). *The influence of the 5-HT specific antidepressant fluvoxamine maleate on suicidal behaviour.* Paper presented at 4th World Congress of Biological Psychiatry, Pennsylvania.

Wernicke J. F., Dunlop S. R., Dornseif B. E., *et al.* (1987). Fixed fluoxetine therapy for depression. *Psychopharmacology Bulletin*, **23**, 164–8.

Zitrin C. M., Klein D. F., Woerner M. G., Ross D. C. (1983). Treatment of phobias. I. Imipramine and placebo. *Archives of General Psychiatry*, **40**, 125–38.

12 Suicide and the management of suicide attempts

KEITH HAWTON

INTRODUCTION

Considerable changes have occurred in the patterns of suicidal behaviour in the UK in recent years. Rates of suicide in England and Wales steadily declined from 1961 until 1976, probably largely because of the introduction of non-toxic North Sea Gas and a massive reduction in the prescribing of barbiturates. The last decade has witnessed a further decline in the suicide rates for women, especially in the younger age groups. By contrast suicide rates for men have risen, this increase occurring among young and middle-aged men. Accompanying this trend there have also been changes in the methods predominantly used for suicide. Fatal drug overdoses have become less common, whereas death by car exhaust fumes and by hanging have increased markedly. Currently there are approximately 4500 official suicides each year in England and Wales.

Attempted suicide rates increased dramatically during the 1960s and early 1970s. In recent years, however, the rates have levelled off and now begun to fall, especially in females (Platt et al., 1988). Nevertheless, deliberate self-poisoning remains the most common medical reason for emergency admission to hospital; among men it is second only to heart attacks. The extent of the problem of attempted suicide (thought to represent as many as 100 000 admissions to general hospitals in this country each year) is thus still a considerable one for the Health Service, and reflects a vast amount of psychiatric and social morbidity. Furthermore, attempts are often repeated (Bancroft and Marsack, 1977) and subsequent suicide occurs in a significant proportion of cases (Hawton and Fagg, 1988).

Among people who kill themselves, or attempt suicide, approximately two-thirds have visited doctors, usually their general practitioners, within the month beforehand, and a third within the week beforehand (Hawton and Blackstock, 1976; Barraclough and Hughes, 1987). Assessment of suicidal potential must therefore be part of the doctor's skills. Furthermore, general practitioners and physicians frequently have to deal with suicide attempters after their attempts. Therefore, the responsibility for the assessment of patients who have taken overdoses or have injured themselves is bound to fall to some extent on non–psychiatrists, even if psychiatry teams, together with general practitioners, have the main responsibility for the management of these patients.

This chapter includes a brief review of official policies on the management of attempted suicide patients, following which the assessment and aftercare of these patients are examined in some detail. Finally, guidelines are provided on factors that should be taken into account when assessing suicide risk, and on the management of those identified as at risk.

POLICIES ON THE MANAGEMENT OF ATTEMPTED SUICIDE

Until recently, official policy with regard to the management of attempted suicide patients was contained in the Hill Report (Central and Scottish Health Services Councils, 1968), which advocated the establishment of poisoning treatment centres in District General Hospitals to which all cases of deliberate self-poisoning should be referred, irrespective of the seriousness of their medical condition. It also recommended that psychiatric emergency cover should be available to the general hospital every day of the week, and that psychiatric and social work assessments should be carried out on all patients.

The recommendations of the Hill Report were never fully met: hardly any poisoning treatment centres were established and the policy on psychiatric assessment was often disregarded, partly because of the vast number of attempted suicide patients who were being referred to general hospitals, and partly because of the many other demands on psychiatrists and social workers. Furthermore, by no means all attempted suicide patients were admitted to general hospitals. As a result, experimental services were established in several centres; most placed greater emphasis on involvement of non-medical staff in the management of suicide attempters, while some involved medical teams more in the assessment. Both types of approach gained support from research studies (Gardner *et al.*, 1978; Gibbons *et al.*, 1978; Newson-Smith and Hirsch, 1979*b*; Catalan *et al.*, 1980; Hawton *et al.*, 1981). These approaches were given official blessing by the Department of Health (Department of Health and Social Security, 1984) following the deliberations of a multi-disciplinary working party. The new guidelines acknowledge the potential role of non–psychiatrists (general physicians, social workers and psychiatric nurses) in the assessment and management of attempted suicide patients, provided they have received adequate training and also have the back-up and supervision of psychiatrists.

While these recent guidelines have been followed in many general hospitals, others still offer inadequate and very limited services for these patients. This is partly due to the cost of establishing an adequate service.

However, the cost may be considerably offset by the marked reduction in bed occupancy by attempted suicide patients that may follow the setting up of a readily available service (Hawton *et al.*, 1979).

ASSESSMENT OF ATTEMPTED SUICIDE PATIENTS

The key questions that should be addressed during the assessment of attempted suicide patients, whether in the casualty department, general medical ward or in the community, are listed in Table 12.1. Before examining how the assessor can approach this, some general points should be made about the assessment procedure.

The assessment should not simply be a fact-finding exercise—it must be remembered that most attempted suicide patients are in a state of crisis and hence are in considerable distress. Therefore the style of the interview is important. The interview should if possible be conducted in a situation which allows privacy; the use of an interview room is best, but this will not always be feasible, either because of the patient's physical state or because a room is simply not available. Adequate time should be allowed—half an hour to an hour will usually be required. The assessment interview should be conducted as soon as possible after the patient has recovered from the medical effects of the attempt or the subsequent treatment. It is pointless trying to assess a drowsy or confused patient. However, if the interview is delayed too long after recovery, important information may become

Table 12.1 Questions to be addressed during the assessment of attempted suicide patients

---

Why did the attempt occur?
Problems
Precipitants

What was the nature of the attempt?
Details of method used (including alcohol)
Suicidal intent
Other motives

Does the patient have a psychiatric disorder?

Is there a risk of:
(a) suicide?
(b) another attempt?

What are the persons coping resources and supports?

How can the person best be helped?

---

inaccessible because of, for example, interactions between the patient and family members.

The attitudes of staff in general hospitals towards attempted suicide patients are often somewhat hostile (Ramon *et al.*, 1975), perhaps because it is thought that a much-needed hospital bed is being occupied unnecessarily. Such attitudes are to some extent understandable, but they are very likely to cause defensiveness if they are conveyed in any way to patients and hence interfere with the assessor's ability to access patients fully and eventually help them.

A semi-structured type of interview is usually best. This avoids the artificiality of a check-list but ensures that the key areas of the assessment are covered. Whie the assessment will need to include several topics which are covered in a routine psychiatric history, the assessor must focus on the attempt itself, both in terms of understanding the reasons for it and its implications.

Whenever possible, additional information should be obtained from sources other than the patient. These include relatives and friends, as well as the patient's general practitioner and anyone else involved in a professional capacity in the patient's care.

Why did the attempt occur?

A useful way of initiating the assessment and of addressing several of the factors in Table 12.1 is to ask for a detailed account of the 48 hours or so leading up to the attempt. During this the interviewer should ask in detail about any aspects which are unclear or not fully explained by the patient. The interviewer should aim to establish a problem list with the patient. It is helpful if the interviewer has in mind a check-list of common problem areas (Table 12.2) to help ensure that nothing is overlooked.

Interpersonal difficulties are the most common problems preceding attempts by adults, and especially problems in the relationship with a partner. Such problems were found in 72 percent of cases in an Oxford study (Bancroft *et al.*, 1977). Work problems, especially unemployment, are also common. Rates of attempted suicide are very high in the unemployed of both sexes, especially in the long-term unemployed (Platt and Kreitman, 1984; Hawton and Rose, 1986; Hawton *et al.*, 1988). However, it is unclear whether this association represents a direct effect of unemployment on domestic life and psychosocial adjustment or whether there are more people at risk among the unemployed for other reasons. Serious problems in the use of alcohol are found in 14–22 percent of male attempters and 4–5 percent of female attempters (Platt *et al.*, 1988). Alcohol use may contribute to both the occurrence of attempts and their danger. Other psychiatric disorders (discussed further below) are present in a substantial proportion of cases. Attempters who are parents, especially mothers, of young children may have considerable difficulties with the children, and in such families there is a very high risk of child abuse or

Table 12.2 Problem areas to be considered during the assessment of attempted suicide patients

1. Relationship with partner or spouse
2. Relationship with other family members, especially young children
3. Employment or studies
4. Finances
5. Housing
6. Legal, including impending court proceedings
7. Social isolation, relationships with friends
8. Use of alcohol and drugs
9. Psychiatric health
10. Physical health
11. Sexual adjustment
12. Bereavement and impending loss

neglect. In an Oxford study, the children of 29 percent of mothers (with children aged 5 years or less) who made attempts had either been physically abused or neglected or were on the at-risk register for abuse or neglect (Hawton *et al.*, 1985). Physical disorders are common in suicide attempters and may act as vulnerability factors, undermining a person's ability to cope with stress. They also contribute to the relatively high eventual mortality of this population (Hawton and Fagg, 1988).

Suicide attempts very often follow life events (Paykel *et al.*, 1975)— serious arguments with, or separation from the partner being the most frequent (Bancroft *et al.*, 1977).

Many adolescent suicide attempters are in considerable conflict with their parents, and approximately half have problems in their relationship with a boyfriend or girlfriend and or, difficulties at school or with employment. Social isolation is another important factor in this group (Hawton *et al.*, 1982).

What was the nature of the attempt?

The interviewer must obtain full details of the actual attempt, including any associated use of alcohol. In Oxford, as elsewhere in the UK, 85–90 percent of cases involve self-poisoning. The most frequent substances used are non-opiate analgesics (especially paracetamol and aspirin), followed by minor tranquillizers and sedatives. There has been a steady decline in overdoses of tranquillizers in recent years, presumably reflecting changes in prescribing habits (Forster and Frost, 1985; Platt *et al.*, 1988). Wrist-cutting is by far the most common form of self-inflicted injury, the cuts often being superficial (Simpson, 1976). More dangerous self-injuries are relatively rare and usually associated with serious suicidal intent.

It is important that the interviewer tries to establish possible motives for the attempt, and especially that the degree of suicidal intent is assessed. Suicidal intent refers to the apparent seriousness or intensity of a patient's wish to terminate his or her life at the time of the attempt. Many attempts involve considerable ambivalence, and therefore suicidal intent represents the balance between the wish to die and the wish to live. Some of the questions that are useful in assessing suicidal intent are shown in Table 12.3. Whenever possible, the interviewer should try to corroborate the patient's account of the circumstances of the attempt when interviewing relatives or friends.

An interviewer-rated questionnaire, the Suicidal Intent Scale (Beck *et al.*, 1974), can be a useful aid when assessing suicidal intent and may help inexperienced interviewers cover the necessary questions. The question-naire includes items relating to the circumstances of the attempt and the patient's self-reported intentions.

Patients themselves often indicate suicidal intent when other people, including the interviewer, do not think there was a serious wish to die. For example, in one study, psychiatric assessors agreed that there was suicidal intent in only half of the cases in which the patients claimed they had wanted to die (Bancroft *et al.*, 1979). In some cases this may have reflected the patient's need to justify his or her behaviour, in others it may have reflected the fact that although the patient felt like dying at the moment of the attempt, death was not the intended outcome.

It should be emphasized that suicidal intent should not be judged from

Table 12.3 Items to cover during the assessment of suicidal intent

1. Whether the attempt was impulsive or planned; if the latter, the duration of the plans

2. Whether the patient was alone, or whether someone was present or within easy access

3. Whether the patient was likely to be found soon after the attempt

4. The nature of any precautions taken to prevent or ensure discovery

5. The drugs taken, including the quantity, and whether other drugs were available but not taken; any alcohol consumed as part of the attempt

6. The patient's expectations regarding the likely effects of the drugs or injury

7. The presence of a suicide note or message

8. The patient's efforts to obtain help after the attempt, and the events leading to admission to hospital

the medical seriousness of an overdose. Thus cases of self-poisoning with low suicidal intent can be associated with high risk of medical complications (Fox and Weissman, 1975) and vice versa. The medical danger of an overdose only contributes to the assessment of intent when the individual is aware of the likely medical consequences of the act (Beck *et al.*, 1975). For example, there is likely to be a clear difference in intent between a nurse who takes an overdose of half a dozen nitrazepam tablets, and a non-medical person who does the same but claims that since two such tablets put a person to sleep then surely six would be fatal.

The motives contributing to overdoses, or self-injuries, are varied, including communication of feelings to other people, an attempt to change someone else's behaviour, temporary escape from a distressing situation or state of mind, and a deliberate effort to get help (Hawton, 1982). If on the basis of the overall assessment it proves impossible to understand the motivation for the behaviour, the interviewer should consider the following possible reasons: some key questions may have been omitted; the patient may have withheld important information, perhaps because of fear of disapproval or continuing suicidal wishes; or the patient may be suffering from a major psychiatric disorder.

It is important to note that the motives for suicide attempts may be fairly complex, and an attempt may have several reasons—for example, an ambivalent wish to die, a need to show other people how hurt the attempter feels, and a wish for temporary oblivion.

Does the patient have a psychiatric disorder?

The majority of suicide attempters report psychiatric symptoms, especially depressed mood, tension, hopelessness, and irritability (Newson-Smith and Hirsch, 1979*a*; Urwin and Gibbons, 1979). Approximately 30 percent are suffering from a psychiatric disorder as defined by the Present State Examination (Index of Definition 6–8; Wing *et al.*, 1974). Most are cases of depression, some patients have anxiety disorders and occasionally patients have schizophrenia (alcoholism has already been considered). A substantial proportion also have personality disorders.

In the majority of cases the psychiatric disorders (especially depression and anxiety) are relatively transient, the proportion with such disorders three months after the attempts having fallen to 8 percent in one study (Newson-Smith and Hirsch, 1979a). This presumably reflects the fact that in many cases the psychiatric symptoms are secondary to life difficulties, which may improve or resolve, sometimes perhaps because of professional or other help. However, there is an important small subgroup of patients who have serious persistent affective or psychotic disorders requiring intensive treatment and among whom are many of those at risk of subsequent suicide.

Assessment of attempted suicide patients must therefore include a thorough assessment of possible psychiatric disorder, based on all the information the interviewer can gather, including from the patient's history, presentation at interview and from other informants.

Is there a risk of suicide?

Studies have consistently shown that approximately one out of every 100 suicide attempters will die by suicide within the year following an attempt, a suicide risk approximately 100 times that of the general population. The risk of suicide remains considerable for at least eight years after an attempt (Table 12.4). Looked at the other way round, of people who kill themselves approximately half have a history of suicide attempts (Ovenstone and Kreitman, 1974). Assessment of suicide risk is therefore of central importance when interviewing suicide attempters. However, one should not underestimate the difficulty of identifying those most at risk (Hawton, 1987).

In assessing risk of suicide following a suicide attempt, the interviewer needs to pay heed to several factors (Table 12.5). The list of demographic, social and clinical factors in Table 12.5 is based largely on the items found by Tuckman and Youngman (1968) to distinguish attempters who subsequently killed themselves from attempters who were still alive several years later. Interestingly, two recent studies also found that attempters who later committed suicide were *less* likely than surviving attempters to have experienced the break-up of a relationship during the year preceding their attempts and/or to have had a major row just before their attempts (Pallis *et al.*, 1982; Hawton and Fagg, 1988). These findings are consistent with those of another study in which depression which followed a break-up of a relationship had a better prognosis than depression for other reasons (Parker *et al.*, 1988).

Attempts with higher suicidal intent are associated with greater risk of eventual suicide (Pierce, 1981). A study of depressed patients with suicidal ideas has demonstrated that in the prediction of suicide the degree of

Table 12.4 Suicide following attempted suicide

	Number of attempted suicide patients	Length of follow-up (year)	Suicides %
Kessel and McCulloch (1966)	511	1	1.6
Hawton and Fagg (1988)	1626	1	1.0
Buglass and Horton (1974)	2809	1	0.8
Buglass and McCulloch (1970)	511	3	3.3
Hawton and Fagg (1988)	1335	8	2.8

Table 12.5 Factors to consider in the assessment of suicide risk

1. Demographic, social and clinical

    (a)   older age

    (b)   male sex

    (c)   unemployment; retired

    (d)   separated, widowed or divorced

    (e)   living alone

    (f)   poor physical health

    (g)   psychiatric disorder, including alcoholism

    (h)   violent method used in attempt

    (i)   suicide note

    (j)   previous attempts

2. Suicidal intent involved in current attempt—was it high, and is it persistent?

3. Attitude to future

4. Are current circumstances likely to change?

5. Available supports

6. Is effective treatment available?

hopelessness experienced by a patient is more important than severity of depression (Beck *et al.*, 1985). Immediate suicide risk will also depend on the extent to which patients believe that their circumstances can change, and whether help is available which can facilitate this. A supportive social network may be a major protective factor against suicide, especially if the patient has at least one readily available confidant.

Is there a risk of a further attempt?

Clearly there is some overlap between risk of further attempts and risk of suicide. Twelve to 15 per cent of patients repeat their attempts within a year, the risk being greatest during the first three months after an attempt (Bancroft and Marsack, 1977). There is a small group of patients who make several, sometimes many, attempts. Such 'chronic' or 'persistent repeaters' pose very difficult management problems for both general medical and psychiatric staff. They have a particularly high risk of eventual suicide (Ovenstone and Kreitman, 1974; Pierce, 1981).

The Risk of Repetition Scale can assist the clinician in the identification of patients at risk of further attempts (Buglass and Horton, 1974). It includes six items, one point being scored for each item that is positive. The items are: (i) problems in the use of alcohol; (ii) diagnosis of socio-pathy ('predominant stress of the patient's situation falls on society');

(iii) previous in-patient psychiatric treatment; (iv) previous out-patient psychiatric treatment; (v) previous suicide attempt resulting in hospital admission; and (vi) not living with relatives. The higher the score the greater the risk of repetition. Patients with scores of zero have a very small probability of repetition, whereas those with scores of 5 or 6 may have approximately a 50 percent chance of repetition within the following year.

Other factors to take into account when assessing risk of a repeat attempt include whether or not there is a good chance of the patient's circumstances changing in the near future, and whether the patient has a history of impulsive or aggressive behaviour. Markedly low self-esteem and hopelessness at the time of an attempt are also associated with increased risk of repetition (Petrie *et al.*, 1988).

What are the person's coping resources and supports?

In planning aftercare, the patient's strength and resources, both past and present, should be assessed. These include:

1. Supportive relationships—friends, relatives and professional helpers (including the general practitioner), and the extent to which these are both available and will be used by the patient.
2. Personal resources—how problems have been managed by the patient in the past; the patient's current assets and strengths, and whether the patient is able to suggest ways of tackling the difficulties.

How can the person best be helped?

At this stage of the assessment it is useful to prepare a problem list (an example is shown in Table 12.6). Often this can be done with the patient. However, a severely distressed patient or one who appears to be concealing information (for example, about alcohol abuse) may not be able to collaborate usefully in this exercise. The problem list serves several purposes: it can help disentangle a mass of difficulties into tangible problems; patients can find it helpful to have their problems clarified; it often points clearly to the nature and focus of appropriate intervention; it can be used to assess progress during treatment; and finally, it provides a useful, clear means of communicating information about a patient to others, including the patient's general practitioner.

AFTERCARE

By way of illustration, the aftercare offered to attempted suicide patients referred to the Emergency Psychiatry team working in the general hospital in Oxford in 1986 is shown in Table 12.7.

Table 12.6 A problem list for someone who took an overdose

Miss M.B., age 22
Overdose of 25 paracetamol, after drinking 6 glasses of wine

Problems	Aftercare
1. Break-up of relationship with long-standing boy-friend following a row 2 days before overdose. Had discovered 6 weeks ago that he was having relationship with another girl	Out-patient appointments to allow ventilation of grief
2. Unemployment: lost job 3 months ago after argument with boss	Explore future work options in out-patient appointment
3. Heavy alcohol consumption during past 4 weeks, secondary to problems 1, 4 and 5	Advice on reducing intake—review progress in out-patient setting
4. Persistent low mood for past 6 weeks, secondary to problems 1 and 5	No specific action— review in out-patient setting
5. Social isolation since lost contact with most of workmates 3 months ago	Explore in out-patient setting how she can begin to re-establish old contacts/make new ones

Psychiatric in-patient care

A fundamental question the clinician needs to address is whether the patient seems capable, with whatever support systems are available, of taking some responsibility for himself or herself, or whether the responsibility for care needs to be taken over temporarily by the clinical service. Specific indications for in-patient care include: severe psychiatric disorder, especially depression or schizophrenia; immediate serious risk of suicide or

Table 12.7 Aftercare offered to attempted suicide patients referred to the Emergency Team in the general hospital in Oxford in 1986 ($n = 687$)

Psychiatric hospital in-patient care	5.1%
Out-patient care	43.8%
Day-patient care	2.5%
Other	13.1%
Return to care of general practitioner	35.5%

repetition of the attempt; and overwhelming crisis, where the patient needs a brief period of intensive care and support.

Occasionally the 1983 Mental Health Act will have to be used to admit a patient to the psychiatric unit. Patients for whom this may be necessary are those refusing admission who are suffering from severe depression with loss of insight, are clearly at serious risk of suicide, or have an acute schizophrenic or organic psychiatric condition. Section 2 (for assessment) is most often used.

Treatment in the in-patient setting will include whichever measures are appropriate for the psychiatric condition (see Hawton and Catalan, (1987); Chapter 7). Unfortunately, suicidal behaviour is not entirely prevented by hospital admission, acute psychiatric in-patient units having suicide rates as much as 50 times higher than the general population (Fernando and Storm, 1984). This is not altogether surprising in view of the fact that approximately one-third of hospital in-patients have a history of suicide attempts (Hawton, 1978). Nevertheless, regular review of suicidal ideation should be part of routine care while patients are at risk, and appropriate ward regimes (including constant or regular observation if necessary) must be agreed for those most at risk. The period of initial recovery from a depressive disorder, when a suicidal patient is becoming less retarded and hence may have more drive to act on suicidal wishes, can be a time of special risk. There is also increased risk of suicide during the period after discharge from hospital (Pokorny, 1964), which emphasizes the need for careful planning of aftercare, including close liaison with the patient's general practitioner and other agencies.

Day-patient care

This may offer a useful intermediate type of aftercare between in-patient and out-patient treatment, particularly if patients are socially isolated or lacking in daytime activities.

Out-patient care

This is the predominant form of psychiatric aftercare that is usually provided. It may be indicated for patients who are prepared to work actively on their problems and/or, where psychotropic drug management needs to be supervised.

A problem-orientated approach to aftercare (Hawton and Catalan, 1987) is suitable for many attempted suicide patients. This is usually brief (two to ten treatment sessions) and entails helping patients use their own resources to tackle some of their current difficulties. In the case of the patient whose problem list is shown in Table 12.6, the therapist helped her to examine ways of renewing and extending her social contacts and of finding new employment, while also allowing her the opportunity within treatment sessions to ventilate her feelings of anger and disappointment about the rejection by her boyfriend.

A problem-orientated treatment approach can also be used for helping couples or families (see Hawton, 1986; Hawton and Catalan, 1987 for full details). Therapeutic interventions based on cognitive behavioural treatment for depression (see Chapter 10) can be very usefully integrated with this type of help.

Psychotropic medication should be reserved for patients with clear clinical disorders, and avoided in those who, for example, have entirely understandable low mood in the face of major interpersonal or other problems. Psychotropic medication will often have been prescribed shortly before an attempt, and will have been a factor in precipitating an overdose in some cases (Hawton and Blackstock, 1977). Thus, treatment more often involves stopping medication rather than initiating its use. However, some attempted suicide patients offered out-patient care will have clinical affective disorders warranting medication, in which case this should be used in full therapeutic doses with special care being taken about the total amount of medication made available, especially for patients with persistent suicidal ideas.

Two controlled evaluative trials of problem-focused aftercare have suggested that it is more helpful to patients in terms of subsequent social adjustment than either routine psychiatric care or simply returning patients to the care of their general practitioners. However, these benefits appear to be confined to women and patients with marital problems (Gibbons *et al.*, 1978; Hawton *et al.*, 1987). The compliance of attempted suicide patients with out-patient care is often relatively poor. Although home-based treatment increases the proportion of cases in which treatment sessions actually occur, it does not appear to convey any extra benefit over out-patient care in terms of eventual outcome (Hawton *et al.*, 1981).

Patients who frequently repeat suicide attempts are notoriously difficult to help. Most have major personality problems and very low tolerance of stress. A preliminary trial of depot flupenthixol for such patients suggested that this approach may be worth trying in some cases (Montgomery and Montgomery, 1982).

Other forms of aftercare

Some patients will most appropriately be helped by Social Services, Marriage Guidance, specialized counselling services (for problems concerning homosexuality, bereavement, and so on), or other agencies. Those with major alcohol problems may require referral to a specialized alcoholism treatment unit. In view of the considerable numbers of attempted suicide patients who have problems in the use of alcohol, there should be close liaison between staff responsible for the care of attempted suicide patients in the general hospital and local alcoholism treatment services.

The second most frequent form of aftercare, as shown in Table 12.7, is returning the patient to the care of the general practitioner. This may be appropriate if the attempt has been very impulsive, the patient's problems are relatively minor, and the patient feels capable of coping with them with perhaps support from relatives or friends. Some general practitioners will in any case wish to provide the aftercare themselves.

SUICIDE RISK

Clinicians should include assessment of suicide risk in the overall assessment of most patients with psychiatric disorder (not just suicide attempters), and certainly all who are depressed.

Assessment of suicide risk is not easy, and represents one of the most stressful tasks to confront doctors. While we have a reasonable understanding of the factors that contribute to the risk of suicide, it is extremely difficult to differentiate patients who are at serious risk from those with relatively low risk (Murphy, 1984; Hawton 1987).

How to assess suicide risk

The following are some guidelines on how suicide risk can be assessed, including factors that should be taken into account. Each factor by itself may not have significant predictive power, but the clinician must draw together all the available information in order to make a global judgement concerning risk. The main concern will be whether or not there is any relatively immediate risk. In this respect patients' current thoughts, including about their future and about suicide as an option, are perhaps the most important factors.

Current suicidal ideas

There is no evidence that discussion of suicide increases the risk that it will actually happen. Many patients with suicidal ideas obtain considerable relief through being able to discuss these with a sympathetic listener. A useful way to broach the topic is to ask patients how they feel about the future, or whether they see things improving. Patients who indicate that they are feeling pessimistic or hopeless should then be asked specifically about whether they ever feel that life is not worth living. Any indication of suicidal ideas should be followed up with enquiry about their extent and nature, including details of any plans that have been made. The clinician should ask about the availability of means of suicide, especially those likely to be lethal. The patient should also be asked if there are any constraints which make it unlikely that suicide will occur (for example, children; other relatives).

Previous suicidal acts

As already noted, attempted suicide greatly increases the risk of eventual suicide. Therefore, the patient should be asked about possible earlier attempts, including any that may not have come to the attention of others.

Supports

Alienation from other people is often a key factor in suicide. Therefore the extent of support available to the patient should be assessed, especially whether there is a readily available confidant with whom the patient is willing to discuss the current difficulties.

Personality traits

Aggressive and impulsive tendencies appear to increase suicide risk, and may be evident from past behaviour, especially when the patient has been under stress.

Other risk factors

In the assessment, account should also be taken of other factors known to increase suicide risk, including: alcohol abuse, unemployment, financial problems, bereavement, chronic physical illness and a family history of suicide.

Principles of management of patients at risk

These are some guidelines worth following when caring for patients thought to be at risk of suicide, whether care is being provided in a psychiatric or general practice setting.

See the patient frequently

Suicidal patients often value having regular frequent appointments. These might be backed up with suggestions as to how the patient can get in contact with the clinician between appointments should the situation become intolerable.

Ensure that the patient has only small amounts of medication available

Prescriptions for only a few days or a week's supply of medication for those receiving psychotropics can both reduce the risk of an overdose and also provide a good reason for regular appointments.

Regularly review suicide risk

Suicidal ideas should be reviewed at each appointment, because these can often change fairly suddenly, especially if the patient's circumstances have altered. It is important not to try forcibly to argue patients out of their pessimistic thoughts or suicidal ideas, but to acknowledge their reality and to try and convey some empathy about the situation. However, sometimes it helps to get the patient to examine the pros and cons of suicide, including the likelihood that the patient's circumstances, mood and so on will change in due course (see Chapter 10 in Beck *et al.*, 1979).

CONCLUSIONS

Suicidal behaviour presents formidable problems for clinicians, partly because it is difficult to predict and partly because it may appear to represent a rejection of the clinician's willingness to try and help patients. Nevertheless, it is essential that general hospital staff and general practitioners inform themselves about suicide and develop the skills necessary to carry out a basic assessment of both suicide risk and the important features of an actual suicide attempt. It is worth reminding ourselves that approximately two-thirds of those who carry out suicidal acts, whether fatal or not, have seen a doctor during the month beforehand. While we should not necessarily respond to this fact as an indictment of our skills, because it tells us nothing about many suicides doctors actually prevent, nevertheless it emphasizes that doctors have at least some potential role in the further prevention of suicidal behaviour.

RECOMMENDED READING

Barraclough B., Hughes J. (1987). *Suicide: Clinical and Epidemiological Studies.* London: Croom Helm.
Hawton K., Catalan J. (1987). *Attempted Suicide: A Practical Guide to its Nature and Management* 2nd edn. Oxford: Oxford University Press.
Morgan H.G. (1979). *Death wishes? The Understanding and Management of Deliberate Self-Harm.* Chichester: Wiley.

REFERENCES

Bancroft J., Hawton K., Simkin S., *et al.* (1979). The reasons people give for taking overdoses: a further enquiry. *British Journal of Medical Psychology*, **52**, 353–65.
Bancroft J., Marsack P. (1977). The repetitiveness of self-poisoning and self-injury. *British Journal of Psychiatry*, **131**, 394–9.
Bancroft J., Shrimshire A., Casson J., *et al.* (1977). People who deliberately poison

or injure themselves: their problems and their contacts with helping agencies. *Psychological Medicine*, 7, 289–303.

Barraclough B., Hughes J. (1987). *Suicide: Clinical and Epidemiological Studies*. London: Croom Helm.

Beck A. T., Schuyler D., Herman J. (1974). Development of suicidal intent scales. In *The Prediction of Suicide* (Beck A. T., Resnik H. L. P., Lettieri D. J., eds.). Maryland: Charles Press.

Beck A. T., Beck R., Kovacs M. (1975). Classification of suicidal behaviors; I. Quantifying intent and medical lethality. *American Journal of Psychiatry*, 132, 285–7.

Beck A. T., Rush A. J., Shaw B. F., Emery G. (1979). *Cognitive Therapy of Depression*. New York: Guilford Press.

Beck A. T., Steer R. A., Kovacs M., Garrison B. (1985). Hopelessness and eventual suicide: a 10 year prospective study of patients hospitalized with suicidal ideation. *American Journal of Psychiatry*, 145, 559–63.

Buglass D., McCulloch J. W. (1970). Further suicidal behaviour: the development and validation of predictive scales. *British Journal of Psychiatry*, 116, 483–91.

Buglass D., Horton J. (1974). A scale for predicting subsequent suicidal behaviour. *British Journal of Psychiatry*, 124, 573–8.

Catalan J., Marsack P., Hawton K. E., *et al*. (1980). Comparison of doctors and nurses in the assessment of deliberate self-poisoning patients. *Psychological Medicine*, 10, 483–91.

Central and Scottish Health Service Councils (1968). *Hospital Treatment of Acute Poisoning*. London: HMSO.

Department of Health and Social Security (1984). *The Management of Deliberate Self-Harm* HN (84) 25. London: Department of Health and Social Security.

Fernando S., Storm V. (1984). Suicide among psychiatric patients of a district general hospital. *Psychological Medicine*, 14, 661–72.

Forster D. P., Frost C. E. B. (1985). Medicinal self-poisoning and prescription frequency. *Acta Psychiatrica Scandinavica*, 71, 657–74.

Fox K., Weissman M. (1975). Suicide attempts and drugs: contradiction between method and intent. *Social Psychiatry*, 10, 31–8.

Gardner R., Hanka R., Evison B., *et al*. (1978). Consultation-liaison scheme for self-poisoned patients in a general hospital. *British Medical Journal*, ii, 1392–4.

Gibbons J. S., Butler P., Urwin P., Gibbons J. L. (1978). Evaluation of a social work service for self-poisoning patients. *British Journal of Psychiatry*, 133, 111–8.

Hawton K. (1978). Deliberate self-poisoning and self-injury in the psychiatric hospital. *British Journal of Medical Psychology*, 51, 253–9.

Hawton K. (1982). How patients and psychiatrists account for overdoses. In *Personal Meanings* (Shepted E., Watson J., eds.). Chichester: Wiley, pp. 103–14.

Hawton K. (1986). *Suicide and Attempted Suicide among Children and Adolescents*. Beverley Hills: Sage.

Hawton K. (1987). Assessment of suicide risk. *British Journal of Psychiatry*, 150, 145–53.

Hawton K., Blackstock E. (1976). General practice aspects of self-poisoning and self-injury. *Psychological Medicine*, 6, 571–5.

Hawton K., Blackstock E. (1977). Deliberate self-poisoning: implications for psychotropic drug prescribing in general practice. *Journal of the Royal College of General Practitioners*, **27**, 560–3

Hawton K., Catalan J. (1987). *Attempted Suicide: A Practical Guide to its Nature and Management* 2nd edn. Oxford: Oxford University Press.

Hawton K., Fagg J. (1988). Suicide and other causes of death following attempted suicide. *British Journal of Psychiatry*, **152**, 359–366.

Hawton K., Rose. N. (1986). Unemployment and attempted suicide among men in Oxford. *Health Trends*, **18**, 29–32.

Hawton K, Gath D. H., Smith E. B. O. (1979). Management of attempted suicide in Oxford. *British Medical Journal*, **ii**, 1040–2.

Hawton K., Bancroft J., Catalan J., *et al.* (1981). Domiciliary and out-patient treatment of self-poisoning patients by medical and non-medical staff. *Psychological Medicine*, **11**, 169–77.

Hawton K., O'Grady J., Osborn M., Cole D. (1982). Adolescents who take overdoses: their characteristics, problems and contacts with helping agencies. *British Journal of Psychiatry*, **140**, 118–23.

Hawton K., Roberts J., Goodwin G., (1985). The risk of child abuse among attempted suicide mothers with young children. *British Journal of Psychiatry*, **146**, 486–9.

Hawton K., McKeown S., Day A., *et al.* (1987). Evaluation of out-patient counselling compared with general practitioner care following overdoses. *Psychological Medicine*, **17**, 756–61.

Hawton K., Fagg J., Simkin S. (1988) Unemployment and attempted suicide among women in Oxford. *British Journal of Psychiatry*, **152**, 632–7.

Kessel N., McCulloch W. (1966). Repeated acts of self-poisinong and self-injury. *Proceedings of the Royal Society of Medicine*, **59**, 89–92.

Montgomery S. A., Montgomery D. (1982). Pharmacological prevention of suicidal behaviour. *Journal of Affective Disorders*, **4**, 291–8.

Murphy G. E. (1984). The prediction of suicide: why is it so difficult? *American Journal of Psychotherapy*, **38**, 341–9.

Newson-Smith J. G. B., Hirsch S. R. (1979a). Psychiatric symptoms in self-poisoning patients. *Psychological Medicine*, **9**, 493–500.

Newson-Smith J. G. B., Hirsch S. R. (1979b). A comparison of social workers and psychiatrist in evaluating parasuicide. *British Journal of Psychiatry*, **134**, 335–42.

Ovenstone I. M. K., Kreitman N. (1974). Two syndromes of suicide. *British Journal of Psychiatry*, **124**, 336–45.

Pallis D. J., Barraclough B. M., Levey A. B., *et al.* (1982). Estimating suicide risk among attempted suicides: I. The development of new clinical scales. *British Journal of Psychiatry*, **141**, 37–44.

Parker G., Blignault I., Manicavasagar V. (1988). Neurotic depression: delineation of symptom profiles and their outcome. *British Journal of Psychiatry*, **152**, 15–23.

Paykel E. S., Prusoff B. A., Myers J. K. (1975). Suicide attempts and recent life events: a controlled comparison. *Archives of General Psychiatry*, **32**, 327–33.

Petrie K., Chamberlain K., Clarke D. (1988). Psychological predictors of future suicidal behaviours in hospitalized suicide attempters. *British Journal of Clinical Psychology*, **27**, 247–57.

Pierce D. W. (1981). Predictive validation of a suicide intent scale. *British Journal of Psychiatry*, **139**, 391–6.

Platt S., Kreitman N. (1984). Trends in parasuicide and unemployment among men in Edinburgh, 1968–82. *British Medical Journal*, **289**, 1029–32.

Platt S., Hawton K., Kreitman N., *et al.* (1988). Recent clinical and epidemiological trends in parasuicide in Edinburgh and Oxford: a tale of two cities. *Psychological Medicine*, **18**, 405–18.

Pokorny A. D. (1964). Suicide rate in various psychiatric disorders. *Journal of Nervous and Mental Disease*, **139**, 499–506.

Ramon S., Bancroft J. H. J., Shrimshire A. M. (1975). Attitudes towards self-poisoning among physicians and nurses in a general hospital. *British Journal of Psychiatry*, **127**, 257–64.

Simpson M. A. (1976). Self-mutilation. *British Journal of Hospital Medicine*, **16**, 430–8.

Tuckman J., Youngman W. F. (1968). A scale for assessing suicide risk of attempted suicides. *Journal of Clinical Psychology*, **24**, 17–9.

Urwin P., Gibbons J. L. (1979). Psychiatric diagnosis in self-poisoning patients. *Psychological Medicine*, **9**, 501–7.

Wing J. K., Cooper J. E., Sartorius N. (1974). *The Measurement and Classification of Psychiatric Symptoms*. Cambridge: Cambridge University Press.

13 The Recognition, Diagnosis and Acknowledgement of Depressive Disorder by General Practitioners

ANDRÉ TYLEE AND PAUL FREELING

INTRODUCTION

An integrative approach to depression in general practice would include: early recognition of available 'cues' to depression; accurate and early diagnosis (or exclusion); acknowledgement and explanation of depression as a syndrome not a symptom; and appropriate management decided upon jointly with the patient. Recognition and acknowledgement are included as distinct steps, because occasionally general practitioners (GPs) say, when asked, that they had recognized someone as possibly depressed but chose not to make a formal diagnosis and be forced to acknowledge it to the patient. Achieving such an integrative approach with all depressed patients at all times will be a stern challenge to any GP's attitudes, skills and knowledge. Skills and knowledge certainly, and attitudes probably, will vary with the frequency with which they have to be deployed.

Rates

There are some difficulties in determining the frequency with which GPs are consulted by depressed patients but such difficulties are not limited to general practice and may reflect the long-running debate about 'caseness' (Bebbington et al., 1981; Wing et al., 1981; Goldberg, 1982).

Blacker and Clare (1987), after reviewing the evidence, suggested that general practice prevalence rates for major and minor depression, as defined by the Research Diagnostic Criteria (RDC) (Spitzer et al., 1978), are probably each about 5 percent. Whatever the true prevalence of depression in the community may be, nearly all of it presents in general practice and very few patients recognized by GPs as having mental illness are referred to a psychiatrist (Fahy, 1974; Grad de Alarcon et al., 1975).

Nearly 13 percent of consecutive attenders aged 15 and over consulting a GP for a new illness have a diagnosable major depressive disorder (Bridges and Goldberg, 1987), yet in the Third National Morbidity Study (Royal College of General Practitioners *et al.*, 1986), GPs from England and Wales, in 1981–82, reported only 28 patients per 1000 per year suffering from depression. In an average GP's list of 2000 patients this would mean about 56 new cases of depression or approximately one every week. This one person per week cannot represent nearly 13 percent of all consecutive attenders aged 15 and over seen with new problems. This large discrepancy may be partly because GPs tend to report to studies only patients for whom they have prescribed drugs (Watson and Barber, 1981; Burton and Freeling, 1982) but choose to manage similar numbers of depressives in ways other than by prescribing antidepressants (Sireling *et al.*, 1985a). The true discrepancy may be larger than the one calculated since the GP-notified figures include patients the GP diagnoses as depressed but who do not conform to psychiatric criteria for the condition, as well as patients who never take the drugs prescribed (Johnson, 1973). Only some half of the patients given antidepressants by their GP received RDC diagnoses of major depression (Sireling *et al.*, 1985a) although 96 percent were categorized as having some kind of psychiatric diagnosis.

INCORRECT ACKNOWLEDGEMENT

Whatever its size most of the discrepancy between diagnosis rates reported by GPs and prevalence rates determined by researchers seems to stem from GPs' failure to acknowledge the depression. Just over half of the major depressives found by screening are not acknowledged as such by their GPs, whether they were consulting for new problems (Bridges and Goldberg, 1987) or for any reason (Skuse and Williams, 1984; Freeling *et al.*, 1985).

Non-acknowledgement is as much a characteristic of American family physicians (Hoeper *et al.*, 1980; Nielsen and Williams, 1980; Hankin and Locke, 1983; Zung *et al.*, 1983; Zung and King, 1983; Zung *et al.*, 1985) and family medicine residents (Moore *et al.*, 1978; Goldberg and Huxley 1980) as it is of British GPs and their vocational trainees.

Most of the studies discussed so far have dealt with samples on which an upper age limit as well as a lower one was imposed. MacDonald (1986) reported low recognition of depression as being less of a problem in the elderly. Although he confirmed a low rate of intervention for depression in this group, he attributed it to failure by GPs to acknowledge and intervene rather than a failure to recognize their patients' depression. MacDonald used a low criterion for classifying a patient's depression as recognized: he asked GPs to rate the extent to which the patient had been depressed over the previous month by ticking boxes which ranged from 'not at all' to 'severely'. The presence of such a form in the notes to be filled in during the consultation may have acted as a cue to the GPs to consider depression.

Some of the caution shown by GPs in making explicit diagnoses of depression may originate from the frequency with which they use drugs to manage such illnesses. In 1985, more than 6.7 million prescriptions for antidepressants were dispensed by the National Health Service (NHS) pharmaceutical services in England and Wales. Patients prescribed anti-depressants were more likely than those whose depression GPs chose to manage in other ways (Sireling *et al.*, 1985a) to be categorized as having case depression on the Index of Definition (Wing, 1976) and had higher Hamilton scores (Hamilton, 1967) and Raskin ratings (Raskin *et al.*, 1970).

Both the group treated by GPs with antidepressants and those managed by them in other ways had significantly lower mean scores than a comparison psychiatric out-patient sample (Sireling *et al.*, 1985b).

ATTITUDES, SKILLS AND KNOWLEDGE

Competence in early recognition, identification, acknowledgement, and management of depression will depend upon the nature of the GP's attitudes, skills and knowledge.

Attitudes

The wide variation among GPs in their detection of psychiatric disorders has been known for over 20 years (Shepherd *et al.*, 1966), and the ways in which this might be explained have been explored in two very contrasting styles. One style focused on the difficulties of defining caseness and categorizing the complex mixtures of affective disorder and psychosocial distress presented to GPs (Shepherd, 1986). The other style, (Balint, 1957) focused on the personalities of the GPs and their understanding, as opposed to categorization, of their patients' problems. By 1979, however, analytical surveys were being conducted which showed that much of the variability among GPs could be accounted for by the personal bias of individual doctors towards or away from such problems (Marks *et al.*, 1979). Over and above such studies there was other more pragmatic evidence available of the importance of GPs' attitudes in accounting for their variability in diagnosing and managing emotional disorder in general and depressive illness in particular.

Practice arrangements

Factors which may be important include practice arrangements within and outside the consulting room. GP attitudes may be apparent in the geographical arrangements within their consulting room. The position of the desk, the doctor and the patient have been reported to be crucial to the development of intimacy (Pietroni, 1976). Certainly, many more GPs today, than in the recent past, routinely arrange the furniture in their consulting rooms so that there is little in the way of physical barrier between them and the patient. Patients have been reported to prefer friendly, less formal consulting rooms without any desk at all (Bevan *et al.*, 1979).

GPs' working arrangements have changed radically over the past decade (Freeling and Fitton, 1983) and the increase in the number and size of group practices and the almost universal adoption of appointment systems makes it increasingly difficult for patients to see their 'personal physician' even in group practices which attempt to maintain personal lists (Pereira Gray, 1979). This seems likely to produce what Balint (1957) described as a 'collusion of anonymity' within a practice, without the original need to refer a patient to a specialist. Ever larger groups of doctors covering each other and sharing lists between themselves, and including in their number transient trainees and even more evanescent students, can deny intimacy to those patients who desire it—although some other patients may welcome its lack. A GP covering an absent partner may be less likely to be 'cued' in to underlying depression in someone unfamiliar who is presenting with a sore throat or, even if a cue is recognized, a *de facto* locum tenens may not be prepared to explore a patient's painful feelings. Equally, it is possible for a GP to become so tolerant of a patient whom he or she knows well that a patient's depressive illness can remain unrecognized (Freeling *et al.*, 1985).

Patients are people

Some personal characteristics of the patient such as age and gender seem to affect a GP's tendency towards preferred diagnoses, with women being more likely to receive diagnoses of affective disorder and prescription for psychotropic drugs, and men being more likely to receive antibiotics (Raynes, 1979). Marks *et al.* (1979) found that demographic characteristics such as unemployment, female sex, and marriages that had ended by separation, divorce, or death, were associated with an increased likelihood of the doctor detecting a psychiatric illness.

On the other hand, in another study, no demographic differences were found between recognized and unrecognized depressed patients although, as is commonly found, females outnumbered men by about 4:1 in both groups (Freeling *et al.*, 1985). One study in the USA suggests that there are some patients who once missed remain that way for a long time (Weissman *et al.*, 1981), although another study has described how some depressives are eventually recognized (Widmer and Cadoret, 1978). In the UK, unrecognized depressives were more likely than recognized ones to have had their illness for more than a year (Freeling *et al.*, 1985).

It does make intuitive sense that marked differences in age, sex, class, and nationality between participants are likely to reduce the effectiveness of their mutual communication. The desired outcome or 'ends' of the doctor and patient may differ. A patient who believes that a diagnosis of depression confers great stigma may resent a doctor with a high bias towards identification of such disorder. Ends desired by the patient may only emerge late in a consultation just as the patient is about to go (the 'while I am here' phenomenon). A doctor with a low bias towards psychiatric diagnoses may choose not to recognie 'cues' to depression but deal only with the presenting complaint, although this may be quite unrelated to the patient's more covert ends. The GP achieves one end by finishing surgery earlier and perhaps another end by avoiding an undesired involvement in the personal feelings of another human being.

Rewards and attitudes

If a doctor believes there to be no effective and acceptable treatment for a condition, then it seems possible that he or she may be reluctant to choose to diagnose that condition when offered an opportunity of avoiding doing so. Attitudes towards the treatment and diagnosis of depression in general practice may be changed by a recent placebo-controlled trial of amitriptyline (Paykel *et al.*, 1988). This study treated general practice depressives for six weeks with amitriptyline, reaching mean doses in the fourth and sixth week of 119 mg and median doses of 125 mg, or placebo. Overall, drug was markedly superior to placebo. Interactions were examined between drug effects and a number of variables including demographic characteristics, history of illness, severity of illness, endogenous symptomatology, and precipitating stress. Only in the area of severity were significant interactions found. Thus amitriptyline was superior to placebo in probable or definite major depression (RDC), but not in minor depression. It was also superior to placebo in subjects with initial scores on the Hamilton rating scale of 13 or more, but not in those with lower scores. It remains important, however, to elicit stresses and life events even if their presence does not predict the effectiveness of drugs. The patient may benefit further from support or even counselling while the effect of the drug is being monitored every week or two. In the Paykel study both drug and placebo groups were seen at weeks 1, 2, 4 and 6, and benefit was seen in the placebo group.

It is clear, of course, that people who complete a placebo-controlled trial may not be representative of all depressed patients consulting GPs. Patients in this study did not differ significantly in most characteristics from a sample reported as being given antidepressants by their GPs (Sireling *et al.*, 1985a). There are, of course, patients in general practice who do not want drug treatment or who drop out of it. The best ways of managing these patients remain to be determined as, indeed they do for acknowledged depressives.

Doctors who judge despair to be understandable and therefore not worthy of drug therapy should reconsider their management. There can be no logic in expecting a depressed patient to be more able to solve the problems of life than one who has benefited from drug treatment, nor is there any particular moral benefit from suffering.

In follow-up studies, unrecognized depressives do slightly worse over three months than recognized depressives (Freeling *et al.*, 1985) even though, as in other studies (Parish, 1971; Johnson, 1973; Tyrer, 1973), the majority of patients treated by GPs did not complete a minimal therapeutic course of antidepressant drugs. Depressed patients about whose outcome their doctors were optimistic, and who were therefore not prescribed antidepressants, fared significantly worse than those who were treated (Zung *et al.*, 1985).

Skills

The interviewing style of the GP encompasses a repertoire of skills used at particular times in the consultation, partly to collect information.

The sequence of history taking, examination, diagnosis and treatment taught at medical school is not always evident in general practice consultations. The patient is not always examined physically before management decisions are made (Bevan *et al.*, 1979). It has been described how GPs tend to make management decisions first and then make a diagnosis to justify those decisions (Howie, 1972). This was nicely caricatured by Marinker (1973) as: 'You are a case of valium, ... I will give you some anxiety.' This style may have developed because a patient often has several simultaneous problems and presents them to the GP as an undifferentiated mixture of physical, psychological, and social symptoms. GPs need therefore to adopt a problem-solving approach (Freeling *et al.*, 1983) whilst the process of their consultations and the nature of the actions terminating them will often reflect the probabilistic nature of their decision making (Crombie, 1963; The Royal College of General Practitioners, 1972). Studies of GPs' decision making in conditions other than psychiatric have used a variety of methods (Freeling, 1967; Anderson *et al.*, 1983). Studies of decision making in psychiatric conditions by GPs (Jenkins *et al.*, 1985) and by GP trainees compared with psychiatric trainees (Wilkinson, 1988) have shown low agreement within and between groups. Self-evidently, it is not simply the possession of an appropriate repertory of interviewing skills which produces accurate decision-making, nor is it simply the possession of factual information about psychiatric dysfunction which is needed to be able to make accurate psychiatric diagnoses in general practice. An understanding of the processes involved seems essential.

Knowledge

A model of the process by which one group of family doctors diagnose depression (Burton and Freeling, 1982) has proved acceptable to other GPs. The study group decided that they had first to be cued to consider depressive illness: they then checked a list of symptoms; and, if doing so indicated depressive illness, they applied two orthogonal sets in order to select treatment.

One was set 'depressive tendencies', which included past or family history of depressive illness, or an adverse upbringing; the other comprised concurrent adverse happenings in their lives.

The most commonly used cue proved to be a single symptom of depression (82 percent); second was the patient saying 'I feel depressed' (52 percent); third was the ill-defined cue that the doctor 'felt' the patient was depressed (53 percent); and fourth was the recurrent presentation of symptoms without identifiable organic cause (44 percent). Only rarely did a single cue trigger the process.

These study doctors had said that if a patient had few recent life events and no obvious depressive tendency they would not prescribe but reconsider the diagnosis, while if a patient had a low depressive tendency but lots of life events they would rely on counselling instead of drugs. When GPs audited what they actually did, every patient that they reported had been prescribed an antidepressant drug, although 36 percent of them were in one of these 'won't prescribe' groups. This group of GPs, like most others studied, showed great variability in that one of them reported nearly a half of all cases reported.

Although unrecognized depressives have been shown to be less depressed than those whose depression is recognized (Freeling *et al.*, 1985), many in the unrecognized group are as ill as those who are recognized. Many of the symptoms overlap and are just as handicapping. These symptoms include: pessimism; guilt; impaired activity; loss of energy; and insomnia. Those symptoms which differ between recognized and unrecognized depressives may give a clue to the process of recognition or cueing in the GP which is involved. It must be said that unrecognized depressives were indeed harder to recognize: they were less likely to admit to or complain of depression and looked and behaved less depressed (Freeling *et al.*, 1985). They were more likely to show a 'distinct quality of mood' (Paykel, 1985), a category of symptom representing a change in internal feelings which is not simply increased sadness but includes descriptions such as 'coldness' or 'deadness' or 'emptiness' inside.

It may be the norm for people to expect their GP to be able to untangle and give meaning to their undifferentiated collection of physical, psychological and social symptoms. This handing over of responsibility may include patients expecting their GP to exclude serious physical conditions first and foremost. It is almost certainly inappropriate for a GP to take an extensive psychiatric history from a patient with probable appendicitis seen at home. The patient expects the GP to have the knowledge necessary to decide on the best course of action although the extent and appropriateness of that knowledge will rarely have been put to the test of a GP's peers unless, perhaps, he or she decides to sit for membership of the Royal College of General Practitioners. Peer assessment for membership does not yet include obervation of the candidates' everyday consultations let alone assessment of their patients' outcome. Does a doctor rated by peers as highly skilled in interviewing, but lacking knowledge, achieve a different outcome for depressed patients than a less skilled doctor who is more knowledgeable? Does it make a difference if the GP is aware that unrecognized depressives are more likely to have a concurrent physical illness making a marked contribution to their depression and tend to be referred to non-psychiatric specialists (Freeling *et al.*, 1985)?

IMPROVING PERFORMANCE

Attempts to 'cue' doctors by providing them with the results of research screening questionnaires applied in the waiting room have not helped (Hoeper *et al.*, 1984), although one GP with a known interest in psychiatry found it helpful (Johnstone and Goldberg, 1976). More effective may be attempts to increase GPs' personal skills and knowledge and to affect their attitudes.

Better interviewing behaviours have been taught and shown to increase the accuracy of American family practice trainees in recognizing psychiatric disorders (Goldberg *et al.*, 1980a, 1980b). Problem-solving techniques taught to a self-selected group of established GPs have improved their skills in psychiatry, which were already good (Gask *et al.*, 1987). Interviewing skills taught to undergraduates persist (Maguire *et al.*, 1986). Communication skills training of GPs has increased patient satisfaction (Evans *et al.*, 1987). It is therefore important to identify interviewing skills which are associated with accurate identification of depression by GPs. Peer assessment of skills is recommended by the Royal College of General Practitioners (1985) as a necessary step forward.

Concern about physical illness is reasonable in any circumstances but some patients who somatize their psychiatric disorder also expect to be fully investigated by a specialist. This may waste time and money in an increasingly stretched NHS in order to get the patient to a point where they can be reassured and the psychosocial aspects of their disorder given more prominence. This is also a feature of the health system in the USA (Katon, 1984; Rodin and Voshart, 1986). Somatizers comprise the majority of the people seeing GPs with new complaints who are missed as suffering from major depressive disorder (Bridges and Goldberg, 1987), although to complicate matters further many had a physical complaint also.

Social and cultural differences cause different norms of patient behaviour and, when doctor and patient differ in these ways, problems in communication may lead to identification problems. Doctors, in social class 1, will have different norms from the majority of their patients and GPs need to know how depressive illness may present in different cultures, ages, social groups and sexes.

A WAY FORWARD

At St George's Hospital Medical School we are studying in considerable detail what it is which actually occurs during consultations between depressed people and their GPs. Our study is funded by the Mental Health Foundation. It seeks to determine any consistent differences in content or interviewing style between videotaped consultations in which major depression (RDC) is acknowledged by instituting some form of management, and those in which it goes unacknowledged; and contrasting these with consultations involving patients who are not depressed. About 40 GPs have been filmed so far, for up to 25 hours each, in order to acquire a subject each for each of the three groups.

Consultation Analysis by Triggers and Symptoms (CATS) is a new instrument developed (Tylee and Freeling, 1987) to code both the content and the use of specific interviewing behaviours from a videotape of a consultation. Physical, psychological or social symptoms mentioned by the patient are recorded in sequence and coded together with the GPs' immediately preceding behaviour, whether verbal or non-verbal. CATS has 200 symptom codings including a category for ill-defined symptoms, which is likely to prove particularly useful in coding the presenting statement by depressed patients. These ill-defined symptoms can be reclassified, or new codings developed at a later stage if, for instance, it becomes apparent that general practice depressives report symptoms different from depressives seen by research psychiatrists. CATS could be modified to study non-psychiatric conditions if desired.

Patients are interviewed within a few days of the recorded interview using a comprehensive interviewing schedule (Sireling *et al.*, 1985a). This schedule provides a 'Gold Standard' for available symptoms with which the symptoms recorded from the videotaped interview can be compared, and it permits classification over and above RDC. Although devised by American research psychiatrists, we have found the RDC definition of major depression easy to memorize and apply in everyday British general practice. The use of such an instrument avoids 'caseness' problems to a large extent, and means that a common language is used for studies until perhaps a more suitable, general practice-generated, alternative is devised. The criteria unfortunately reflect some of the difficulties encountered by GPs because they include some symptoms which are expected in physical conditions such as poor appetite, poor sleep and fatigue.

A consultation must be judged as a whole and not simply as the sum of its parts. Therefore, a companion rating scale, Consultation Analysis by Behaviour and Style (CABS), has been devised. It is intended to assess doctors' behaviour and style more globally (Tylee and Freeling, 1987). CABS draws on what is known about 'desirable' doctor interviewing behaviours in general rather than only those most suitable for the purposes of diagnosing psychiatric illness. It assesses these behaviours mainly on 4-point scales. This technique has been easily taught to and applied by a consensus criterion group of GPs and a GP trainee group. CABS assesses interviewing skills; problem definition; and the selection, naming, solving or management of key problems. The emotional tone of the consultation, degree of empathy and use of authority are assessed also.

PRELIMINARY FINDINGS

Some early findings are available from videotapes of this study. The tables below focus on two aspects: presenting symptoms; and the position in the consultation sequence of the first symptom mentioned which could be a cue to a depressive illness. One table has been used for each of the three groups of patients studied.

The controls (Table 13.1)

The range of presenting symptoms for the control consultations demonstrates the variety of everyday general practice. None of them starts with a symptom directly cueing a GP to consider depressive illness, although in a third of the consultations such symptoms were presented later. These may well relate to the presenting physical problem: they cannot relate to an underlying depression. An example is the person with period problems

Table 13.1 Symptoms and cues to depression at consultation—controls without depression

Presentation symptom	First verbal cue	Cue position
1. Thumb pain	—	—
2. Tetanus booster	—	—
3. Knee swelling	—	—
4. Coil change	—	—
5. Cough	—	—
6. Breast tenderness	—	—
7. Nasty taste	—	—
8. Ankle sprain	—	—
9. Voice loss	—	—
10. Lump in wound	—	—
11. Sheath burst	—	—
12. Hand numb	—	—
13. Vaginal burning	Night waking	17
14. A bit sick	Night waking	2
15. Migraine	Gets on my nerves	9
16. Period trouble	Tiredness	4
17. Itch all over	Little sleep	6
18. Itch on leg	No energy	5
19. Dull arm ache	Feel so depressed	10

who is tired; could this be due to an anaemia caused by menorrhagia? The last consultation contained a statement of depressed mood despite that person scoring below the accepted threshold of the screening instrument.

Acknowledged group (Table 13.2)

Symptoms which cue for depression appeared within the first three statements of 13 of the 21 consultations. The very first statement made by the patient was a depression cue in 8 consultations. Three other consultations had relatively early first cues to depression. Of interest are the two consultations that resulted in the patient being newly acknowledged by their GP as depressed without any symptoms of depression being discussed at all! These patients may represent the 'doctor felt the patient was depressed' cue of the earlier study of process by Burton and Freeling (1982).

Unacknowledged group (Table 13.3)

Only 5 (of 21) consultations contained a possible cue in the first three statements, compared with 13 in the acknowledged group. On the other hand four of these cues were the first statement made by the patient and

13.2 Consultations with acknowledged major depression

	Presentation symptom	*First verbal cue*	*Position of cue*
1.	Depressed		1
2.	So nervous		1
3.	Redundancy worry		1
4.	Can't cope		1
5.	Problem sleeping		1
6.	Nerves gone		1
7.	In a nervous state		1
8.	Unable to lose weight		1
9.	Sore biopsy site	Tired	3
10.	Funny thumb	Miserable	3
11.	Leg pain	Can't be bothered	3
12.	Breathing trouble	Frightened	3
13.	Bad leg	Weight problem	3
14.	Change of life	Depressed	4
15.	Hip pain	Tension	5
16.	Vomiting	Run down	7
17.	Leg pulsation	Extremely tired	8
18.	Abdominal pains	Worry	10
19.	Bad sinusitis	Not happy	12
20.	Neck cyst		
21.	Weak leg		

Table 13.3 Consultations with unacknowledged major depression

Presenting symptom	First verbal cue	Position of cue
1. Contractions		
2. Fell off motor bike		
3. Burning abdo pain		
4. Bronchial		
5. Stomach pain		
6. Foot rash		
7. Catarrh		
8. Knee pains		
9. Pain passing urine	I feel low	24
10. Bellyaches	Miserable	14
11. Stomach cramps	Work worry	14
12. Bad throat	Feel down	10
13. Need antacid	Home stress	7
14. Skin rash	Lot of stress	5
15. At point zero		1
16. Not eating		1
17. Constipated		1
18. Extremely run down		1
19. Pill	No brighter	2
20. Hot flushes	Bad tempers	4
21. Bad throat	No energy	4

there is one consultation in which depression is not acknowledged by the GP despite an opening statement of 'I am really at point zero'. The GP in this case discussed the failure of physiotherapy to alleviate the patient's neck pain and referred her to an orthopaedic surgeon. In 8 consultations no symptoms at all were mentioned which might suggest depression to the doctor.

Whilst these early findings may prove to be unrepresentative of all consultations eventually filmed, they remain interesting. They certainly suggest that symptoms mentioned early in consultations influence whether depression is acknowledged by GPs. Further analyses will examine what syndromes of symptoms GPs use to make the diagnosis of depressive illness and what symptoms are present when they do not acknowledge depression. By comparing such findings with the symptoms elicited in the extensive diagnostic interview, criteria which are commonly used by GPs to recognize depression may emerge. Conversely, it may be that GPs do not demand the presence of the same number of symptoms as do psychiatrists to make a diagnosis of depression. This combination of fewer symptoms required and fewer symptoms utilized by GPs would explain the presence of both false positive and false negative diagnoses when GPs are assessed against research 'Gold Standards' which themselves have been validated against the clinical work of specialist psychiatrists. It may be, also, that repetition of a symptom may weigh more heavily with a GP as an indication of severity than it does to a psychiatrist.

It is intended to establish whether particular consulting styles are related to accurate identification and acknowledgement of depression. One study found a strong correlation between patients' scores on a psychiatric screening questionnaire and the number of cues to psychological disturbance given in the consultation (Davenport *et al.*, 1987). The authors concluded that the reason why some doctors are better able than others to detect psychiatric illness is that they are more likely to allow patients to express verbal cues about lowered mood as well as somehow permitting 'vocal' (termed by others to be paraverbal) cues such as sighing.

THE FUTURE

As studies begin to determine what distinguishes acknowledged from unacknowledged depressive illness, so more general practice-based research becomes necessary. Whilst we know something about the marked benefits to acknowledged patients of treatment with tricyclic antidepressants in recommended dosages we have yet to determine the appropriate management for patients reluctant to take, or not benefiting from, such medication. We do not know for sure that unacknowledged patients will benefit from the same treatments as acknowledged ones, indeed we do not know what benefits these patients may receive simply from being acknowledged. An integrative approach to the management of our depressed patients adopted now is likely to benefit them. Further research is required before we can be sure that we have described all that needs be integrated for their benefit.

REFERENCES

Anderson H. R., Freeling P., Patel S. P. (1983). Decision making in adult asthma. *Journal of the Royal College of General Practitioners*, 33, 105–8.

Balint M. (1957). *The Doctor, the Patient, and the Illness*. London: Pitman Medical.

Bebbington P. E., Tennant C., Hurry J. (1981). Adversity and the nature of psychiatric disorder in the community. *Journal of Affective Disorders*, 3, 345–66.

Bevan J., Cunningham D. and Floyd C. (1979). *Doctors on the Move*. Exeter: Royal College of General Practitioners.

Blacker C. V. R., Clare A. W. (1987). Depressive disorder in primary care. *British Journal of Psychiatry*, 150, 737–51.

Bridges K., Goldberg D. (1987). Somatic presentation of depressive illness in primary care. In *The Presentation of Depression: Current Approaches* (Freeling P., Downey L. J., Malkin J. C., eds.). London: The Royal College of General Practitioners, pp. 9–11.

Burton R. H., Freeling P. (1982). How general practitioners manage depressive illness: developing a method of audit. *Journal of the Royal College of General Practitioners*, **32**, 558–61.

Crombie D. L. (1963). Diagnostic methods. *Journal of the Royal College of General Practitioners*, **6**, 579–89.

Davenport S., Goldberg D., Millar T. (1987). How psychiatric disorders are missed during medical consultations. *Lancet*, **2**, 439–40.

Evans J., Kiellerup F. D., Stanley R. O., *et al.* (1987). A communication skills programme for increasing patients' satisfaction with general practice consultations. *British Journal of Medical Psychology*, **60**, 373–8.

Fahy T. J. (1974). Pathways of specialist referral of depressed patients from general practice. *British Journal of Psychiatry*, **124**, 231–9.

Freeling P. (1967). The significance of symptoms. *Proceedings of the Royal Society of Medicine*, **60**, 34–7.

Freeling P., Fitton P. (1983). Teaching practices revisited. *British Medical Journal*, **287**, 353–7.

Freeling P., Burton R., Chegwidden R., *et al.* (1983). *A Workbook for Trainees in General Practice*. Bristol: Wright PSG.

Freeling P., Rao B. M., Paykel E. S., *et al.* (1985). *British Medical Journal*, **290**, 1880–3.

Gask L., McGrath G., Goldberg D., Millar T. (1987). Improving the psychiatric skills of established general practitioners: evaluation of group teaching. *Medical Education*, **21**, 362–8.

Goldberg D. (1982). The concept of a psychiatric 'case' in general practice. *Social Psychiatry*, **17**, 61–5.

Goldberg D., Huxley P. (1980). *Mental Illness in the Community — The Pathway to Psychiatric Care*. London: Tavistock Publications.

Goldberg D. P., Steele J. J., Smith C. (1980a). Teaching psychiatric interviewing skills to family doctors. *Acta psychiatrica Scandinavica*, **62**, 41–7.

Goldberg D. P., Steele J. J., Smith C., Spivey L. (1980b). Training family doctors to recognize psychiatric illness with increased accuracy. *Lancet*, **ii**, 521–3.

Grad de Alarcon J., Sainsbury P., Costain W. R. (1975). Incidence of referred mental illness in Chichester and Salisbury. *Psychological Medicine*, **5**, 32–54.

Hankin J. R., Locke B. Z. (1983). Extent of depressive symptomatology among patients seeking care in a prepaid group practice. *Psychological Medicine*, **13**, 121–9.

Hamilton M. (1967). Development of a rating scale for primary depressive illness. *British Journal of Social and Clinical Psychology*, **6**, 278–96.

Hoeper E. W., Nycz G. R., Regier D. A. (1980). Diagnosis of mental disorder in adults and increased use of health services in four out-patient settings. *American Journal of Psychiatry*, **137**, 207–10.

Hoeper E. W., Kessler L. G., Burke J. D., Pierce W. (1984). The usefulness of screening for mental illness. *Lancet*, **i**, 33–5.

Howie J. G. R. (1972). Diagnosis — the Achilles heel. *Journal of the Royal College of General Practitioners*, **22**, 310–15.

Jenkins R., Smeeton N., Marinker M., Shepherd M. (1985). A study of the classification of mental ill health in general practice. *Psychological Medicine*, **15**, 403–9.

Johnson D. A. W. (1973). Treatment of depression in general practice. *British Medical Journal*, **2**, 1061–4.

Johnstone A., Goldberg D. (1976). Psychiatric screening in general practice: a controlled trial. *Lancet*, **i**, 605–8.

Katon W. (1984). Depression: relationship to somatisation and chronic illness. *Journal of Clinical Psychiatry*, **45**, 4–11.

MacDonald A. J. D. (1986). Do general practitioners 'miss' depression in elderly patients? *British Medical Journal*, **292**, 1365–7.

Maguire G., Fairbairn S., Fletcher C. (1986). Benefit of feedback training in interviewing as students persist. *British Medical Journal*, **1**, 268–70.

Marinker M. (1973). The doctors role in prescribing. In *The Medical Use of Psychotropic Drugs* suppl. 2, vol. 23. London: Royal College of General Practitioners.

Marks J. N., Goldberg D., Hillier V. F. (1979). Determinants of the ability of general practitioners to detect psychiatric illness. *Psychological Medicine*, **9**, 337–53.

Moore J. T., Silimperi D. R., Bobula J. A. (1978). Recognition of depression by family medicine residents: the impact of screening. *Journal of Family Practice*, **3**, 509–13.

Nielsen A. C., Williams T. A. (1980). Depression in ambulatory medical patients, prevalence by self-report questionnaire and recognition by non-psychiatric physicians. *Archives of General Psychiatry*, **37**, 999–1004.

Parish P. A. (1971). The prescription of psychotropic drugs in general practice. *Journal of the Royal College of General Practitioners*, **21**, (suppl. 4), 1–77.

Paykel E. S. (1985). The clinical interview for depression: development and validity. *Journal of Affective Disorders*, **9**, 85–96.

Paykel E. S., Hollyman J. A., Freeling P., Sedwick P. (1988). Predictors of therapeutic benefit from amitriptyline in mild depression: a general practice placebo-controlled trial. *Journal of Affective Disorders*, **14**, 83–95.

Pereira Gray D. J. (1979). The key to personal care. *Journal of the Royal College of General Practitioners*, **29**, 666–78.

Pietroni P. (1976). Non-verbal communication in the general practice surgery. In *Language and Communication in General Practice* (Tanner B., ed.). London: Hodder and Stoughton.

Raskin A., Schulterbrandt J., Reatig N., McKeon J. J. (1970). Differential response to chlorpromazine, imipramine and placebo. A study of sub-groups of hospitalized depressed patients. *Archives of General Psychiatry*, **23**, 164–73.

Raynes N. V. (1979). Factors affecting the prescribing of psychotropic drugs in general practice consultations. *Psychological Medicine*, **9**, 671–9.

Rodin G., Voshart K. (1986). Depression in the medically ill: an overview. *Americal Journal of Psychiatry*, **143**, 696–705.

Royal College of General Practitioners (1972). *The Future General Practitioner— Learning and Teaching*. London: British Medical Journal.

Royal College of General Practitioners (1985). *What Sort of Doctor. Assessing Quality of Care in General Practice*. Exeter: Royal College of General Practitioners.

Royal College of General Practitioners, Office of Population Censuses and Surveys, and Department of Health and Social Security (1986). *Morbidity Statistics from General Practice. Third National Study, 1981–1982*. London: HMSO.

Shepherd M. (1986). Chairman's closing remarks in *Mental Illness in Primary*

Care Settings (Shepherd M., Wilkinson G., Williams P., eds.). London: Tavistock Publications.

Shepherd M., Cooper M., Brown A. C., Kalton G. (1966). *Psychiatric Illness in General Practice*. Oxford: Oxford University Press.

Sireling L. I., Paykel E. S., Freeling P., *et al.* (1985a). Depression in general practice: case thresholds and diagnosis. *British Journal of Psychiatry*, **147**, 113–9.

Sireling L. I., Freeling P., Paykel E. S., Rao B. M. (1985b). Depression in general practice: clinical features and comparison with out-patients. *British Journal of Psychiatry*, **147**, 119–25.

Skuse D., Williams P. (1984). Screening for psychiatric disorder in general practice. *Psychological Medicine*, **14**, 365–77.

Spitzer R. L., Endicott J., Robins E. (1978). Research Diagnostic Criteria; rationale and reliability. *Archives of General Psychiatry*, **35**, 773–82.

Tylee A. T., Freeling P. (1987). Consultation Analysis by Triggers and Symptoms (CATS). A new objective technique for studying consultations. *Family Practice*, **4**, 260–5.

Tyrer P. (1973). Drug treatments of depression in general practice. *British Medical Journal*, **2**, 18–20.

Watson J. M., Barber J. H. (1981). Depressive illness in general practice: a pilot study. *Health Bulletin*, **39**, 112–6.

Weissman M. M., Myers J. K., Thompson W. D. (1981). Depression and its treatment in a US urban community 1975–76. *Archives of General Psychiatry*, **38**, 417–21.

Widmer R. B., Cadoret R. J. (1978). Depression in primary care: changes in pattern of patient visits and complaints during a developing depression. *Journal of Family Practice*, **7**, 293–302.

Wilkinson G. (1988). A comparison of psychiatric decision-making by trainee general practitioners and trainee psychiatrists using a simulated consultation model. *Psychological Medicine*, **18**, 167–77.

Wing J. K. (1976). A technique for studying psychiatric morbidity in in-patient and outpatient series and in general population samples. *Psychological Medicine*, **6**, 665–71.

Wing J. K., Cooper J. E., Sartorius N. (1974). *The Measurement and Classification of Psychiatric Symptoms*. Cambridge: Cambridge University Press.

Wing J. K., Bebbington P. E., Hurry J., *et al.* (1981). The prevalence in the general population of disorders familiar to psychiatrists in hospital practice. In *What is a Case* (Wing J. K., Bebbington P. E., Robins L. N., eds.). London: Grant McIntyre.

Zung W. W. K., King R. E. (1983). Identification and treatment of masked depression in a general medical practice. *Journal of Clinical Psychiatry*, **44**, 365–8.

Zung W. W. K., Magill M., Moore J. T., George D. T. (1983). Recognition and treatment of depression in a family medicine practice. *Journal of Clinical Psychiatry*, **44**, 3–6.

Zung W. W. K., Zung E. M., Moore J., Scott J. (1985). Decision making in the treatment of depression by family medicine physicians. *Comprehensive Therapy*, **11**, 19–23.

14 *The role of self-help groups in the management of depression*

JUDY WILSON

INTRODUCTION

'I wept when I first met B. I couldn't believe there was anyone else like me.'
'It gives you a marker. If you see others worse than yourself, then you get some idea of how you are.'
'It makes me feel I can't be that bad if I managed to do something for somebody else.'
'I see the group as a safety net. I can go back to it if my depression returns.'

Members of self-help groups based on depression quoted above were reflecting on their experience of belonging to a group run, not by professional workers, but by people who are themselves depressed. They had all decided to do something about their situation, and for them, membership of a group of fellow sufferers was part of their strategy.

Groups based on depression form only a very small proportion of the self-help groups that are in existence. While it is valuable to examine the contribution of such groups, this chapter will cover the whole field of self-help groups based on health, social and personal problems. Nearly all self-help groups (and in surprising numbers), address the problem of depression that their members either experience already or are liable to experience as part of their problems. Prevention of depression, not simply its management, is part of their contribution.

What is a self-help group? It is important to distinguish between what they *are* and what they *do*. A key point in the definition of a self-help group is that its members, themselves experiencing the problem that brings the group together, are in charge and control of the group. A useful general definition, suggested in a study of members of four national self-help organizations, is that self-help groups are 'groups of people who feel they have a common problem and have joined together to do something about it' (Richardson and Goodman, 1983). This, though helpful, and probably the best definition offered in this country, does not sufficiently clarify the essential points of membership and leadership. It implies too that the motivation for joining a group is always to solve a current problem. In practice, some people join or form a group because of a wish to be helpful to people who are currently facing difficulties which they themselves have faced in the past, and with which they may still also be trying to cope. There is no formal distinction in a self-help group between givers and receivers of help.

None of these points—direction of the group by its members, motivation to help others, and lack of distinction between givers and receivers—would apply to mutual support groups run by professionals, but their activities might be very similar. Exactly what self-help groups do will depend on what their members decide, but activities often include giving mutual support, providing practical information and helping members to cope with everyday life. It is not intended, in this chapter, to compare and evaluate the two very different forms of groups—those run by members themselves and those led by professionals—but it is important to have in mind their differences. Nor is this a comprehensive study of self-help groups, either generally or in their role in managing depression. It draws largely on the experience of a local health service-funded scheme, now called the Nottingham Self Help Team, which was set up in 1982 to provide support and information to a very wide range of self-help groups, and to people looking for them. The evidence from this and other sources suggests that a high proportion of these groups are already covertly helping with the management of depression. It will be seen, too, that with appropriate attitudes, support and resources, many others can be established to contribute further to the prevention as well as the management of depression.

A REVIEW OF THE LITERATURE

There is little literature in this country on self-help groups relating to depression and not a great deal on self-help groups generally. Compared to the United States and to Germany, it is a field to which little attention has been given. In Hamburg, for example, a 5-year research study revealed the existence of 570 groups and established the generally favourable attitude of professional workers towards them (Deneke, 1983). In the USA, many years of substantial research programmes, some of which are quoted below, have led to a clear policy decision by the Surgeon General on the value of self-help groups (Riessman and Gartner, 1987). A review of self-help by Pancoast *et al.* (1983) includes six essays on professional relationships with self-help groups. Despite very different systems of health care, it is possible and useful to learn from the experience of other countries. That review, and another major collection (Hatch and Kickbusch, 1983), contribute to our understanding of self-help in the UK.

Some UK research, though valuable at the time, is now somewhat dated (for example, Robinson and Robinson, 1979). This is such a quickly developing field that one must have reservations about relying on research

234 Depression: An integrative approach

done over a decade ago. Levy (1982) traced this rapid development in a survey of national self-help organizations, but there has been a substantial increase since his work, as confirmed by Lock (1986).

Richardson and Goodman (1983) provide valuable evidence of the diversity of self-help groups. They draw attention, too, to the way the character of groups is heavily influenced by the one factor they can do little about—namely the nature of the problem for which they were formed. This is of particular importance when considering the role of self-help groups for people who are depressed, when lack of motivation to do anything, let alone get to a group, is a common situation. Richardson and Goodman demonstrated that members of self-help groups covered a range of occupations and, by extension, social classes. Thus self-help is not simply a middle-class preoccupation. Finally, the research showed that the self-help experience was by no means an identical one. Members were not all alike and their motivation and length and degree of involvement in their group varied a great deal.

Individual groups

Studies of individual groups, some of which are referred to below, provide useful complementary material to more general research. Accounts found in a wide variety of journals show that many different professionals are interested in self-help and how they might work with groups. One such account, which was carefully researched, demonstrates the value of self-help groups based on depression and how leadership can, with forethought and ample time, be transferred to the group itself even if this was not appropriate at the beginning (Northern Ireland Association of Mental Health, 1986).

A study of widows' groups in the US compared members of self-help groups to similarly bereaved psychotherapy patients, and to those who sought no formal help. 'Significant positive changes' were found to have occurred only for those who had participated actively in the self-help groups (Lieberman and Videka–Sherman, 1986). Handford's account (1985) of postpartum depression is of a treatment model in Canada based on the guiding principle that women themselves are the experts on this condition. All three sources affirm the value of self-help groups for their members.

Women

One continuing theme in all the literature on self-help, as with depression, is that a large proportion of people involved are women (Starr, 1985). A common thread is women's lack of self-confidence and feelings of low self-esteem. A research project funded by the Equal Opportunities Commission, setting women's self-help and health into a general women's context, began to look into this question (Foley, 1985). An American view is that:

'self-help groups seek to restore women's sense of autonomy over their own lives, to restore their self-reliance, and to lessen their dependency on institutions that define the lives of women' (Gartner, 1985).

It is also valuable to look rather wider, to a field which is perhaps 'pre-self-help', namely adult education. Courses and study groups in women's health both overlap with and can lead to self-help groups. Teaching material produced with these in mind has already proved invaluable to the work of some self-help groups based on women's health issues (Workers' Educational Association, 1986). This approach also takes account of the fact that not everyone may be ready and confident enough for a single-issue, self-help group and may need to go through another stage first. Groups based on 'women's health' generally avoid labelling. Acceptance of a particular condition is often necessary before people decide to go to a single-issue group. The experience of a worker on a women and mental health, self-help project in Bristol confirms that this is a particular issue in the mental health field and may prevent some people joining specific-issue groups (Trevithick, 1988).

Self-care

It is not always easy to look at self-help groups as a discreet area of operation. There are a number of overlaps. The literature demonstrates one overlap between individual self-care and self-help groups. Many groups see their role as providing information about self-care to their members. They rarely, however, promote one particular solution. Instead, they give choices about what is available and feedback from members on what they have found helpful. There is now a wide selection of titles on the self-management of depression. Two titles in particular (Rowe, 1983; Weekes, 1983) are quoted regularly in contributions from members in the newsletters of the Fellowship of Depressives Anonymous (FDA). Rowe, the first author to open up discussion on depression outside the medical sphere, is one of few authors to make the link between self-care and self-help groups, encouraging sufferers to find and join groups as part of a coping strategy.

Newsletters of national organizations like FDA are valuable sources of information on self-care literature. The Manic Depression Fellowship, too, regularly reviews books in its members' newsletter, as does Depressives Associated (DASS). All these national, specialist organizations provide an extremely useful role in providing outlets for information about depression—a vital part of self-care. It may be that this is, ultimately, of greater significance than actual membership of groups based on depression. FDA, for example has only 20 groups and links with 12 more. DASS reports that 28 local groups are meeting regularly. Their newsletters, as with the individual studies, affirm the value of groups, but also give evidence of their vulnerability and limits—a topic to be addressed later in this chapter. But one must not dismiss the importance of their work. They do work for their members; they provide information and, most important, evidence to fellow sufferers that life can continue and that there are ways to cope.

World Health Organization

It is important to see the role of self-help groups in the management of depression in a worldwide context. The World Health Organization (WHO), for example, in its *Targets for Health for All by the Year 2000* (World Health Organization, 1985), demonstrates that current broad views of health policy include non-medical methods, and indeed that a totally professional approach to treatment is unrealistic. The important collection of writings on self-help (Hatch and Kickbusch, 1983) is based on this approach. The growing body of knowledge on self-help has been brought together by WHO-sponsored workshops on self-help. Some solution of the problem of definitions is helped, for example, by a summary included in a collection of reports on the ten WHO workshops on self-help (International Information Centre on Self-Help and Health, undated).

Why this upsurge of activity? Dean (1985) distinguishes between groups 'next' to the system and those opposed to the system. She suggests that many needs are not satisfied in personal social networks or—a significant point for medical practitioners—by publicly created services. The expansion of mutual aid groups—a term often in use in America—is due, she feels, to the nature of many contemporary problems which are better resolved by this form of caring; to malfunctioning in existing health services; and to unavailable services for specific types of problem or for specific populations.

The literature does not provide a coherent picture of self-help groups and their relationship to professional care. Much more research is needed before the undoubtedly interesting strands identified here can be linked together any more. Even then, a clear picture may well not emerge. It is tempting to approach and evaluate self-help as if it were a professional service; it is not. Some people would maintain in fact that only members of groups themselves can evaluate their work. What one can do, however, is evaluate systems of support that have been set up to further the work of self-help groups. A piece of action research illuminates some of the key issues around the development of self-help and describes a possible model for enabling it to expand. A selection of its findings are now summarized (Wilson, 1987).

THE NOTTINGHAM EXPERIENCE

Nottingham, a Midlands city of just under 300 000 people, has a population structure broadly similar to both the Trent region, and to England as a whole. One may see it as a fairly average sort of city and results here could, it is suggested, be expected in other similar urban areas. The material presented here draws largely on a thesis (Wilson, 1987), based on research undertaken in 1982/3.

The self-help picture in 1987 in Nottingham

The number of groups doubled between 1982 and 1987, from 60 to 120. An analysis of the 120 groups in the 1987 Directory of Self Help Groups (Self Help Team 1987a), reveals a high proportion of groups (72 percent) based on problems in which there is likely to be a large component of depression (Fig 14.1).

The groups included in the 72 percent are based on issues such as bereavement, having a handicapped child, tranquillizer addiction, suffering from a chronic illness or coping with a major disability. Those not associated with depression (13 percent) are generally more practical in their approach: aiming to pass on skills, like breastfeeding; providing an information service; helping people to stop smoking; providing a service; or campaigning for change as a major part of their work.

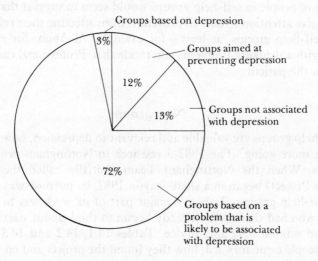

Fig. 14.1 *An analysis of the 120 groups listed in the 1987 directory of self-help groups in Nottingham*

Prevention of depression

A number of groups were set up consciously—in part at least—to prevent depression from setting in: those based on loneliness, being widowed at a young age, being a single parent, being a stroke victim, mothers apart from their children, and some of the groups based on a disability. The initiator of the Partially Sighted Society was shocked into starting a group:

I'd come to terms reasonably well with my own loss of sight when I met S. She had lost most sight in one eye and had been told she could expect deterioration in the other. I invited her to my house, tried to give her hope and tell her about all the help that was available and that people rarely lost all their sight. It was no good—the next week she took her own life.

Families

An increasing number of groups are for people who don't have a problem themselves but are close to people, perhaps caring full-time for them, who do. For sometimes it is the depression of other members of the family which has affected people to a great degree:

It's three years since my husband took his life. I still ask myself why? Suicide is such a difficult subject to talk about publicly. My family don't want me going on about it. I feel I must start a group for people who are in the same situation and perhaps we can prevent some of the pain I've experienced.

Management of depression does not stop with the patient. The experience of people in self-help groups would seem to suggest that there is a need to give attention to how to prevent it from affecting their relatives too. Some self-help groups, at least—for example, Al Anon, for relatives of people with a drinking problem—do tackle this. Professional care tends to focus on the patient.

New groups

If self-help groups are valuable and relevant to depression, how then might one get more going? The 1982/3 research in Nottingham provides some answers. When the Nottingham Team (initially called the Self Help Groups Project) began in a small way in 1982, its purpose was not to start new self-help groups. Rather, a major part of its work was to respond to people who had themselves already begun to think about starting a group and who wanted help and advice. Tables 14.1, 14.2 and 14.3 show how many people came forward, how they found the project and on what issues the potential groups were based.

The deliberately reactive approach of the Team meant that the methods used for giving help were similar to those that are common in neighbourhood community work, namely, some practical services; access to other helpful individuals and agencies and to information; developing people's skills and confidence; and helping groups find an appropriate structure. Support of this kind was given for an average of five months. Too brisk an encounter, it was found, did not allow the personal relationships and confidence of group members to grow. Too long a link risked inhibiting the development of skills and responsibility and dependence on the project rather than the autonomy which was the goal from the start.

Table 14.1 Approaches made to Nottingham Self Help Groups Project during 1982–3 for help with starting a new group

Approaches	1982	1983	Total
Approaches which led to a group starting, and still being in existence at the end of 1983.	7	11	18
Approaches which led to a group starting and then finishing.	1	1	2
Approaches which led to a group being partly operative by the end of 1983.	3	10	13
Approaches which did not led to the formation of a group.	6	7	13
Total number of approaches	17	29	46

One surprising finding emerged in the analysis of the work: the lack of support from national organizations. Less than a quarter of the new groups had help from national bodies when they began and some of the help that they received was often insensitive and inflexible. (Though these com-

Table 14.2 Agencies/publicity outlets which acted as a link between Nottingham Self Help Groups Project and people wanting help with new groups

Link	1982	1983	Total
Professional workers	3	6	9
Local voluntary organizations	6	2	8
NCVS*	1	2	3
NCVS media project	0	3	3
Central TV	0	3	3
Nottingham Evening Post	2	3	5
Other self-help groups	1	2	3
Shopping Centre exhibition	0	1	1
Contacts from past job of worker	4	1	5
General knowledge of the project	0	6	6
Total	17	29	46

* Nottingham Council for Voluntary Service.

Table 14.3 Problems on which groups or potential groups, which contacted the project for help, were based

---

Alzheimer's disease	Marie Charcot Tooth disease
Asthma	Migraine
	Myositis ossificans progressiva
Back pain	
Blind children	Partial sight
Burns	Phobias (3)
	Psychiatric problems
Caesarean birth	Physical handicap
Cancer	Postnatal support
Crohn's disease	Plastic surgery
	Premenstrual stress
Depression (2)	
	Relatives of the elderly
Eating problems	
Epilepsy	Scoliosis
	Single parents (2)
Food allergies	Step-parents
	Stopping smoking
Glue sniffing	
	Tranquillizer dependency
Handicapped children (5)	Twins
Head injuries—(young members)	Triplets, quads and quins
Hearing loss	
Heart pacemakers	Widowhood
Infertility	

---

ments, it should be made clear, do not apply to the national organizations based on depression mentioned earlier.) The importance of a flexible, local source of help for new groups came to be seen as even greater by contrast. Less surprising was the proportion of women among the initiators: 91 percent. For as Table 14.3 demonstrates, many of the issues on which groups were based were those affecting women or people women cared for.

Good practice

Success in a self-help group is not totally measurable. For example, even when groups did not actually get going (which was the case in about one-third of the initial contacts), there was nearly always some achievement to be noted. It proved difficult to be precise about the meaning of success. But one did come to identify what seemed to make new groups work and what was likely to inhibit their development. This is shown in Table 14.4 and 14.5.

Table 14.4 Factors which contributed to the success of new groups

---

- A serious problem as a basis for the group
- Motivation by 'veterans' to help people currently experiencing the problem
- Sensitive professional support to the group
- Back up by other agencies and links with them
- Links with other self-help groups
- Sensitive back up by national organizations
- A key charismatic personality as originator, but one who does not dominate the group
- Constructive use of the media
- Good choice of meeting room
- Regularity of meetings
- Availability of practical resources relevant to the group and the first members
- Contribution by people already experienced in organizing
- Commitment by people who might be inexperienced in organizing but have the capacity to grow in skills and in willingness to take on responsibility
- Key initiators with settled homes and families
- Good outside speakers at early meetings
- Opportunities for members to be helpers straight away
- A framework of organization, built on the concept of sharing out jobs
- Newsletter or members letter
- Leaflet or card produced by the group

Table 14.5 Factors which are likely to bring problems to new groups or contribute to their failure

---

- Key initiators being too close to their problem
- Major physical disabilities or mental condition which make organizing a group very difficult
- Very small number of sufferers
- Over-ambitious plan
- Unsympathetic/dreary personality of initiator
- Lack of realization of the need for some structure and organization
- Lack of realization of need to share out jobs and involve people immediately
- A working-class neighbourhood as a base
- Over-control by professionals
- Insensitive, overbearing help from a national organization
- Erratic life of initiators
- Unpredictable personal or health problems
- Lack of a nucleus of key committed people
- Unsuitable meeting place
- Continuous change of meeting arrangements
- No printed material
- Very small number of members
- A dominating controlling key initiator
- A programme that doesn't appeal to members
- Lack of commitment after initial enthusiasm

Professional workers

As Table 14.2 shows, nearly 20 percent of the links between the project and new groups were made by professional workers employed in the health and social services. In eight of these cases, there was ongoing work with individual professional workers, backing them up in their enabling, facilitating role, rather than undertaking detailed work with the group directly. It was only towards the end of the 2-year research period that the complexity of this task for professional workers became apparent. It emerged that not only do members of groups experience lack of confidence when initiating groups—so do professionals who take on the role of background support rather than leadership. Nor does professional training equip them with the appropriate skills. Moreover, the whole question of client or patient/professional relationship makes it difficult for many workers to step outside their controlling role.

There appeared to be three different categories of professionals:

instinctive enablers	30 percent
enablers in principle	50 percent
traditionalists	20 percent

'Instinctive enablers' found it relatively easy to take on the facilitating role, but often wanted confirmation that what they were doing was acceptable. 'Enablers in principle' were much more confused. Professional training seemed to provide a straitjacket, making them assume there would be specific outcomes—a dangerous assumption when working with self-help groups. 'Traditionalists' found it almost impossible to cross the patient/professional boundary. Analysis of their work brought some further conclusions on good practice (Table 14.6).

Professionals' information role

However, professionals do not only have a role to play with self-help groups as they begin. Perhaps even more important, and more attainable, is their role as information providers. In a later stage of the work of the Nottingham Self Help Team, further research was carried out, this time by a neutral outsider (Unell, 1987). As part of her evaluation, Unell undertook a survey of hospital and community-based nursing staff, covering paediatrics, psychiatry and community nursing, and achieving a 70 percent response rate. Seventy-one percent of the respondents said they had linked patients with groups in the past. This was usually done by supplying information, though 34 percent of the sample had effected a direct introduction. The directory of self-help groups produced by the Self Help Team emeged as the most popular information source among district nurses and health visitors, although other agencies, and the media, as well as word of mouth were also important sources.

Table 14.6 Factors which indicate that a professional may successfully facilitate a self-help group

---

- An allocation of a substantial amount of time:
  (i) in pre-planning;
  (ii) of several hours per week, often at unusual times;
  (iii) over a period of some years, if needed
- A warm, outgoing personality
- The ability to be informal and 'unprofessional'
- Back up by senior officers
- The use of an experienced supervisor or outside consultant for advice and as a sounding board
- The availability and use of practical resources within the worker's department (as long as these are offered and used sensitively to back up, not to dominate the group)
- A willingness to let the group develop differently than had been thought at the outset
- Cooperation with professionals in other disciplines
- A recognition of potential in lay people
- A willingness to take risks
- A conscious continuous evaluation of the development of the group and the professional's role within it
- A desire from the beginning to be the person who introduces people and then acts as an outside supporter, rather than leader
- An appreciation of the likely need for permanent links with the group and ongoing back up to it
- Perceiving the value of an outsider in helping the group to identify and decide on their aims

---

Note These factors are not listed in any specific order.

Unell's survey revealed a great deal of interest and understanding of self-help among professionals. Knowledge about groups was extensive and this was matched by a readiness to link patients with appropriate groups. Attitudes were generally very sympathetic with some carefully argued reservations about the effectiveness of self-help, occasionally tinged with anxiety about threats to professional authority.

But few people in the sample were prepared to become directly involved in the support of self-help groups, and fewer still in their initiation. Fundamental changes, Unell concludes, in the attitudes and priorities of management and in the content of professional training are probably needed before support to self-help becomes part of the working repertoire of front-line, health care staff.

Intermediary role

Would this encouraging and useful work have happened without the work of the Self Help Team? The intermediary role was, and is, crucial to the pattern of partnership that has now evolved between a substantial number of health professionals and self-help groups in Nottingham (The Self Help Team, 1987b). A general practitioner was very clear about the need for an informed and credible intermediary when he approached the Team for help with seminars at the Medical School in 1983, saying: 'My eyes lit up when I came across your project. I felt that we should really be doing something about self-help, but I didn't know where to start.'

Continuing evaluation of the Team's work has confirmed the importance of the Team's role as a clearing house for information. Growing involvement with professional training, as far as small resources permit, has also demonstrated the value of a trusted intermediary. The research in 1982 and 1983, however, led to conclusions on the limits as well as the strengths of our work. It was easy to set unrealistic targets and the research revealed that our aims had been over-ambitious in the early days. Constant monitoring, evaluation and change has since helped the Team to operate within reasonable boundaries. The satisfaction of the Health Authority with its work is demonstrated by increased and permanent funding of 90 percent of the Team's costs. Management and base, however, have remained outside the health service. The intermediary role, it has been concluded, can best be played from just outside the system.

STRENGTHS AND LIMITATIONS OF SELF-HELP GROUPS

Strengths

The evidence so far from research, from WHO endorsement, and from the personal testimony of members, would suggest that for most of their members, self-help groups work. People would not make the enormous effort that is sometimes needed to attend and to give to groups if they did not feel groups helped them. Nor would the idea be spreading in the way it is, if they did not work. One can identify a number of particular strengths.

First, they build on a wish by people to do something about their own problems. This does not necessarily mean that professional care is then rejected. For most people the two go side by side. But self-care can be a lonely business. Groups bring together people with similar motivation and a shared deep-down conviction that part of the way to cope with their problems lies within them as individuals.

Second, groups offer the opportunity to be helpful. Conventional voluntary work often demands a level of self-confidence and personal stability which is rarely to be found among people with major problems in their lives. Involvement in self-help groups means people can be helpful, in itself therapeutic, without having to put on a volunteer label. Their help, coming from someone who has experienced the same situation, is also often the most acceptable. And a whole wealth of community talent, at present unappreciated, can be harnessed.

Third, groups provide a link. For some, this is a link with information, which is increasingly being seen as a valuable tool in helping people cope and recover. For others, it is a stepping stone to normal life. While some people remain group members for many years, others move on, having regained confidence and learned new skills. They may well, however, retain contact with the group. Groups also offer a link between helpful services and people who need them, confirmed by studies of groups of parents of handicapped children (Hatch and Hinton, 1986).

Fourth, groups help prevent problems from becoming acute. The account by a young widow of her emergence to normal life is typical of hundreds of people involved in Nottingham groups (Dawson, 1987). The link that so many groups (Figure 14.1) have with depression, means that it is highly likely that when people attend them regularly some depression can be prevented.

Last, groups offer a valuable resource to professionals in helping them to understand what it is really like to experience a problem and how professional care can best be given. An increasing number of Nottingham groups are being asked to give talks or organize study days for a wide range of professionals and students. Less directly, often through the media, they can also have an effect on the understanding of the general public and contribute to the destigmatizing of conditions.

Limitations

The same sources also reveal the limits to groups. Endorsing their work does not mean that they are the ultimate answer to all needs, nor that they are right for everyone.

Group members would be the first to agree that membership of self-help groups does not necessarily follow just because one has a particular problem. It must feel right for the individual and come at the right time. Nor are they normally the only strategy for coping. People must feel free to choose what is right for them. Probably only a small minority of people experiencing a problem will actually join a relevant self-help group.

Even for those who wish to, there is not always a group nearby. Even with common problems, there is rarely national coverage. Strategies are being evolved for getting over the problem—newsletters, pen-friend schemes, telephone links, regional meetings—but accessibility is always going to be a problem. It would be rash to approach the contribution of self-help groups with the expectation that systematic coverage is possible or even desirable. Their very nature may make this unrealistic and inappropriate.

A further limit comes again from the very fact—one of the characteristics, of course, of self-help groups—that all their members are experiencing the same problem. Medical practitioners sometimes fear that patients will be dragged down by being in contact with people in the same situation, perhaps worse than they are. This is a particular issue in progressive conditions. Members of such groups accept that this is indeed a problem. The experience of people who give self-help a chance, that is they go regularly and over some time, is that this can be got over. Where members are as likely to improve—depression is an example—as to get worse, then contact with other members may in fact be a help rather than a problem. A further risk—for perhaps that is the way to see it—is that groups may hand out inappropriate advice. This may happen occasionally, but in practice seems to be rare.

A more problematic area comes from the way groups are organized. Many groups experience limits because they find it difficult to organize themselves, particularly if there is no appropriate national organization or local support centre. In a very small minority of cases groups can also get taken over and inappropriately led.

Finally, and associated with the last point, the very condition on which the group is based is likely to bring problems of organization, recruitment of members and communication. Each group needs to approach this realistically and evolve ways of solving the problem or of operating within the limits they have.

Constraints imposed by professionals

Constraints on the effectiveness of groups do not come solely from group members or arise from the problem on which they are based. Professional attitudes and practices also inhibit what they do. Further research could well investigate the following:

lack of trust by professionals in lay people's ability and potential;
the issue of professional power and reluctance to develop partnership;
lack of effort to obtain and pass on information;
poor use of resources which could be useful to groups;
exclusion of the topic from training;
professionals' over-involvement in self-help;
unrealistic expectations by doctors of being able to control their patients' total environment.

Professionals may well need to examine, evaluate and change their own attitudes and practice.

CONCLUSIONS

The evidence we have so far is not extensive, but from what literature there is, particularly from other countries and from the undoubted spread of self-help groups in Nottingham and in the rest of the UK, one may claim that a significant number of people find self-help helpful. Further research is needed before one can attempt to quantify how many people are involved in this country, but in the US, an estimate of 3 million has been quoted (Paskert and Madara, 1985). As has been made clear, one needs to see the contribution of self-help groups to the management and prevention of depression in a wide context, not only by looking at groups operating obviously in the mental health field.

But if they are a 'good thing', as described by a senior medical officer at the DHSS, how can one get more of them? How might their contribution be strengthened? How could they be made more accessible? The answer is not a large scale top–down strategy. Instead a flexible, gradual, three-pronged approach needs to be adopted.

Expansion of local support

First, the value of locally based centres for self-help groups, such as the Nottingham Self Help Team, is now well recognized. Replication of the idea, which rightly is usually adopted in part, not in total, to meet the needs of each area, has been going on since 1983. Some schemes are as general as Nottingham's, others work in a specialist area of health. Resources were expanded rapidly in 1986 when a DHSS-sponsored funding programme 'The Self Help Alliance' began. This project, part of the DHSS 'Helping the Community to Care Programme', has provided 3-year funding to 18 schemes around the country, and is being evaluated by the Tavistock Institute.

One may question the motives of the government's desire to encourage self-help groups but, whatever the reasons at government level, extension of such schemes and long-term funding for them by local health authorities, could lead to further expansion of groups relevant to depression. A reactive, facilitating approach, however, is as important as actual resources, and a willingness to accept patchy and perhaps erratic development is needed. This bottom–up strategy could, in fact avoid the danger of politicians implementing support to self-help as a cost-cutting exercise.

Changes in professional attitudes

Second, there needs to be more done to ensure that professionals play a sensitive role in strengthening the work of groups and making it possible for potential members to get to them. Self-help centres in their intermediary role can contribute to this but, as small and relatively powerless bodies, cannot achieve all the change that is needed. More research is needed, preferably commissioned by individual professions on the lines outlined above, to help identify what changes are needed and how they might be brought about.

Awareness of self-help groups' role

Third and last, one needs to see the contribution of self-help groups in context. It is only part of a programme of self-care. There may need to be 'pre-self help' activities. Self-help groups may well fit alongside professional care or be apart from it. One needs to approach them as interwoven with other concepts and services, while being aware of the unique contribution which self-help groups make. It does self-help no good to over-applaud it. Self-help groups are not a panacea. But they are a growing and important part of a pattern of health care.

REFERENCES

Dawson P. (1987). Young Widowed. *Self Help News*, No. 87/2, 1–2.

Dean K. (1985). Lay care in illness. *Social Science and Medicine*, **22**, 275–84

Deneke C. (1983). How professionals view self-help. In *Rediscovering Self-Help.* (Pancoast D. L., Parker P., Froland C., eds.). Beverly Hills: Sage Publications.

Foley R. (1985). *Women and Health Care: Self Help Health Groups in Britain.* London: Howe Publications.

Gartner A. (1985). A typology of women's self-help groups. *Social Policy*, **15** (No. 3), 25–30.

Handford P. (1981). Postpartum depression: what is it, what helps? *Canadian Nurse*, January (1), 30–3.

Hatch S., Hinton T. (1986). *Self-help in Practice: A Study of Contact-a-Family, Community Work and Family Support.* University of Sheffield, Joint Unit for Social Services Research.

Hatch S., Kickbusch I. (1983). *Self-Help and Health in Europe: New Approaches in Health Care.* Geneva: World Health Organization.

International Information Centre on Self-Help and Health (undated). *WHO and Self-Help: A Summary of the Most Important Papers on Self-Help and Health with WHO Involvement.*

Levy L. (1982). Mutual support groups in Great Britain. *Social Science and Medicine*, **16**, 1265–75.

Lieberman M. A., Videka–Sherman L. (1986). The impact of self-help groups on the mental health of widows and widowers. *American Journal of Orthopsychiatry*, **56**, 435–49.

Lock S. (1986). Self-help groups: the fourth estate in medicine. *British Medical Journal*, **293**, 1596–1600.

Northern Ireland Association for Mental Health (1986). *Self-help and Depression.*

Pancoast D. L., Parker P., Froland C. (1983). *Rediscovering Self-Help: Its Role in Social Care.* Beverly Hills: Sage Publications.

Paskert J., Madara E. J. (1985). Introducing and tapping self-help mutual aid resources. *Health Education*, **16**, 25–9.

Richardson A., Goodman M. (1983). *Self-help and Social Care: Mutual Aid Organisations in Practice.* London: Policy Studies Institute.

Riessman F., Gartner A. (1987). The Surgeon General and the self-help ethos. *Social Policy*, **18**, 23–5.

Robinson D., Robinson Y. (1979). *From Self Help to Health: A Guide to Self-Help Groups.* London: Concord Books.

Rowe D. (1983). *Depression: The Way Out of your Prison.* London: Routledge and Kegan Paul.

The Self Help Team (1987a). *Self Help Groups in Nottingham and District.*

The Self Help Team (1987b). *Promoting Partnership*. Nottingham, The Self Help Team.

Starr I. (1985). The depressed sex? *Social Work Today*. **16**, 16–7.

Trevithick P. (1988). Womankind. *MASH (Mutual Aid and Self Help: the bulletin of the National Self Help Support Centre*, Spring issue, No. 7., 3.

Unell J. (1987). *Help for Self Help: A Study of a Local Support Service*. London: Bedford Square Press.

Weekes C. (1983). *Self Help for Your Nerves*. London: Angus and Robertson.

Wilson J. (1987). *Supporting Self Help Groups*, Loughborough University, unpublished thesis submitted for the degree of Master of Philosophy.

Workers' Educational Association (1986). *Women and Health: Activities and Materials for Use in Women's Health Courses and Discussion Groups*. London: WEA/Health Education Council.

World Health Organization (1985). *Targets for Health for All: Targets in Support of the European Regional Strategy for Health for All*. Copenhagen: WHO Regional Office for Europe.

SOME USEFUL ADDRESSES

Depressives Associated,
PO Box 5,
Castle Town,
Portland,
Dorset DT5 1BQ
(SAE with all enquiries)

Fellowship of Depressives Anonymous,
36, Chestnut Avenue,
Beverley,
N. Humberside HU17 9QU
(SAE with all enquiries).

Manic Depression Fellowship,
51, Sheen Road,
Richmond upon Thames,
Surrey IW9 1YO.

National Self Help Support Centre,
26, Bedford Sq.,
London WC1 3HU.

The Self Help Team,
20, Pelham Rd.,
Sherwood Rise,
Nottingham NG5 1AP.

Index

Abuse, drugs of, 98, 115
Adenylate cyclase system, 189
Adinazolam, 182
Admission to hospital, 3
Adolescent depression, 109–21
  affective psychosis, 116
  chronics, 120–1
  examination, 116–18
    diagnostic assessment, 117–18
    initial contact, 116-17
    interviewing, 117–18
  external causes related, 114–15
  masked depression, 115
    recurrent, 120–1
  maturational stress related, 114
  patterns, 113–16
  prevalence, 112-13
  therapy, 118–19
    parental/family, 120
Alpha-adrenoceptors:
  blockade, 57
  neuroendocrine function measures, 55–6
  neuroendocrine function tests, 54
Alpha-adrenoceptor antagonism, 188
Adoption studies, 68
Adrenocorticotrophic hormone (ACTH), 43–4
Adversity, 66–7
Affective disorder (psychosis):
  adolescent, 116
  biopsychosocial models, 65
Age, 7
Akinetic mutism, 141
Al Anon, 238
Alcohol, 94

Alcoholics, suicide incidence, 94
Alprazolam, 95, 182
Amantadine, 97
American Psychiatric Association
  Diagnostic and Statistical Manual,
  DSM III, 6, 11–12
Amitryptiline, 187 (table), 191, 220
  and neuroleptic, 153
Amphetamines, 54, 98
Antidepressants, 179–93
  adverse reactions, 182–3
  dopaminergic effects, 189
  elderly patients, 152–4
  for:
    anxiety, 179–80
    recurrent depression, 191
    recurrent transient mood
      changes, 192–3
  receptor changes induced, 58–9
  reducing wish of death from
    overdosage, 184
  long-term treatment, 190–2
  toxicity in overdose, 183–5
  tricyclic, 56–7, 58, 88
    anticholinergic effects, 153
    depression induced by, 97–8
    elderly patients, 153
Antihypertensive drugs, 85–9
Antimalarial drugs, 95
Antimicrobial agents, 95–6
Anxiety and Depression Scale, 133
Anxiolytic-sedatives, 94–5
Apomorphine, growth hormone
  response, 55
Appetite suppressants, 97
Associations, 7–9
Attempted suicide, *see* Suicide

Automatic thoughts questionnaire, 177

Barbiturates, 94
  withdrawal, 94
Beck Depression Inventory, 133
Bedford College Diagnostic Scheme, 22
Bedford College Life Event and Difficulty Schedule, 23
Benzodiazepines, 94–5, 153, 181–2
  dependence, 181–2
Bethanidine, 87 (table)
Biopsychosocial models of affective disorder, 65
Brupropion, 189
Bulimia nervosa, 187
Buspirone, 188
Butyrophenones, 99

CATEGO, 5–6
Center for Epidemiological Studies Depression Scale (CES-D), 5
Childbirth, 128–30
  rite de passage, 130
Chlomipramine, 56
Chlordiazepoxide, 180
m-chlorphenylpiperazine, 56, 188
Chlorpromazine, 99
Choline, 98
Cimetidine, 98
Classification, 9–14
  DSM III, 11–12
  International Classification of Disease, 13–14
  psychotic/neurotic distinction, 10–11
  unipolar/bipolar illness, 9–10
Clomipramine, 183 (table), 184
  placebo-controlled studies, 187 (table)
Clonidine, 55–6, 58, 87 (table), 88
Cognitive therapy, 165–77
  assessment, 165–6
    thoughts/images, 166–7
  effectiveness evaluation, 171–5
    acute treatment, 172–4
    relapse prevention, 174–5
  evaluation of thoughts as hypotheses, 167–8

suitable patients, 175–6
  techniques, 170–1
    alternative therapy, 171
    cognitive rehearsal, 170–1
    task assignment, 170
  transferable aspects, 176–7
  underlying assumptions, 169–70
  underlying fears, 168–9
Concern, 26
Consultation Analysis by Behaviour and Style, 224–5
Consultation Analysis by Triggers and Symptoms, 224
Contextual measure, 26
Coping with Depression (I. M. Blackburn), 176–7
Corticosteroids, 96
Corticotrophin-releasing factor (CRF), 53–4
  overproduction, 54
Cortisol, 53
  response to methylamphetamines, 54
Cushing's syndrome, 96
Cyclic adenosine monophosphate (cAMP), 189
Cyclothymia, 12
Cystic fibrosis, 49
Cytotoxic drugs, 96

Dacarbazine, 96
Debrisoquine, 87 (table)
Delusional depression, 69
Dementia:
  distinguishing depression from, 142–3
  multi-infarct, 143
L-deprenyl, 190
Depressives Associated, 235–6, 249
Depressive stupor, 141
Desipramine, 57, 58
Deviant personalities, 48
Dexamethasone resistance, 55
Dexamethasone suppression test, 11, 66, 69
  elderly people, 148
Diagnostic Interview Schedule, 6
Diazepam, 94, 153, 180
Diethylpropion, 97
Distress *vs* disease, 40–1

Disulfiram, 98
Dothiepin, 183 (table)
Doxepin, 183 (table)
Drug abuse, 98, 115
Drug-related depression, 81–99
  cause/effect, 82–3
  phenomenology, 81–2
  reporting methods, 83–4
  see also specific drugs
Duchenne muscular dystrophy, 48–9
Dysfunctional Attitude Scale, 169
Dysthymia, 12

Edinburgh Postnatal Depression
  Scale, 134
Elderly, depression in, 140
  biological factors in causation,
    147–50
    neuroendocrine, 148
    neurophysiological, 149–50
    neuroradiological, 148–9
    neurotransmitter, 147–8
  characteristics, 141–4
    acute phobic anxiety, 142
    akinetic mutism, 141
    behaviour disturbance, 143–4
    depressive stupor, 141
    hypochondriasis, 143
    mild forms of depression, 141–2
    pain, 143
    pseudodementia, 143
  drug therapy, 152–4
  electroconvulsive therapy, 154
  epidemiology, 144–7
    institutional patients, 146–7
  mortality, 154–5
  physical illness associated, 150
  prevalence, *see* Prevalence
  prognosis, 154–6
    long-term, 155–6
  psychosocial factors in causation,
    150–2
    life events, 151–2
    social isolation, 152
  treatment, 152–4
    drug, 152–4
    ECT, 154
    psychological, 154
Electroconvulsive therapy, elderly
  patients, 154

Endocrine changes, 69–71
Endogenous depression, 67, 68
  frequency of depression in 1st
    degree relatives, 73–5
  life events and onset, 72–3
'Endogenous' symptoms, 66
Epidemiology, 3–9
Epistasis, 48
Equal Opportunities Commission, 234
Evolutionary theories of manic
  depression, 47–8

Familial factors, 71–7
Familiarity, 68
Fellowship of Depressives
  Anonymous, 235, 249
Fenfluramine, 97
Flunarazine, 98
Fluoxetine, 184, 185–6
Flupenthixol, 193
Fluphenazine decanoate, 91–2
Fluphenazine enanthate, 91–2
Fluvoxamine, 184, 185–6, 187

GBR12909, 189
General population surveys, 4–7
General practitioner, 216–28
  acknowledged major depression,
    226
  attitudes, 218, 219–21
  improving performance, 223
  frequency of consultations, 216–17
  knowledge, 221–3
  non-acknowledgement of
    depression, 217–18
  practice arrangements, 218–19
  skills, 221
  suicide patient, 210
  symptoms/cues to depression,
    221–2, 225 (table)
  unacknowledged major depression,
    226–7
Genetics, 45–50, 67–8
Gepirone, 56, 188
Granulomatous disease, chronic, 48,
  49
Griseofulvin, 95
Growth hormone (GH), 55
Guanethidine, 87 (table)

Hamilton Rating Scale for
Depression, 88, 182
Hudson Generalized Contentment
Scale, 88
5-hydroxytryptamine (5-HT):
receptor function, neuroendocrine
tests, 56
specific antagonists/agonists, 187–8
uptake inhibitors, 184–7
Hypercortisolaemia, 53
Hypochondriasis, 143
Hypothalamic-pituitary-adrenal axis,
53–4, 69, 71

Idazoxan, 188
Imipramine, 59, 99, 180
fatal poisoning, 183 (table)
prophylactic ability, 191
Index of Definition, 5–6
Index of Negativity of Core
Relationships, 33–5
Index of Past Adversity, 39
Indomethacin, 97
Infanticide Act (1938), 125
Interactions, 65, 69
Interactive models, 65–77
International Classification of Disease,
13–14
Iproniazid, 99
Isoniazid, 95

Levodopa, 96–7
Life events role, 22
Lithium, 99, 153–4, 191
prophylactic ability, 191
Lorazepam, 153
Lysergic acid diethylamide (LSD), 98

Major depression, 11–12
Mania, switch rate to depression, 94
Manic depression:
clinical heterogeneity, 46–7
evolutionary theories, 47–8
genotypic forms, 46–7
mutations causing, 48–50
X-linked genetic transmission, 8,
45–6
Manic Depression Fellowship, 235,
249
Maprotilene, 183 (table)

Masked depression, 115–16
Maturational stress, 114
Melancholia, 12
Melatonin, 57, 59
Meperidine, 99
Metaclopramide, 98
Methadone, 98
Methergoline, 56
Methoxamine, 54
Methylamphetamines, 54
Methyldopa, 87 (table), 88
Metronidazole, 95
Mianserin, 153, 187–8, 193
fatal poisoning, 183 (table)
Minaprine, 189
Missed depression, 4
Moclobemide, 190
Monoamine oxidase inhibitors, 59,
153, 189–90
tyramine pressor response (cheese
effect), 190
Montgomery–Asberg Depression
Rating Scale, 134
Mood disorders (DSM IIIR), 12 (table)
Mother, early loss of, 38–9
Mother and Baby In-Patient Unit
(Manchester), 135
'Move on' depression, 47

Nalidixic acid, 95
National Self Help Support Centre,
249
Neuroendocrine status, 70
Neuroleptics, 91–4
low-dose, 193
Neurotic depression, 10–11
frequency of depression in 1st
degree relatives, 73–5
life events and onset, 72–3
prevalence, 4
women, 8
Nifedipine, 98
Nomifensine, 184, 189
'Non-endogenous' depressives, 68
Nonsteroidal anti-inflammatory
analgesics, 97
Noradrenaline, 57, 189
uptake inhibition, 58
Norfluoxetine, 186
Norzimelidine, 186

Oral contraceptives, 89–91
  low-dose oestrogen, 91
Oxaprotiline, 57
Oxprenolol, 87 (table)

Panic, 180
Parent and Baby Day Unit (Stoke-on-
  Trent), 135
Parkinson's disease, 97
Paroxetine, 185–6
Partially Sighted Society, 237
Perlindole, 190
Personality disorders, recurrent
  transient mood changes, 142–3
Phentermine, 97
Phenylbutazone, 97
Phobic anxiety, acute, 142
Phosphodiesterase inhibitors, 59,
  189
Physical diseases causing depression,
  83
Pineal gland, melatonin secretion in,
  59
Pizotifen, 98
Postnatal depression, *see* Puerperal
  depression
Postpartum disorder, 8
Prazosin, 57
Premarital pregnancy, 38–9
Premenstrual syndrome (tension), 8,
  89
Prescription Event Monitoring, 84
Present State Examination, 5
Prevalence, 3–4, 6–7
  adolescent depression, 112–13
  Basque-speaking community, 21
  Camberwell women, 23–6
  elderly people, 140, 144–7
    institutional patients, 146–7
  Islington women, 26–7
  Japanese elderly, 21
  puerperal depression, 125
Prior psychiatric symptomatology, 32
Procainamide, 99
Prolactin, 56
Propanolol, 87, 88
Provoking agent, 23
Pseudodementia, 142–3
Pseudo-depression, 86, 88
Psychotherapy, elderly patients, 154

Psychotic depression 10–11
  prevalence, 4
  women, 8
Puerperal depression, 124–36
  clinical facilities, 134–5
  detection, 133–5
  family implications, 130–1
  health personnel training, 131–3
  prevalence, 125–8
  self-report scale, 134
Pyridoxine, 91
  deficiency, 91

Ranitidine, 98
Raskin three-area scale, 134
Ranwolfia alkaloids, 86
Reactive depression, 67, 68
Recovery from depression, 40
'Release' phenomenon, psychosis, as,
  47–8
Research Diagnostic Criteria, 6
Reserpine, 85, 86
Ritanserin, 188
Rolipram, 189

Schizophrenia:
  depression as symptom, 93
  suicide risk, 93
Self-esteem, low, 22, 29
Self-Evaluation and Social Support
  Schedule, 33
Self-help groups, 232–48
  limitations, 245–6
  literature, 233–6
    individual groups, 234
    self-care, 235–6
    women, 234–5
    World Health Organization, 236
  Nottingham experience, 236–44
    agencies/publicity outlets, 239
      (table)
    families, 238
    new groups, 238–40, 241 (tables)
    prevention of depression, 237–8
    problems encountered, 240
      (table)
  professional workers, 242–3
    changes in attitudes, 247
    constraints imposed, 246
    strengths, 244–5

Self-Help Team, 249
Sex incidence, 7–8
Single mothers, 26
Social class, 8–9
Social disadvantages, 8
Social dominance hierarchy, 47
Social factors, 21–9, 65–6, 69–77
Social isolation in old age, 152
Social support, 29–31, 32–8
Somatizers, 223
'Stay put' depression, 47
Stimulants, 97
Subclinical symptomatology, chronic, 22
Suicide (attempted suicide), 9, 197–212
    adolescent, 118
    aftercare, 206–10
        day-patient, 208
        general practitioner, 210
        out-patient, 208–9
        psychiatric in-patient, 207–8
    alcoholics, 94
    assessment of attempted suicide patients, 199–206
        help for person, 206, 207 (table)
        nature of attempt, 201–3
        person's resources/supports, 206
        psychiatric disorder presence, 203–4
        purpose of attempt, 200–1
        risk of further attempt, 205–6
        risk of suicide, 204–5
    child, antisocial behaviour preceeding, 115
    incidence, 197
    male preponderance, 8
    management of attempted suicide, 198–9
    reducing risk of death from antidepressant overdosage, 184

risk, 210–12
    assessment, 210–11
    management, 211–12
transient mood changes precipitating, 192–3
women, attempts by, 8
Sulphonamides, 95

Temazepam, 153
Thiazide diuretics, 97
Thiothixene, 193
Thymoxamine, 54
Tizanidine, 98
Transient mood changes, 192–3
Trazadone, 153, 187–8
Triazolam, 153
Tricyclic antidepressants, *see under* Antidepressants
Trimipramine, 183 (table)
Tryptophan, 91
    metabolism pathways, 92 (fig.)
Twin studies, 68

Vinblastine, 96
Vulnerability, 28–9

Women, 23–7
    early loss of mother, 38
    loss of core person, 27
    past adversity, 38–9
    recovery from depression, 40
    severe events affecting, 26–9
    single mothers, 26
    social support, 29–31, 32–8
    suicide attempts, 8
    working class, 26
World Health Organization, 236

X-linked manic depression, 45–6

Zimelidine, 184, 185–6, 191–2
Zimelidine syndrome, 186